GERMAN MEDICAL DATA SCIENCES:
VISIONS AND BRIDGES

Studies in Health Technology and Informatics

This book series was started in 1990 to promote research conducted under the auspices of the EC programmes' Advanced Informatics in Medicine (AIM) and Biomedical and Health Research (BHR) bioengineering branch. A driving aspect of international health informatics is that telecommunication technology, rehabilitative technology, intelligent home technology and many other components are moving together and form one integrated world of information and communication media. The series has been accepted by MEDLINE/PubMed, SciVerse Scopus, EMCare, Book Citation Index – Science and Thomson Reuters' Conference Proceedings Citation Index.

Volume 243

Recently published in this series

ISSN 0926-9630 (print)
ISSN 1879-8365 (online)

German Medical Data Sciences: Visions and Bridges

Proceedings of the 62nd Annual Meeting of the German
Association of Medical Informatics, Biometry and Epidemiology
(gmds e.V.) 2017 in Oldenburg (Oldenburg) – GMDS 2017

Edited by

Rainer Röhrig

Medical Informatics – Carl von Ossietzky Universität Oldenburg, Germany
Conference Chair

Antje Timmer

Epidemiology and Biometry – Carl von Ossietzky Universität Oldenburg,
Germany
Chair Scientific Program Committee; Epidemiology

Harald Binder

Institute for Medical Biometry and Statistics, Albert-Ludwigs University,
Freiburg, Germany
Biometry

and

Ulrich Sax

Medical Informatics, University Medical Center Göttingen, Göttingen, Germany
Medical Informatics

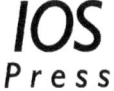

IOS
Press

Amsterdam • Berlin • Washington, DC

ISBN 978-1-61499-807-5 (print)
ISBN 978-1-61499-808-2 (online)
Library of Congress Control Number: 2017951833

Cover Image by University of Oldenburg, David Saß, Marius Butt and Rainer Röhrig

Publisher
IOS Press BV
Nieuwe Hemweg 6B
1013 BG Amsterdam
Netherlands
fax: +31 20 687 0019
e-mail: order@iospress.nl

For book sales in the USA and Canada:
IOS Press, Inc.
6751 Tepper Drive
Clifton, VA 20124
USA
Tel.: +1 703 830 6300
Fax: +1 703 830 2300
sales@iospress.com

Visions and Bridges

Preface by the Editors

We are living in the information age, characterized by the shift from traditional industry to an economy based on information computerization. Ten years after the first iPhone appeared on the market, digitization has become habitual: there is hardly any professional or private area in this world not affected by digitization. This also applies to health care.

Our vision for healthcare in the information age is to improve clinical decision making and the effectiveness and efficiency of health systems by data methods and technology:

- Integrate available data and information for biomedical research.
- Access and provide information, knowledge and decision support to patients and healthcare professionals.

As medical data scientists, we develop methods for clinical research and provide them to clinical researchers, manufacturers and clinicians. In the information age, we are important actors in the health care systems.

Ubiquitous information technology profoundly changes the sociotechnical system of health care: Patients are empowered by information technology, health care professionals are overwhelmed by the complexity and the magnitude of the data, not being trained to deal with it. This accelerates shared decision-making, requiring other skills from physicians as well as new ways to how medical knowledge is provided. As of now, availability of information is not the crucial point. Rather, selecting relevant information and assessing the quality of the information remains a challenge.

Information technology also has an impact on hierarchy and communication paths in the hospitals. Similar to the development, introduction and evaluation of new medical procedures, we must understand all effects on the target system in the application of information technology. This is an obligatory prerequisite to determine the benefit of what and to be able to control the risks of side effects. We have to face the fact that the increasing impact of information technology on patient care is directly linked to our own commitment to apply the principles of evidence-based medicine.

We can only master this challenge together: It is necessary for all stakeholders, scientist, clinicians and patients to work together in research and health care. We need to bridge!

- Bridging the various disciplines in the Data Sciences
- Bridging data scientists and clinicians
- Bridging different healthcare professionals
- Bridging science and society
- Bridging providers and patients!

GMDS 2017 catalyzes constructing these bridges.

Finally some data: Two-hundred-and-forty contributions were submitted, among 77 full papers. These were reviewed in a two stage interdisciplinary peer-reviewing process: A total of 766 reviews, some of which were very comprehensive, were produced by 186 reviewers. 42 full papers are accepted for publication in this volume of *Studies in Health Technology and Informatics*. We cordially thank all authors and reviewers for this work at the scientific core of the conference.

Rainer Röhrig
Antje Timmer
Harald Binder
Ulrich Sax

German Medical Data Sciences

Preamble by Ulrich Mansmann
President of GMDS

Congratulations to the editorial board (Dr. Rainer Röhrig, Dr. Antje Timmer, Dr. Harald Binder, and Dr. Ulrich Sax) for this impressive volume of scientific contributions to the annual meeting of the German Society of Medical Information Sciences, Biometry, and Epidemiology (GMDS). It documents the wide spectrum of research interests and activities within as well as the interactions between the three scientific fields which shape the GMDS. Actually, it is the first internationally published volume of extended papers presented on our national annual meeting.

The volume presents work which reflects a manifold of aspects around the digitalization of medicine. It represents work of specialists of high value for physicians as well as health systems analysts. The conference offers an intensive dialogue between the GMDS community and the actors in our health care systems to handle and shape the digitalization of medicine. There is an urgent need to develop this dialogue and to prepare people to be knowledgeable enough to make this dialogue productive. The structured education of medical data scientists is a prerequisite to drive this development and one of the leading topics of the conference.

Digitalization of Medicine also implies a good infrastructure for health related information (creation, storage, and use) which is more as software and hardware. Essential aspects are related to organizational structures, standards, competences, and processes. In July 2017, the Federal Ministry of Education and Research just initiated a comprehensive program to implement this development for German University Hospitals. The conference will present the concepts behind the Medical Informatics Initiative (MI-I). Some of the contributions presented in this volume are inspired by the preparing work for the MI-I. I hope that they will steer a discussion which strengthen the process to build on our infrastructure for health related information, to make people interested, and to motivate them to increase their personal competences.

Finally, good research is the result of data which is carefully documented, processed according the state-of-the-art, analyzed with appropriate strategies, and published following the established reporting guidelines as well as being able to be reproduced. The process of research should be transparent, impartial, and aware of the context in which it takes place. Good research is more than good data. The GMDS sees its task in providing the extras which are needed to produce good research. Therefore, the conference is an important event and the papers presented prove that editors and scientific program committee did an excellent job.

I thank the organizers of the conference for this great work, good luck and a big success.

Ulrich Mansmann
GMDS president

Reviewers for GMDS 2017

Adelmann, Sarah
Ahlbrandt, Janko
Albrecht, Urs-Vito
Altmann, Udo
Ammenwerth, Elske
Andersohn, Frank
Askevold, Ingolf
Bauer, Christian R
Baum, Benjamin
Becker, Kurt
Behrends, Marianne
Beißbarth, Tim
Bender, Ralf
Benner, Axel
Binder, Harald
Bitzer, Eva Maria
Blobel, Bernd
Böckmann, Britta
Boeker, Martin
Boldt, Ralf
Bott, Oliver Johannes
Böttger, Sebastian
Brammen, Dominik
Breil, Bernhard
Breitschwerdt, Rüdiger
Brenck, Florian
Breu, Ruth
Bruland, Philipp
Bürkle, Thomas
De Bruin, Jeroen
de Laffolie, Jan
de Sordi, Dominik
Deisz, Robert
Denecke, Kerstin
Deserno, Thomas
Dörks, Michael
Drepper, Johannes
Drichel, Dmitriy
Drösler, Saskia
Drösler, Saskia E
Duftschmid, Georg
Dugas, Martin
Duhm-Harbeck, Petra
Egbert, Nicole

Esdar, Moritz
Fischer, Burkhard
Fischer, Stefanie
Flemming, Daniel
Friedl, Sven
Fudickar, Sebastian
Gacek, Stefanie
Ganslandt, Thomas
Ganzinger, Matthias
Graubner, Bernd
Griebel, Lena
Groß, Martin
Gudenkauf, Stefan
Haag, Martin
Haarbrandt, Birger
Haas, Peter
Häber, Anke
Handels, Heinz
Hardt, Juliane
Hartz, Tobias
Haux, Reinhold
Hein, Andreas
Heinze, Oliver
Herff, Christian
Heuten, Wilko
Hoffmann, Barbara
Hoffmann, Falk
Hübler, Axel
Hübner, Ursula
Hueske-Kraus, Dirk
Ingenerf, Josef
Ittner, Karl
Jahn, Franziska
Jöckel, Karl-Heinz
Johner, Christian
Juhra, Christian
Jürgens, Verena
Kappen, Sanny
Karch, André
Karopka, Thomas
Katalinic, Alexander
Kieschke, Joachim
Kitzig, Andreas
Klausen, Andreas

Knaup-Gregori, Petra
Koch, Christian
Kock, Ann-Kristin
Koppelin, Frauke
Kouematchoua, Ghislain
Krahn, Tobias
Kraus, Stefan
Krawczak, Michael
Krumkamp, Ralf
Lablans, Martin
Langanke, Martin
Lange, Kathrin
Langkafel, Peter
Lenz, Richard
Liebe, Jan-David
Lindoerfer, Doris
Linnen, Heidi
Lipprandt, Myriam
Löbe, Matthias
Lüpkes, Christian
Lux, Thomas
Majeed, Raphael W.
Marschollek, Michael
Martens, Alke
Meyer, Thorsten
Moll, Peter
Moreno, Beatrice
Müller, Hermann
Müller-Mielitz, Stefan
Naziyok, Tolga P.
Neubert, Antje
Neumuth, Thomas
Nöllke, Peter
Nussbeck, Sara Yasemin
Oemig, Frank
Özyurt, Jale
Palm, Christoph
Piro, Neltje E.
Plischke, Maik
Pobiruchin, Monika
Prasser, Fabian
Rauch, Geraldine
Rauch, Jens
Röhrig, Rainer
Rüther, Alric
Sauer, Jürgen
Sax, Ulrich
Scherag, André
Schlattmann, Peter

Schmedt, Niklas
Schmidt, Carsten Oliver
Schmidtmann, Irene
Schneider, Henning
Schöler, Anke
Schreiweis, Björn
Schulze, Mareike
Schütze, Bernd
Sedlmayr, Brita
Sedlmayr, Martin
Seeger, Insa
Seggewies, Christof
Seifert, Sascha
Sellemann, Björn
Singer, Susanne
Skonetzki, Stefan
Snieder, Harold
Sobotka, Fabian
Sohrabi, Keywan
Soto-Rey, Iñaki
Speer, Ronald
Spreckelsen, Cord
Staemmler, Martin
Stang, Andreas
Stäubert, Sebastian
Stenzhorn, Holger
Stöhr, Mark R.
Stolpe, Susanne
Storck, Michael
Strahwald, Brigitte
Thiemann, Volker
Thoben, Wilfried
Thun, Sylvia
Timmer, Antje
Toddenroth, Dennis
Tolxdorff, Thomas
Trinczek, Benjamin
Umbach, Nadine
Wiesner, Martin
Wilken, Marc
Winter, Alfred
Wolf, Ivo
Xu, Tingyan
Zaiß, Albrecht
Zapf, Antonia
Zeleke, Atinkut Alamirrew
Zenker, Sven
Zöllner, Iris

Contents

5. Health Care Information Systems

6. Interoperability – Standards, Terminologies, Classification

7. Biomedical Informatics, Innovative Algorithms and Signal Processing

1. Teaching & Training

German Medical Data Sciences: Visions and Bridges
R. Röhrig et al. (Eds.)
© *2017 German Association for Medical Informatics, Biometry and Epidemiology (gmds) e.V. and IOS Press.*
This article is published online with Open Access by IOS Press and distributed under the terms
of the Creative Commons Attribution Non-Commercial License 4.0 (CC BY-NC 4.0).
doi:10.3233/978-1-61499-808-2-3

3

How to Teach Health IT Evaluation: Recommendations for Health IT Evaluation Courses

Elske AMMENWERTH[a,1], Nicolet DE KEIZER[b], Jytte BRENDER McNAIR[c],
Catherine K. CRAVEN[d], Eric EISENSTEIN[e], Andrew GEORGIOU[f], Saif KHAIRAT[g],
Farah MAGRABI[h], Pirkko NYKÄNEN[i], Paula OTERO[j], Michael RIGBY[k],
Philip SCOTT[l], Charlene WEIR[m]

[a] *Institute of Medical Informatics, UMIT – University for Health Sciences,
Medical Informatics and Technology, Hall in Tirol, Austria*
[b] *Academic Medical Center, University of Amsterdam, Netherlands*
[c] *Department of Health Science & Technology, Aalborg University, Denmark*
[d] *Informatics Institute, University of Missouri, Columbia, USA*
[e] *Duke University, Durham, North Carolina, USA*
[f] *Centre for Health Systems & Safety Research, Australian Institute of Health
Innovation, Macquarie University, Sydney, Australia*
[g] *University of North Carolina-Chapel Hill, Chapel Hill, North Carolina, USA*
[h] *Centre for Health Informatics, Australian Institute of Health Innovation,
Macquarie University, Sydney, Australia*
[i] *University of Tampere, Faculty of Natural Science, Tampere, Finland*
[j] *Hospital Italiano de Buenos Aires, Buenos Aires, Argentina*
[k] *Keele University, Keele, Staffordshire, ST5 5BG, U.K.*
[l] *Centre for Healthcare Modelling and Informatics, University of Portsmouth, United
Kingdom*
[m] *University of Utah, Salt Lake City, Utah, USA*

Abstract. Systematic health IT evaluation studies are needed to ensure system quality and safety and to provide the basis for evidence-based health informatics. Well-trained health informatics specialists are required to guarantee that health IT evaluation studies are conducted in accordance with robust standards. Also, policy makers and managers need to appreciate how good evidence is obtained by scientific process and used as an essential justification for policy decisions. In a consensus-based approach with over 80 experts in health IT evaluation, recommendations for the structure, scope and content of health IT evaluation courses on the master or postgraduate level have been developed, supported by a structured analysis of available courses and of available literature. The recommendations comprise 15 mandatory topics and 15 optional topics for a health IT evaluation course.

Keywords. Evaluation studies, curriculum

---

[1] Corresponding Author: Prof. Dr. Elske Ammenwerth, Institute of Medical Informatics, UMIT – University for Health Sciences, Medical Informatics and Technology, Eduard Wallnöfer Zentrum 1, 6060 Hall in Tirol, Austria, e-mail: elske.ammenwerth@umit.at

1. Introduction

High-quality and efficient health care seems not possible nowadays without the support of information technology (IT) [1]. Health IT has been shown to improve the quality and efficiency of clinical processes and health outcome, and to reduce morbidity, mortality and costs [2]. However, the impact of health IT may not be optimal, and it can also pose risks to patient safety. To verify that appropriate benefits are forthcoming and unintended side effects of health IT are avoided, systematic evaluation studies are needed to ensure system quality and safety, as part of an evidence-based health informatics approach [3, 4].

To guarantee that health IT evaluation studies are conducted in accordance with appropriate scientific and professional standards, well-trained health informatics specialists are needed. The recently updated recommendations of IMIA, the International Medical Informatics Association, on health informatics education [5] state that the topic "evaluation and assessment of information systems" should be part of health informatics curricula; arguably aspects of it should also be in wider health management and policy curricula so as to ensure achievement of an evidence-based approach in practice. However, the IMIA recommendations do not give details on what should be taught with respect to evaluation as part of a health informatics curriculum.

The objective of this contribution is to provide recommendations for the structure, scope and content of health IT evaluation courses.

2. Methods

The overall approach consisted of an iterative process, coordinated by the working groups on health IT evaluation of EFMI (European Federation for Health Informatics), IMIA (International Medical Informatics Association) and AMIA (American Medical Informatics Association).

First, structure, scope and content of successfully running health IT evaluation courses from ten university courses in Europe, the United States and Australia were collected (openly available at [6]). Also, core literature on health IT evaluation (e.g. [4, 7, 8]) was analysed regarding content. Then, an open workshop at Medical Informatics Europe (MIE2014) in Istanbul with 30 participants collected ideas for recommended core content in a structured way. Results from the course analysis, literature analysis as well as from this workshop were then aggregated to form a preliminary list of initial recommendations comprising 33 content items as well as the structure and scope of the course. This list was verified by discussion among the authors of this contribution.

In a follow-up open workshop at Medical Informatics Europe (MIE2015) in Madrid, the 25 participants were then asked to judge the importance of each of these content item (high, medium, low), and to identify possible missing items. Overall, five new items were proposed. In an updated version of the recommendations, items were now separated into mandatory content (for those considered important by the majority of participants) and optional content (for the rest).

The updated recommendations were then validated in an open workshop at Medinfo 2015 in Sao Paolo. The 16 participants discussed whether they were clear and comprehensive. The resulting version of the recommendations consisted of 14 mandatory and 12 optional content items.

A follow-up open workshop at AMIA 2015 in San Francisco with 15 participants was used to further validate the recommendations. Suggestions for optional content were added, alongside suggested clarifications. After this workshop, the final version of the recommendations consisted of 15 mandatory and 15 optional content items.

3. Recommendations for health IT evaluation courses

3.1. Structure and scope of the course

- **Focus of the course**[2]: Theoretical & practical introduction into health IT evaluation.
- **Level of the course**: Master or postgraduate level.
- **Course objective:** Students should be able to: i) plan their own (smaller) evaluation study; ii) select and apply selected evaluation methods, iii) perform a study and report its results; and iv) appraise the quality and the results of published health IT evaluation studies.
- **Scale of the course:** The mandatory core topics can be taught in a course of 6 ECTS (European Credit Transfer and Accumulation System[3]) which is equivalent to 4 U.S. credit hours[4]. U.S. programs may choose to offer the more standard 3-credit hour, semester long course. The duration of the course can be longer if optional content or extended practical training is added.
- **Format of the course:** Courses may be given in various module formats and structures (e.g. traditional class room courses, blended learning courses, or fully online courses that follow best practices).
- **Participants:** The recommendations address multidisciplinary groups of students, with backgrounds for example in computer science, health informatics, medicine, nursing, social science, information sciences, or business.
- **Practical training:** The recommendations suggest that practical evaluation training is included; this training can focus on different aspects, depending on the learning objectives, the level of participants, and the available time.
- **Prerequisites:** Before joining the health IT evaluation course, the students should have obtained sufficient background knowledge in the following basic research topics: Philosophy of science, scientific evidence, literature searching and critical appraisal, designing a research study, ethical principles of research, quantitative research methods and statistics, qualitative research methods, management of research projects, and clinical care delivery processes and health IT. If students do not have this knowledge beforehand, this needs to be added to a health IT evaluation course.

---

[2] In these recommendations, the term "course" refers to an identifiable part of an overall degree programme, such as a module or a unit.

[3] ECTS is a standard for comparing the study attainment and performance of students of higher education across Europe; 6 ECTS are equivalent to 150 - 180 hours of overall student workload (both classroom time and homework). Six ECTS is roughly equivalent to 10% of an academic year.

[4] 1 credit hour = 50 minutes spent in class.

3.2. Content of the course

Table 1 presents the recommended core content.

Table 1. Recommendations for mandatory and optional content of health IT evaluation courses.

Mandatory core topics	
Theory	
A1	Need for evidence-based health informatics (i.e. health IT and patient safety, efficiency, quality, user satisfaction), and reasons for undertaking evaluations
A2	Theories of evaluation (e.g. inductive or deductive, formative or summative)
Practice	
A3	Building an evaluation study (e.g. information needs, stakeholder analysis, tailor the evaluation, steps of an evaluation study, obtain permissions)
A4	Study designs for health IT evaluation studies (e.g. experimental, quasi-experimental, observational)
A5	Indicators for health IT quality (structure, process, outcome quality) and their relation to clinical indicators
A6	Practical training in health IT evaluation (e.g. write an evaluation plan based on a realistic case study; conduct a real evaluation project; discuss and criticize a published evaluation study)
Methods and metrics	
A7	Measurement principles (e.g. objectivity, reliability, validity of measurements, types of bias)
A8	Quantitative data collection methods in health IT evaluation
A9	Qualitative data collection methods in health IT evaluation
A10	Multi-methods approaches and triangulation
A11	Quality of health IT evaluation studies
Reporting	
A12	Reporting and publishing of an evaluation study
A13	Finding, appraising and interpreting the evidence from published evaluation studies
A14	Answering "so what…" questions: What do evaluation results mean for IT management and for the quality and safety of clinical processes? How can evaluation results impact health IT practice?
Ethics	
A15	Obtaining ethical approval and other required permissions for evaluation projects
B Optional topics (examples to be chosen based on available time and background of participants)	
B1	Evaluation frameworks for health IT evaluation
B2	Evaluation of user and technology acceptance
B3	Evaluation of usability
B4	Technical evaluation (software testing)
B5	Evaluation of people and organizational issues
B6	Evaluation of clinical impact
B7	Economic evaluation
B8	Socio-technical and implementation-science approaches to evaluation
B9	Evaluation as part of quality and safety management and improvement frameworks
B10	Evaluation of data quality and data analytics
B11	Evaluation of health IT implementation
B12	Health Technology Assessment
B13	Systematic reviews and meta-analysis
B14	Simulation studies as an approach to evaluate health IT
B15	Regulatory issues impacting health IT evaluation (e.g. medical device regulations, FDA)

4. Discussion and conclusion

This paper presents recommendations for a health IT evaluation course as part of a master or postgraduate programme. Their development was coordinated by health IT evaluation experts from North America, Europe and Australia, all with teaching experience in academic settings. In addition, around 80 workshop participants contributed with their expertise to the recommendations.

The recommended content should not be seen as a cookbook. It does not specify how many hours of lecturing should be invested in each sub-topic. This has to be decided by lecturers and course planners based on overall programme objectives, learning objectives for the evaluation course, background of the students, content of previous education, and available time. It also does not describe specific learning outcomes.

The recommendations assume that all items are taught on an introductory level. Extended knowledge, e.g. in qualitative methods, could be covered in specialized lectures, as well as the listed optional topics. It is also possible to split the content into a basic course (3 ECTS) and an advanced course (3 ECTS).

Riding a bike cannot be taught by theory alone. Thus, we recommend including interdisciplinary practical training – either on an individual basis or even better in interdisciplinary groups of students. When real evaluation projects are conducted by students, a good balance between the available time, the complexities of real-life evaluations and the need to provide meaningful evaluation results is often a challenge.

Follow-on activities which are desirable as part of this continuous educational development program are consulting a wider stakeholder group on the recommendations and validating it through use and review in academic practice.

We invite all teachers of health IT evaluation courses to use these recommendations when designing an evaluation course, to add their course description to [6], and to report on their experiences. We also invite feedback on the use of the principles of this module as a means of instilling an evidence-based approach to health informatics application in wider health policy and health care delivery contexts.

Acknowledgment

We appreciate the support of Regis Beuscart, Damina Borbolla, Nadia Davoody, George Demiris, Vasilis Hervatis, Sabine Koch, John Mantas and Christian Nøhr in providing course descriptions or supporting the organization of the workshops.

References

[1] Haux R, Medical informatics: past, present, future, *Int J Med Inform*, **79**(9) (2010),599-610.
[2] Lau F, Kuziemsky C, Price M, Gardner J, A review on systematic reviews of health information system studies, *J Am Med Inform Assoc*, **17**(6) (2010),637-45.
[3] Rigby M, Ammenwerth E, Beuscart-Zephir M, Brender J, Hyppönen H, Melia S, et al., Evidence Based Health Informatics: 10 years of efforts to promote the principle, *Yearb Med Inform*, **8**(1) (2013),34-46.
[4] Ammenwerth E, Rigby M, editors. Evidence-Based Health Informatics. Amsterdam: IOS Press; 2016.
[5] Mantas J, Ammenwerth E, Demiris G, Hasman A, Haux R, Hersh W, et al., Recommendations of the International Medical Informatics Association (IMIA) on Education in Biomedical and Health Informatics. First Revision, *Methods Inf Med*, **49**(2) (2010),105-20.
[6] EFMI WG Eval. Curricula of Health IT Evaluation Courses [Available from: https://iig.umit.at/efmi/curricula.htm]. Last access: 10.10.2016.
[7] Friedman C, Wyatt JC, *Evaluation Methods in Medical Informatics*, 2nd ed, New York: Springer, 2006.
[8] Brender J, *Handbook of Evaluation Methods for Health Informatics*, Burlington, MA: Elsevier Academic Press, 2006.

German Medical Data Sciences: Visions and Bridges
R. Röhrig et al. (Eds.)
© 2017 German Association for Medical Informatics, Biometry and Epidemiology (gmds) e.V. and IOS Press.
This article is published online with Open Access by IOS Press and distributed under the terms
of the Creative Commons Attribution Non-Commercial License 4.0 (CC BY-NC 4.0).
doi:10.3233/978-1-61499-808-2-8

Developing and Evaluating Collaborative Online-Based Instructional Designs in Health Information Management

Elske AMMENWERTH[a,1], Werner O. HACKL[a],
Michael FELDERER[c], and Alexander HOERBST[b]

[a] *Institute of Medical Informatics, UMIT – University for Health Sciences,
Medical Informatics and Technology, Hall in Tirol, Austria*
[b] *eHealth Research and Innovation Unit, UMIT – University for Health Sciences,
Medical Informatics and Technology, Hall in Tirol, Austria*
[c] *Institute of Computer Science, University of Innsbruck, Austria*

Abstract. The number of students enrolled in online courses is increasing steadily. Distance education offers many advantages, but also has inherent challenges. Successful distance education needs a thoughtfully designed instructional strategy where students are supported to actively create knowledge. We present the design and evaluation of three online-based courses in health informatics. The courses were based on a collaborative instructional strategy. The evaluation comprised workload analysis, student evaluation, student interviews and student reflections. Students expressed high satisfaction with online learning, despite a high workload, and high perceived learning outcomes. Using the Community of Inquiry framework as reference, we found very high levels of teaching presence, social presence and cognitive presence. Summarizing, we found that the chosen instructional strategy supported student-centered, collaborative learning. We conclude by presenting lesson learned for online-based instructional design.

Keywords. Learning; Education, distance; Cooperative behavior

1. Introduction

The number of students enrolled in online courses is increasing steadily. One in four U.S. students takes at least one distance education course, with 2.8 million U.S. students taking all of their courses at distance [1]. Online courses offer advantages, including self-directed and self-paced learning and learning "anywhere" and "anytime".

From a constructivist point of view, learning is a process that works best in interaction with other persons [2]. Collaborative learning is thus considered a key element for successful learning in online settings [3]. Online courses should support students to "gradually construct systems of shared meanings" [4]. Studies show advantages of collaboration in online learning activities, such as more engaged learning, increased motivation, more active processing of information, improvement of meta-cognitive and social skills and overall better knowledge acquisition and retention [5, 6].

---

[1] Corresponding author, Elske Ammenwerth, Eduard Wallnöfer Zentrum 1, A - 6060 Hall in Tirol, elske.ammenwerth@umit.at.

However, to facilitate interaction, online instructors need to address specific challenges of online learning such as reduced possibility of transmitting socio-emotional information, more complicated coordination of asynchronous activities and the challenge of lurking, i.e. passive participation in online activities [7]. Collaborative online teaching thus needs a thoughtfully planned instructional strategy to facilitate students' interactions as well as monitoring of quantity and quality of the interactions.

In this paper, we present the evaluation of three online courses. The aim of the evaluation was to ascertain whether the chosen collaborate instructional strategy was successful with regard to workload, student satisfaction and learning processes.

2. Instructional strategy for the online modules

We used a constructivist instructional design that was influenced by the instructional design principles of David Merrill [8] (stressing the need to active students and to focus on real-world applications), the ARCS model of motivational design [9] (e.g. focusing on how to gain attention of students, how to integrate their past experiences) the expository 3-2-1-design framework by Michael Kerres [10] (taking e.g. the idea of learning activities to fulfill learning processes) and the concept of E-tivities by Gilly Salmon [7] (offering a structure for learning activities and group processes).

All courses consisted of meta-information (learning objectives, estimated workload, instructional approach, the instructor's role etc.) and of learning activities. Each learning activity comprised a structured description of learning objectives, tasks to be done, expected reaction to the solutions of other participants and materials to solve the learning activity. These learning activities were not meant to test competencies, but to allow the students – alone and in interaction with the others – to accomplish the intended learning process and to develop new knowledge and skills.

Each week comprised of a set of learning activities. These activities comprised, among others, reading literature and discussing concepts; analyzing case studies; developing presentations for other students; present arguments; reflect on alternatives develop a project plan; conduct a data analysis; or develop specifications and concepts. At the end of each week, participants were asked to reflect on their learning progress. For each learning activity, needed materials (presentation, paper, book chapters, or web sites) were directly provided, or a starting point for students' individual research was given. Moodle was used as electronic learning platform. The instructor was present throughout the course to give input and to facilitate the discussions. To be successful, participants had to complete all learning activities and had to get involved into thoughtful discussions with other participant. Also, weekly reflections were mandatory.

In 2016, three pilot online courses were conducted with 15 – 20 participants: A four-week course on project management; a six-week course on clinical data analysis; and a six-week course on eHealth. Participants came from various health care professions. They mostly did not know each other before the course. Participation was voluntary and free of charge. Successful participants got a certificate. Success criteria were active participation in group discussions and successful completion of all learning activities, such as conducting a statistical analysis or presentation of a project plan.

All instructors got an introduction into the chosen instructional design and completed a four-week online-based training on e-moderation. Instructors regularly discussed the progress of their courses among each other, to allow ongoing feedback and professional development.

3. Evaluation methods

To evaluate feasibility and success of the pilot courses from various perspectives, we combined several evaluation methods. First, students documented their workload on a daily basis to allow us to verify whether the intended workload of 10 – 15 hours/week was reached. Students also were asked to self-assess their personal learning process based on a rubric that focused among others on level of participation, reading of learning materials, individual learning progress and contribution to the group. Interaction patterns were analyzed and visualized from log data taken from the learning platform Moodle; results on this are presented elsewhere [11]. The Community of Inquiry (CoI) Survey [12] was translated into German, using a controlled forward and backward translation approach, and applied at the end of the third course to assess the level of teaching presence, social presence and cognitive presence. CoI is a widely accepted conceptual framework that describes critical prerequisite factors for deep and meaningful learning in online learning environments [13]. At the end of the course, a university-wide standardized and fully anonymized student evaluation was conducted. Finally, semi-structured interviews after the end of the courses were conducted with all (successful and non-successful participants), to explore perceived learning process and learning outcome as well as – where applicable – reasons for drop-out.

4. Results

Table 1 presented selected indicators of the three courses. Students were online in around 80% of all days and actively contribute to the course in two-thirds of all days (for details, see [11]). All unsuccessful students (with the exception of one student) dropped out before end of the course.

Table 1. Selected indicators of the three online courses.

	Course 1	Course 2	Course 3
Number of learning activities	29	25	30
Threads	364	242	438
Total number of posts (instructor / participants)	234 / 1,235	231 / 1,101	146 / 1,568
Average number of words per post (instructor / participants)	87 / 72	56 / 67	72 / 89
Success rate	9/16 (59%)	8/16 (50%)	13/21 (62%)
Student workload	18 ± 6 hours/week	13 ± 3 hours/week	14 ± 2 hours/week
Student evaluation (1 = very good, 5 = not good at all)	1,1 (n=9)	1,0 (n=7)	1,2 (n=14)

Table 2 shows the perceived teaching presence, social presence and cognitive presence for course 3. All three scores as well as the resulting CoI score show quite high marks (> 4.2 out of 5). In the interviews, students reported a good cohesion and interaction within their group, an open and supportive discussion culture and an increase in knowledge due to the interaction and cooperation in the diverse group. Students appreciated the flexibility of online learning. Several students reported to be surprised how well this form of collaborative learning worked. On the critical side, the high workload and the need to be online nearly daily were highlighted as challenges. Another challenge for students was to rejoin ongoing activities after longer absences (i.e. due to illness). Overall, in the interviews, students were very positive about this way of learning and several students stated to be willing to join future courses.

Table 2. Results from the Community of Inquiry survey in course 3 (n=16). 1 = Minimum, 5 = Maximum.

	Mean	Standard Dev.
Teaching presence	4.20	0.80
Social presence	4.17	0.91
Cognitive presence	4.47	0.68
Overall CoI score	4.40	0.70

5. Discussion

The chosen instructional strategy seemed successful in facilitating a trustful interactive and collaborative learning environment. This is visible both in quantitative data (e.g. good evaluation, high number of student's posts, high CoI results) as well as in the qualitative data (e.g. interviews). Learning processes seemed to be quite intensive and engaged. As we did not perform a summative assessment at the end, these results need to be confirmed in further courses.

The chosen instructional design specifically addressed the needs of part-time students, such as exploitation of previous knowledge, application of new knowledge, interaction with other students and learning independent of time and place [14]. Workload was high with around 15 hours per week. Some students were not able to follow the course due to other commitments and dropped out mostly in the first two weeks. However, nearly all of these drop-outs stated that they appreciated the chosen instructional design and found it very helpful for learning. We consider the success rates as high for these voluntary pilot courses and for the quite high workload.

Compared to traditional instructor-centered courses, the chosen instructional design affected both students' roles and instructors' roles. Instead of being passive receivers of the instructor's knowledge, students had to be active constructors of their own learning processes. This both active as well as interactive learning was quite intensive, as workload showed. Also the role of the instructor changed from expert ("sage on the stage") to learning coach ("guide by the side"), a role also called the „new teacher" [15]. In our case, all instructors had to modify their instructional designs and materials that they had successfully applied in face-to-face-teaching for many years and had to develop realistic and challenging learning activities that fostered interaction and deep thinking. To be successful in this new role, instructors need pedagogical knowledge and technical knowledge besides their usual content knowledge [16]. Supporting training on both pedagogical and technical issues of online-learning was thus offered mandatory to all participating instructors.

Based on the results of the evaluation, the following modifications in the instructional design are planned: Applicants are better informed on the chosen instructional design, the expected workload, the need for continuous and collaborative participation and the role of the instructor, as some students dropped-out because of the unexpected high workload;. Summative tests will be added to test acquired competencies, as this will allow verifying that online participants achieve the same competency level as participants in the traditional face-to-face courses. As learning outcomes are based on the learning process, we will also more formally assess the quality of participation and contribution of each student as part of the overall grade.

6. Conclusion

A new fully online master program in health information management is planned to start in October 2017 at UMIT (http://www.umit.at/him). Based on the results of the pilot modules, the chosen instructional design will be finalized. As part of an ongoing scientific evaluation of the chosen instruction strategy, we will continue to collect data on participation, interaction, workload, learning process and learning outcome, to identify factors that can predict the satisfaction and the success of students in online courses and to design instructing guidelines for future courses.

7. Conflict of Interest

The authors are responsible for the online programme in health information management.

References

[1]   Babson Survey Research. 2015 Online Report Card - Tracking Online Education in the United States 2015 [Available from: https://onlinelearningconsortium.org/read/online-report-card-tracking-online-education-united-states-2015/]

[2]   Vygotzky L, *The Development of Higher Psychological Processes*, Cambridge, Massachusetts: Harvard University Press, 1978.

[3]   Anderson T. Towards a Theory of Online Learning. In: Anderson T, Elloumi F, editors. Theory and Practice of Online Learning. Athabasca University, 2008.

[4]   Coll C, Engel A, Bustos A, Distributed Teaching Presence and Participants' Activity Profiles: a theoretical approach to the structural analysis of Asynchronous Learning Networks, *European Journal of Education*, **44**(4) (2009),512-38.

[5]   Chou C. A Comparative Content Analysis of Student Interaction in Synchronous and Asynchronous Learning Networks. Proceedings of the 35th Hawaii International Conference on System Sciences. 10.1109/HICSS.2002.9940932002.

[6]   Lenning O, Ebbers L, The powerful potential of learning communities: Improving education for the future, *ASHE-ERIC Higher Education Report*, **26**(16) (1999),1-173.

[7]   Salmon G, *Etivities – The key to active online learning*, New York: Routledge, 2013.

[8]   Merrill M, First principles of instruction, *Educational Technology Research and Development*, **50**(3) (2002),43-59.

[9]   Keller J, *Motivational Design for Learning and Performance: The ARCS model approach*, New York: Springer, 2010.

[10] Kerres M, *Mediendidaktik. Konzeption und Entwicklung mediengestützter Lernangebote*, München: Oldenbourg, 2013. S. 331 ff.

[11] Ammenwerth E, Hackl W, Monitoring of students' interaction in online learning settings by structural network analysis and indicators, Proceedings of Informatics for Health Conference, Manchester (2016).

[12] Arbaugh J, Clevland-Innes M, Diaz S, Garrison D, Ice P, Richardson J, et al., Developing a community of inquiry instrument: Testing a measure of the Community of Inquiry framework using a multi-institutional sample, *Internet and Higher Education*, **11**(133-8) (2000).

[13] Garrison R, Anderson A, Archer W, Critical Inquiry in a Text-based Environment: Computer Conferencing in Higher Education The Internet and Higher Education, *The Internet and Higher Education*, **2**(3) (2000).

[14] Knowles M, *Andragogy in Action*, San Francisco: Jossey-Bass, 1984.

[15] Kalantzis M, Cope B, The Teacher as Designer: pedagogy in the new media age, *E-Learning and Digital Media*, **7**(3) (2010).

[16] Mishra P, Koehler P, Technological Pedagogical Content Knowledge: A Framework for Teacher Knowledge, *Teachers college Record*, **108**(6) (2006),1017-54.

German Medical Data Sciences: Visions and Bridges
R. Röhrig et al. (Eds.)
© 2017 German Association for Medical Informatics, Biometry and Epidemiology (gmds) e.V. and IOS Press.
This article is published online with Open Access by IOS Press and distributed under the terms
of the Creative Commons Attribution Non-Commercial License 4.0 (CC BY-NC 4.0).
doi:10.3233/978-1-61499-808-2-13

User Experience Evaluations in Rehabilitation Video Games for Children: A Systematic Mapping of the Literature

Carolina RICO-OLARTE[a], Diego M. LÓPEZ[a,1], Bernd BLOBEL[b,c], Sara KEPPLINGER[d]

[a] Telematics Engineering Research Group, University of Cauca, Colombia.
[b] eHealth Competence Center Bavaria, Deggendorf Institute of Technology, Germany.
[c] Medical Faculty, University of Regensburg, Germany
[d] Human-centered Media Technologies (HMT), Fraunhofer IDMT, Germany

Abstract. Background: In recent years, the interest in user experience (UX) evaluation methods for assessing technology solutions, especially in health systems for children with special needs like cognitive disabilities, has increased. Objective: Conduct a systematic mapping study to provide an overview in the field of UX evaluations in rehabilitation video games for children. Methods: The definition of research questions, the search for primary studies and the extraction of those studies by inclusion and exclusion criteria lead to the mapping of primary papers according to a classification scheme. Results: Main findings from this study include the detection of the target population of the selected studies, the recognition of two different ways of evaluating UX: (i) user evaluation and (ii) system evaluation, and UX measurements and devices used. Conclusions: This systematic mapping specifies the research gaps identified for future research works in the area.

Keywords. Systematic mapping study; user experience evaluation; children; cognitive disabilities.

1. Introduction

User Experience (UX) can be defined as "a person's perception and responses that result from the use or anticipated use of a product, system or service" [1]. UX evaluation is particularly important for solutions in the health context, since users/patients need to maintain the motivation to keep using the technology. There are several UX evaluation methods [2], and they are classified depending on the data collected, the measures taken, and the way the data are collected [3]. Classification is also depending on the properties of UX that can be reliably and repeatedly measured and those that cannot, like the psychophysiological measures of an individual [4]. In recent years, the interest in the topic has increased [5]. Notwithstanding this growth, we have not found a comprehensive overview about the UX evaluation methods, particularly methods for evaluating health technologies for children with special needs.

---

[1] Corresponding Author, Diego López, PhD, Full Professor, Universidad del Cauca, Calle 5 N° 4-70, Popayán, Colombia; E-mail: dmlopez@unicauca.edu.co

We conducted a Systematic Mapping Study (SMS) to aggregate and categorize primary studies, creating an overview of the research area/topic in question [6]. The results from this SMS include the identification of several important factors, and the devices and measurements used to evaluate the user state explicitly or implicitly. We discuss the implications from the type of studies found and finally, we draw some conclusions regarding the study and the challenges it presented for the future work. Part of the motivation for doing this SMS came from the current scenario from the HapHop-Physio project [7]. It supports the rehabilitation of children with intellectual and cognitive disabilities, focusing on memory and concentration therapies. While developing the game, it was challenging to measure satisfaction in children: whether they would be able to play with the game, have fun while using it and undergo the therapies. However, we could not identify enough adapted tools to evaluate the whole experience that children can have while using this game.

2. Methods

A SMS was conducted to provide an information structure about the topic at hand. SMS is a five-step process, starting with the definition of the research questions, followed by a search for primary studies, thereafter screening the found papers for including them in or excluding them from the study. As a fourth step, key-wording of the abstracts is completed to finally perform data extraction and mapping of the selected papers [6]. There are two core components of a SMS: the research questions and the systematic map. For analyzing the scope of research provided by publications on the topic to see trends over time, the following research questions (RQs) were raised:

RQ1: Are there video games, exer-learning games, serious games and/or games for health supporting cognitive therapies for children with cognitive disabilities?

RQ2: Which video games supporting cognitive therapies have been designed and/or evaluated by UX?

RQ3: Has UX evaluation of video games (exer-learning, serious, for health) been performed in an implicit or explicit way?

Conducting the search for primary studies and screening papers for inclusion is a technical aspect and is not detailed here. After the selection of the papers meeting the criteria established for the purpose of this study, the next step was to look for key-words and concepts for building a set of categories to classify the selected papers. As a result, the following categories were defined to classify the studies by their type, according to an existing classification of research approaches [8]:

1. Guidelines papers: Studies that sketch new methods and frameworks proposed to structure the implementation of video games according to their final purpose.

2. Design proposals: In this category, all studies that propose the design of an interactive system to fulfill requirements for certain disability and population are included, following pre-stablish or validated models of their own.

3. Solution proposals: This category includes studies that describe the construction of a specific solution for the treatment, rehabilitation or improvement in health or social interactions of a population with a disability.

4. Validation papers: These studies use several resources to measure the user experience of video games, through design and development stages.

Besides identifying the type of research that was carried out and reported in the selected studies, it is also important to characterize the research objectives of these primary studies. Therefore, the second classification comprises:

A. Evaluating games: These studies verify through different evaluation methods, how the users perceived the designed/developed game.

B. Verifying benefits: The authors from these studies measure how the game impacts the health of the user.

C. Rehabilitation: These studies present the games as the mean to rehabilitate people with cognitive disabilities.

D. Improving skills: The studies present games for developing the cognitive skills of healthy people.

E. Building good games: These studies propose some guidelines to make good games fulfilling its rehabilitation purpose.

F. Creating methods: The authors of these studies propose new evaluation methods for evaluating as well as possible a rehabilitation game.

G. Improving games: These studies show how a previous game was changed due to performed evaluations.

3. Results

We extracted and analyzed data from the abstract and key-words in 49 papers. The first outcome of the systematic mapping study is an overview from literature about video games used for supporting rehabilitation therapies, especially for children with cognitive impairments.

Regarding RQ1, we found seven types of games (Figure 1), but nothing on exer-learning games. Different type of games found in the studies and classified as interactive games, web platforms, technology solution systems, robots, Brain-Computer Interface systems, and haptic systems, were set as Human-Computer Interaction (HCI) systems.

Regarding the age of target users, we found not only children (47%), but also elderly people (13%). 40% of the studies did not report the target audience. When talking about the children being the target users, not all the studies were designed/developed for children with cognitive impairments. 41% of the studies were looking for improving cognitive skills for children in their developmental stage. Among the disabilities found (59%), there are Down syndrome, obsessive-compulsive disorder, Attention Deficit Hyperactivity Disorder, and delays in speech.

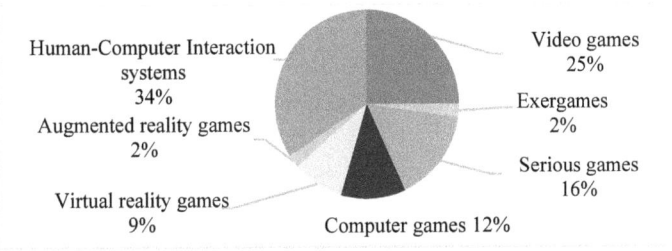

Figure 1. Video games types

RQ2 has two parts for answering it: Regarding the studies belonging to the design proposal category from the classification scheme, only 10% of the studies were designed from UX, and the remainder 90% used other methods. Regarding the UX evaluation from the HCI field, it is important to recognize two perspectives of this evaluation: (i) the evaluation of a system for improving it (user's opinion on the system) or, (ii) the evaluation of the user to improve the system (system's impact to the user). Just 17 of the studies use UX evaluation methods (5 for user evaluation and 12 for system evaluation) to assess the designed/developed system, while the 21 deploys their own evaluation methods (14 for user evaluation and 7 for system evaluation). The evaluations of the user we identified in the studies were, among others, controlled trials, taking neuropsychological measures, obtaining psychophysiological data, and recording audios and videos. In the other hand, the system evaluations included case studies, comparative studies, and feasibility studies. Regarding RQ3, 82% of the UX evaluation studies used explicit evaluation methods, while 18% deployed implicit ones. Regarding No UX evaluations, this ratio is 52% to 48%. Those studies performing the implicit evaluations, independently if they were UX or No-UX evaluations, used multiple devices for obtaining physiological measures in order to get objective data. Some of the devices/wearables used were electroencephalography neuroheadsets, Kinect from Xbox One, 3-axis accelerometers, 3D sensors, Microsoft Band 2, MYO sensors. Several of the physiological measures mentioned in the studies include EEG brainwaves, electrodermal activity, stress levels, contraction of facial muscles, movement and postural attitudes, galvanic skin response, skin temperature, heart rate, interbeat interval, heart rate variability, and respiratory rate. There has been a recently growing research interest on developing games for health environments in a personalized way, taking into account user centered methods such as the UX for the improvement of the system, and at the same time, the improvement of user's health.

The final result of the SMS is a systematic map characterizing the type of research that was carried out and the research objectives of these primary studies, as defined in the methods section. For representing this, we generate a bubble plot over the classification schemes with the studies (Figure 2) bearing in mind that the size of the bubbles is determined by the amount of studies that have been classified in the pair of defined categories. This x-y plot is the map of our research on video games for rehabilitation of cognitive disabilities in children. The categories with most studies were solution proposals for evaluating the therapeutic video games (8 papers) and validation papers for creating new evaluation methods for these kind of video games (8 papers). The research objectives categories for evaluating games and creating methods had several studies in it, with 13 and 11 studies respectively.

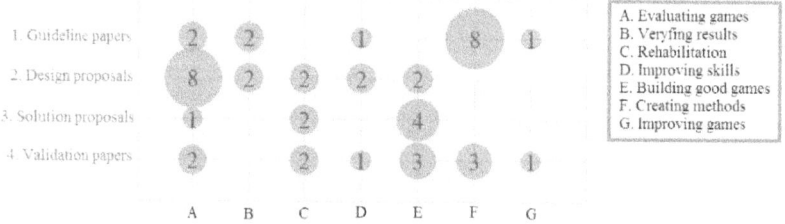

Figure 2. Distribution of the research by research objectives (x-axis) and study type (y-axis)

4. Discussion and Conclusions

Performing a SMS, we could create an overview about the topic video games to support cognitive therapies for children and how to evaluate them using UX methods. There is no clear methodology regarding parameters to be assessed both for user and for system evaluation. We followed the SMS process by defining three research questions to be answered with the findings of the study. One of the contributions of this study was the categories classification according to the research objectives; these categories gave us implications about the types of research conducted in the area, mostly evaluation of the rehabilitation systems (not their improvement) and the creation of new evaluation methods for the therapeutic systems (not standardized ones). With the map of the study built from the classification scheme, we could identify the way the video games have been developed and evaluated for the rehabilitation therapies contexts, thereby determining research gaps and future research opportunities. An unbiased selection process is difficult to ensure. However, some precautions were taken, e.g., the RQs and the inclusion and exclusion criteria were established before conducting the SMS. Another threat to the validity of the study consists of whether we selected all relevant studies in the area or not; we minimize this threat by taking into account several important scientific databases, both from the health and computer disciplines, and also considering the synonyms of the searched key-words. The final threat could be the classification scheme; nevertheless, the proper way to categorize the resulting studies relies on the perspective of the researcher in the consulted topic. As future work, we will investigate the gaps identified in this study regarding the UX evaluation concerns, to have a conceptual and developmental standard framework for estimating the implicit UX in rehabilitation video games for children.

Acknowledgments

This work was founded by the General System of Royalties (SGR) in Colombia under the "InnovAccion" Program and project HapHop-Fisio (VRI ID 4441)

References

[1]   "ISO 9241-210:2010(en), Ergonomics of human-system interaction — Part 210: Human-centred design for interactive systems." [Online]. Available: https://www.iso.org/obp/ui/#iso:std:iso:9241:-210:ed-1:v1:en. [Accessed: 01-Jun-2017].

[2]   "All About UX." [Online]. Available: http://www.allaboutux.org/. [Accessed: 31-Oct-2016].

[3]   V. Roto, A. Vermeeren, K. Väänänen-Vainio-Mattila, and E. Law, "User Experience Evaluation – Which Method to Choose?," in *Human-Computer Interaction – INTERACT 2011*, P. Campos, N. Graham, J. Jorge, N. Nunes, P. Palanque, and M. Winckler, Eds. Springer Berlin Heidelberg, 2011, pp. 714–715.

[4]   P. Kashfi, R. Feldt, A. Nilsson, and R. B. Svensson, "A Conceptual UX-Aware Model of Requirements," in *Human-Centered and Error-Resilient Systems Development*, Springer, Cham, 2016, pp. 234–245.

[5]   C. L. B. Maia and E. S. Furtado, "A Systematic Review About User Experience Evaluation," in *Design, User Experience, and Usability: Design Thinking and Methods*, A. Marcus, Ed. Springer International Publishing, 2016, pp. 445–455.

[6]   K. Petersen, R. Feldt, S. Mujtaba, and M. Mattsson, "Systematic Mapping Studies in Software Engineering," in *Proceedings of the 12th International Conference on Evaluation and Assessment in Software Engineering*, Swinton, UK, UK, 2008, pp. 68–77.

[7]   C. Rico-Olarte, S. Narváez, C. Farinango, D. M. López, and P. S. Pharow, "HapHop-Physio A Computer Game to Support Cognitive Therapies in Children," *Psychol. Res. Behav. Manag.*, vol. 10, pp. 1–9, 2017.

[8]   R. Wieringa, N. Maiden, N. Mead, and C. Rolland, "Requirements Engineering Paper Classification and Evaluation Criteria: A Proposal and a Discussion," *Requir Eng*, vol. 11, no. 1, pp. 102–107, Dec. 2005.

18

German Medical Data Sciences: Visions and Bridges
R. Röhrig et al. (Eds.)
© *2017 German Association for Medical Informatics, Biometry and Epidemiology (gmds) e.V. and IOS Press.*
This article is published online with Open Access by IOS Press and distributed under the terms
of the Creative Commons Attribution Non-Commercial License 4.0 (CC BY-NC 4.0).
doi:10.3233/978-1-61499-808-2-18

The Implementation of Medical Informatics in the National Competence Based Catalogue of Learning Objectives for Undergraduate Medical Education (NKLM)

Marianne BEHRENDS [a, 1], Sandra STEFFENS [b] and Michael MARSCHOLLEK [a]

[a] *Peter L. Reichertz Institute for Medical Informatics, Hannover Medical School, Hannover, Germany*
[b] *Dean's Office, Hannover Medical School, Hannover, Germany*

Abstract. *Introduction:* The National Competence Based Catalogue of Learning Objectives for Undergraduate Medical Education (NKLM) describes medical skills and attitudes without being ordered by subjects or organs. Thus, the NKLM enables systematic curriculum mapping and supports curricular transparency. In this paper we describe where learning objectives related to Medical Informatics (MI) in Hannover coincide with other subjects and where they are taught exclusively in MI.
Methods: An instance of the web-based MER*LIN*-database was used for the mapping process.
Results: In total 52 learning objectives overlapping with 38 other subjects could be allocated to MI. No overlap exists for six learning objectives describing explicitly topics of information technology or data management for scientific research. Most of the overlap was found for learning objectives relating to documentation and aspects of data privacy.
Discussion: The identification of numerous shared learning objectives with other subjects does not mean that other subjects teach the same content as MI. Identifying common learning objectives rather opens up the possibility for teaching cooperations which could lead to an important exchange and hopefully an improvement in medical education.
Conclusion: Mapping of a whole medical curriculum offers the opportunity to identify common ground between MI and other medical subjects. Furthermore, in regard to MI, the interaction with other medical subjects can strengthen its role in medical education.

Keywords. Medical Education, Medical Informatics, Teaching, Curriculum

1. Introduction

For German medical education, the National Competence Based Catalogue of Learning Objectives for Undergraduate Medical Education strives to define competencies students should have acquired by the time they graduate [1]. The catalogue is divided

---

[1] Marianne Behrends, Peter L. Reichertz Institute for Medical Informatics, University of Braunschweig - Institute of Technology and Hannover Medical School, Carl-Neuberg-Strasse 1, 30625 Hannover, Germany; E-mail: Behrends.Marianne@mh-hannover.de

into three sections with 19 chapters and 1958 learning objectives [2]. The first section consists of seven chapters representing the different physicians' roles (e.g. medical expert, communicator, manager, etc.). The second section includes medical knowledge, clinical expertise and professional attitudes. The third section lists a number of typical patient encounters and diseases.

The NKLM presents a medical 'core curriculum' that goes beyond the established order of medical subjects or organs. The approach is rather to teach important medical competencies and skills. This offers the possibility for all subjects in a medical faculty to compare their learning content with NKLM learning objectives (so-called 'mapping'). In this way, the mapping of a whole curriculum provides a certain degree of transparency. Thereby also small subjects – like Medical Informatics (MI) – can demonstrate their contribution to Undergraduate Medical Education.

This paper discusses the 'mapping-experience' of MI at Hannover Medical School (MHH) and shows where learning objectives related to the MI overlap with other subjects and where MI exclusively teaches them.

The overlap of learning objectives shows where interdisciplinary teaching cooperations could be meaningful. Since the learning content of MI in Hannover is based on the catalogue of competency-based learning objectives „Medical Informatics" for undergraduate medical education of the gmds [3], the results could also be relevant for other faculties.

2. Methods

At MHH mapping the curriculum in comparison to the NKLM was done by using the web-based MERLIN-database [4]. The MER*LIN*-database is a web application realized with PHP and MySQL and developed in the joint project *Medical Education Research - Lehrforschung im Netz BW* which was funded by the German Federal Ministry of Education and Research [5]. MI was mapped by the module coordinator and two teachers. Using the MER*LIN*-database all subjects could be identified that have learning objectives in common with MI. Furthermore, learning objectives that were exclusively taught by MI could be identified. In a second step, the selected NKLM competencies were assigned to main topics of MI.

3. Results

In total, 52 learning objectives from ten different chapters could be assigned to MI (figure 1). Predominantly, learning objectives associated to the physicians' roles 'scholar', 'collaborator', 'health advocate" and 'professional' and 'medical-scientific skills' were identified. Furthermore, learning objectives from 'diagnostic procedures', 'therapeutic principles', 'ethics, history and law of medicine' and 'health promotion and prevention' and the role 'medical expert' were assigned to MI.

With regard to other medical subjects, an overlap with 38 other subjects exists. The strongest overlap exists with Hygiene (22 learning objectives) followed by Clinical Medicine, General Medicine, Gynecology/Obstetrics and Pain Management (figure 2).

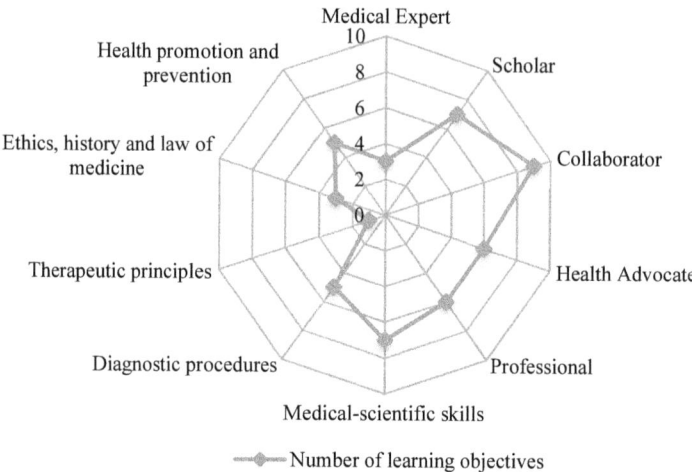

Figure 1. Distribution of learning objectives of MI according to the NKLM.

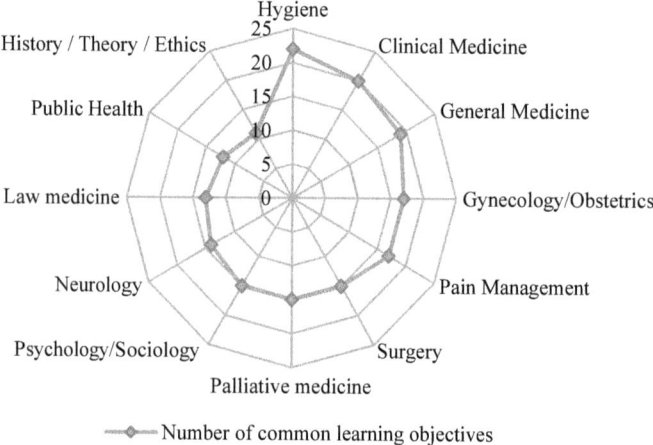

Figure 2. Medical subjects with more then ten overlaps with MI.

Table 1 contains the NKLM reference number [2] of all learning objectives of MI sorted by the number of overlap with other medical subject. Column three contains the main MI topics of the learning objectives.

Table 1. Learning Objectives of the Medical Informatics in the NKLM.

No of other subjects	No of learning objective in NKLM	Main topics of Medical Informatics
none	10.7.1.1, 10.7.1.3, 10.7.1.4, 10.7.1.5, 14a.2.2.13, 14c.6.3.3	hospital information systems, electronic patient records, storage and transmission of medical data, telemedicine, management of scientific research
1-2	6.3.1.1, 6.3.1.3 , 6.4.3.3, 8.4.1.3, 10.7.1.2, 14c.6.3.2, 15.12.2.1, 19.1.10.3,	medical learning and teaching systems, project management in research, medical information systems, clinical workplace systems, assisting health technologies, consumer health informatics
3-14	5.2.2, 6.3.1.2, 6.3.2.1, 6.3.2.2, 6.3.2.3, 8.2.2.1, 8.2.2.2, 8.2.2.3, 8.3.2.1, 8.4.1.1, 8.4.1.2, 8.4.2.1, 8.4.2.2, 10.1.1.1, 11.1.2.1, 11.2.3.1, 11.2.3.2, 11.1.3.1, 11.4.3.5, 14a.2.2.1, 14a.2.2.12, 14a.3.1.1, 14c.6.3.1, 15.1.1.3, 15.1.1.7, 15.1.1.8, 15.3.1.2, 16.5.3, 18.1.1.5, 18.3.1.2., 18.3.2.3, 19.1.6.2, 19.1.9, 19.1.10.1, 19.1.10.2,	interdisciplinary cooperation, telematics services, data privacy and protection in science, decision support systems, data handling, medical classification systems, special aspects of data privacy, documentation of medical data, image and image signal processing, and other
27	5.1.2, 5.3.4, 11.1.1.3	documentation of medical data, special aspects of data privacy

In terms of content, no overlap exists with regard to learning objectives that explicitly describe the handling and usage of information technology or data management for scientific research (table 1), e.g. hospital information systems, electronic patient records, storage and transmission of medical data, telemedicine, (table 1).

Learning objectives regarding topics like medical learning and teaching systems, project management in research, medical information systems, clinical workplace systems, health-enabling technologies and consumer health informatics are taught only by a maximum of two other subjects.

Learning objectives relating to documentation of medical data and special aspects of data privacy are taught by 27 other subjects (table 1).

4. Discussion

The NKLM offers the possibility to map a whole curriculum, thus revealing common learning objectives. For MI, we could identify a number of shared learning objectives with other subjects. However, the overlap of learning objectives does not necessarily mean that other subjects teach topics of MI. For example, learning objectives describing themes of information technology are exclusively conveyed by MI. However, the strong overlap of learning objectives with the Hygiene was not expected.

A limitation of this work is that in some cases the NKLM learning objectives are open for interpretation. Therefore, the assignment of MI topics to the learning objectives can, to some extent, only provide a rough orientation. Nevertheless, it can help MI to identify common ground with other medical subjects which could lead to an important exchange and hopefully an improvement in medical education.

5. Conclusion

Mapping of a whole medical curriculum offers the opportunity to identify common ground between MI and other medical subjects. By using MER*LIN*-database and the support of the deans' office it was possible to conduct the analysis with a reasonable investment of time and effort. One of the next steps will be the interdisciplinary exchange about common learning objectives, hopefully involving synergy effects and streamlining for students. After all, interdisciplinary teaching of medical core competences is one of the central approaches of the NKLM and might hopefully lead to an improvement of undergraduate medical education. Furthermore, in regard to MI, the interaction with other medical subjects can strengthen its role in medical education.

6. Conflict of Interest

The authors state that they have no conflict of interests.

References

[1]   M.R. Fischer, D. Bauer, K. Mohn. Finally finished! National Competence Based Catalogues of Learning Objectives for Undergraduate Medical Education (NKLM) and Dental Education (NKLZ) ready for trial. GMS Z Med Ausbild. 2015;32(3):Doc35.
[2]   http://www.nklm.de (2017-03-16)
[3]   R. Röhrig, J. Stausberg, M. Dugas, GMDS project group „Medical Informatics Education in Medicine", Development of national competency-based learning objectives "Medical Informatics" for undergraduate medical education, *Methods Inf Med.* **52** (3) 2013, 184–188.
[4]   O. Fritze, M. Boecker, M. Gornostayeva, S. Durante, J. Griewatz, W. Öchsner, E. Narziß, A. Wosnik, M. Lammerding-Köppel. Kompetenzorientiertes Curriculummapping im MERlin-Projekt: eine Online-Datenbank als Tool zur gezielten curricularen Weiterentwicklung. *Jahrestagung der Gesellschaft für Medizinische Ausbildung (GMA). Hamburg, 25.-27.09.2014.* Düsseldorf: German Medical Science GMS Publishing House; 2014. DocV232. DOI: 10.3205/14gma255
[5]   http://www.merlin-bw.de/ (2017-05-16)

2. Epidemiological Surveillance, Screening and Registration

German Medical Data Sciences: Visions and Bridges
R. Röhrig et al. (Eds.)

doi:10.3233/978-1-61499-808-2-25

Implications of Low Levels of the UV Index for Sun Protection

Maria LEHMANN[a,1], Annette B. PFAHLBERG[a], Henner SANDMANN[b],
Wolfgang UTER[a] and Olaf GEFELLER[a]

[a] *Dept. Med. Inf., Biometry and Epidemiology, University of Erlangen, Germany*
[b] *German Federal Office for Radiation Protection, Oberschleißheim, Germany*

Abstract. A Global Solar Ultraviolet Index (UVI) value of 2 is generally linked to the health message 'You can safely stay outside!' To examine whether this is sound advice for all skin types and even for prolonged periods spent outside we used erythemal irradiance data of all 136 days during the study period from 2014 till 2016 with such a UVI measured by the German Federal Office for Radiation Protection (BfS) in Munich, Germany. A comparison between the ambient erythemal doses calculated for various time intervals and minimal erythemal doses (MEDs) of the Caucasian skin types I-IV led us to a critical reappraisal of the above health message. Specifically, the message might be misleading if people with a fair complexion want to spend several hours outside, because without any protective measures the doses received can be sufficient to induce erythema. We thus recommend an amendment of the health message related to a safe level of the UVI and, moreover, generally tailoring UVI-related health messages to different skin types. Currently, these messages do not seem to be strictly evidence based, which might be one reason for the unexpected result of our analysis.

Keywords. Ultraviolet rays, health promotion, radiation monitoring

1. Introduction

The Global Solar Ultraviolet Index (UVI) describes the maximum intensity of erythemally weighted solar ultraviolet (UV) radiation received during a particular day on the earth's surface [1]. For this purpose, the highest 30-min moving average, presented as a single value rounded to the nearest whole number, is defined as the measured daily maximum UVI [2]. The UVI was introduced in 1995 by the World Health Organization (WHO), the World Meteorological Organization, the United Nations Environment Programme and the International Commission for Non-Ionizing Radiation Protection (ICNIRP) [3].

In a practical guide [2] published in 2002 these organizations described how the UVI should be used as a public awareness tool. Possible values of the UVI cover the interval 0 to 11+. This value range was divided into 5 exposure categories which were linked to specific health messages. The exposure category 'low', defined as the range from 0 to 2, is connected to the simple messages 'No protection required' and 'You can safely stay outside!' As these messages do not contain any time limitation, one could

---

[1] Corresponding Author: maria.lehmann@fau.de
The present work was performed in partial fulfillment of the requirements for obtaining the degree
"Dr. rer. biol. hum." at the University of Erlangen-Nuremberg.

expect that staying outside all day with a UVI value of 2 will not lead to harm through UV radiation. In 2012, however, a report from the UVI working group of ICNIRP [1] stated that, although the threshold for recommending sun protection at UVI levels of 3 and above was reconfirmed, sun protection might be recommended for people burning easily and planning to stay outdoors for prolonged periods. It remained unclear what evidence led to this ICNIRP statement. In particular, the reconfirmation of the UVI threshold for a safe outdoor stay and the change of general health messages concerning UVI into more complex skin type specific messages need to be scrutinized. The aim of our study is thus to quantify UV exposure on days with a UVI value of 2 using ambient UV erythemal irradiance data. We compare the resulting erythemal doses for different time intervals with minimal erythemal doses (MEDs) focusing on the Caucasian skin types I to IV as described by Fitzpatrick [4]. Thus we examine whether staying outside on days with a UVI of 2 is indeed free of UV-related risk in different skin photo types.

2. Methods

Ambient UV erythemal irradiance data measured at the German Federal Office for Radiation Protection (BfS) facility in Munich-Neuherberg (48.21°N, 11.58°E, altitude 493m a.s.l.) were used. This measuring station is part of the German solar UV-monitoring network (described in detail in [5]), led-managed by the BfS. At that site, a double monochromator Bentham DTM300 is used as a spectral radiometer. Incident radiation is transmitted from a horizontal detector to that device via an optical fiber. Inside of the spectral radiometer, radiation is split by wavelength with the use of a diffraction grating and mapped onto a photomultiplier. The resulting photocurrent is converted to spectral irradiance (unit $Wm^{-2}nm^{-1}$) by applying a calibration function. Spectral irradiance is then weighted with the International Commission on Illumination (CIE) erythemal reference action spectrum, leading to erythemal irradiance (unit Wm^{-2}). Measurements are conducted every 6 minutes between sunrise and sunset. Quality control is assured through the additional use of erymeters and comparison to modelled values. The calibration of the measuring device is traceable to the German National Metrological Institute. Erythemal irradiance data from 2014 until 2016 of all available days with a UVI value of 2 from the Munich measuring station were used.

Erythemal irradiance data were linearly interpolated and integrated over ten different time intervals to calculate erythemal doses received therein. We defined noon as 13:00 local time, irrespective of the actual solar noon occurring on average at 12:20 local time on measurement days when standard time was in effect and at 13:07 local time on measurement days when daylight saving time was in effect, respectively. We assumed that people spending their lunch break outdoors would do this mostly around this time, no matter if daylight saving time was in effect or not. The considered intervals were 12:45-13:15, 12:30-13:30, 12:00-14:00, 11:30-14:30, and 11:00-15:00, corresponding to 0.5, 1, 2, 3, and 4h around noon, respectively. Ambient erythemal doses were also calculated for the intervals 9:00-11:00, 15:00-17:00, 8:30-11:30 and 14:30-17:30, being equivalent to 2h and 3h, each before and after noon, respectively. Additionally, the total ambient daily erythemal doses, from sunrise to sunset, were calculated. Data were analyzed using the statistical software package R (www.R-project.org).

Table 1. Average minimal erythemal doses (MEDs) of Fitzpatrick skin types [4]. (SED = Standard Erythema Dose = 100 J/m² effective)

Fitzpatrick skin type	Minimal Erythemal Dose (SED)
I	2.0
II	2.5
III	3.0
IV	4.5

Average erythemal doses received on the detector are reported as mean ± standard deviation with minimum and maximum. They were compared to average MEDs of Fitzpatrick skin types I through IV as shown in Table 1. One MED is the amount of solar UV exposure that produces minimal perceptible redness of the skin 24h after exposure. It can therefore be considered a short-time maximum dose that should not be exceeded to prevent detrimental effects of UV radiation [6].

3. Results

The sample consisted of erythemal irradiance data of 136 days with a UVI value of 2. Most of these days fell into the winter period (n=54), followed by fall (n=45). Thus these two seasons provided 73% of our data. Only few days fell into spring (n=22) and summer (n=15), because a UVI of 2 in spring/summer in Munich occurs only on days with a dense cloud cover. Seasons were defined astronomically. Altogether, 53% (n=72) of the days occurred when standard time was in effect and 47% (n=64) of the days occurred during the period of daylight saving time.

Table 2. Ambient erythemal UV exposure calculated for different time intervals on days with a UVI value of 2. (SED = Standard Erythema Dose = 100 J/m² effective)

Time interval (local time, duration)	UV exposure			
	Mean (SED)	Standard deviation (SED)	Maximum (SED)	Minimum (SED)
Before noon				
09:00-11:00, 2h	1.5	0.5	2.9	0.1
08:30-11:30, 3h	2.3	0.7	4.6	0.6
Around noon (13:00)				
12:45-13:15, ½h	0.7	0.2	1.2	0.2
12:30-13:30, 1h	1.4	0.4	2.3	0.4
12:00-14:00, 2h	2.8	0.7	4.4	1.0
11:30-14:30, 3h	4.0	1.0	6.4	1.4
11:00-15:00, 4h	5.1	1.2	8.1	2.0
After noon				
15:00-17:00, 2h	1.0	0.6	3.9	0.1
14:30-17:30, 3h	1.6	0.9	5.3	0.2
Total day				
Sunrise – sunset	8.1	2.0	16.6	4.5

Ambient erythemal doses and the time intervals during which they are received are shown in Table 2. In the two shortest considered time intervals, half an hour and one hour around noon, the mean received erythemal doses are 0.7 ± 0.2 standard erythema doses (SED, equivalent to 100 J/m² effective after weighting with the CIE action spectrum) and 1.4 ± 0.4 SED, respectively. Both doses are smaller than the MEDs of all Caucasian skin types. The mean erythemal dose received in the 2h-interval around noon is 2.8 ± 0.7 SED, which is greater than one MED of skin types I and II. MEDs of skin types III and IV are exceeded after 3h and 4h of exposure around noon (4.0 ± 1.0 SED and 5.1 ± 1.2 SED), respectively.

When we take a look at exposure loads that are received either before or after noon, we notice that these 2h-intervals expectedly yield less erythemal dose than an interval of the same duration around noon. Mean doses in both intervals are smaller than the MEDs of the Caucasian skin types. A 3h exposure before noon leads to a mean ambient erythemal dose of 2.3 ± 0.7 SED which is larger than one MED for skin type I. An interval of the same duration, but during afternoon, leads to a mean dose of 1.6 ± 0.9 SED which is well below the MEDs of skin types I to IV.

Maximum doses are significantly higher than the mean doses for all intervals and therefore start exceeding MEDs in much smaller intervals (details see Table 2).

The mean total ambient daily erythemal dose is 8.1 ± 2.0 SED which exceeds the MED of skin type I 4.1-fold, the MED of skin type II 3.2-fold, the MED of skin type III 2.7-fold and the MED of skin type IV 1.8-fold. Even the minimum dose (4.5 SED) exceeds the MEDs of skin types I to III and is equivalent to one MED of skin type IV.

4. Discussion

The WHO health message 'You can safely stay outside!' for days with a UVI of 2 could not be confirmed entirely when comparing calculated ambient erythemal doses for various time intervals with the MEDs of Caucasian skin types. Our evaluation of UV hazard on days with a UVI value of 2 used irradiance data from 136 of such days in Munich in the years 2014-2016. Our focus on data from Munich does not imply that our results cannot be generalized to other regions, as the UVI is a standardized quantity irrespective of geographical location.

If we look at the mean erythemal doses, the MED of skin type I is exceeded after an exposure of 3h before noon or even less than 2h around noon. The latter exposure time of 2h around noon also yields exposure loads greater than the MED of skin type II. After 3h of exposure around noon also skin type III would have received more than one MED and 4h of exposure even exceed one MED for skin type IV. In rare cases, MEDs can be exceeded in significantly shorter time intervals. Differences in received doses between time intervals of equal length before and after noon are likely due to the fact that we considered 13:00 local time as noon, irrespective of the solar noon which is averagely 40 minutes before this for the 53% of our sample using standard time and 7 minutes after this for the 47% of our sample using daylight saving time. The cumulated daily ambient erythemal dose is distinctly greater than the MEDs of all Caucasian skin types.

Our study has some limitations. (i) By calculating erythemal doses for time intervals of various lengths up to total daily irradiation and comparing these to MEDs we assume that the Bunsen-Roscoe reciprocity law is valid in these ranges. This means that UV-induced damage in human skin is directly proportional to the total energy dose, irrespective of the exposure duration needed to deliver this dose. Unfortunately, research on this topic, particularly in a clinical context, is scarce. As other authors also use MEDs to evaluate UV effects not only for short-time exposure, but for e.g. daily doses [6], we consider this a valid option for the time being. (ii) The ambient erythemal doses we used are a potentially weak proxy for individual exposure as they are measured on a horizontal detector and most human skin surfaces are not oriented horizontally. On the one hand, skin surfaces facing the sun can receive significantly higher irradiances (up to 40%) during periods with clear sky and small solar elevation angle [7]. This is likely true for the vast majority of days in our sample as they belong to the fall and winter period. On the other hand, under cloudy conditions, UV on these tilted surfaces can also be reduced by 50% in comparison to horizontal-incidence UV [7]. This is likely true for the days in our sample belonging to the spring and summer period. Aside from that, many studies examined the ratio between personal and ambient daily exposure, frequently called exposure ratio (ER). For outdoor workers (who obviously spend a large fraction of the day outside) a review from 2011 reported ranges of average values of ER of 8-66% (arms and wrists), 11-85% (vertex) and 11-70% (shoulder) [8]. The high variability of these data even for the same body site demonstrates that ER is highly dependent on individual behavior, e.g. use of shade, intermittent indoor activities and bodily posture. In conclusion we think that our study represents an appropriate 'worst-case-scenario' concerning the maximum doses on days with a UVI of 2 received without any protective measures.

As ICNIRP has already stated, the health messages for low UVI values might need to be changed. This is supported by our analysis which indicates that UV hazard from prolonged periods spent outside on days with a UVI of 2 is not as harmless as assumed, especially for the fair skin types I and II. We therefore suggest a time limitation to be added to the related UVI health message. In accordance with Zaratti et al. [9] we also recommend that UVI health messages should be adapted to the most sensitive major sub-group of a country or region. Different recommendations for different skin types are contrary to the notion of keeping messages for the public simple, but marked differences in susceptibility to UV damages are well known. These differences manifest in factors of up to 2.25 between the MEDs of the different Caucasian skin types and lead to pronounced heterogeneity in our analysis of MEDs received by different skin types in the same time interval.

To the best of our knowledge, objective and evidence-based criteria for the health messages concerning the UVI have never been defined or at least not been published. WHO and its partner organizations are thus, in line with [9], encouraged to remedy this lack of transparency to enable the evaluation of such preventive advice given to the public.

References

[1] Allinson, S., et al., Validity and use of the UV index: report from the UVI working group, Schloss Hohenkammer, Germany, 5-7 December 2011. *Health Physics.* **103** (2012), 301-306.
[2] World Health Organization, Global Solar UV Index: A Practical Guide. 2002: Geneva, Switzerland.
[3] International Commission on Non-Ionizing Radiation Protection, Global Solar UV Index - A joint recommendation of the WHO, WMO, UNEP and the ICNIRP. 1995: Oberschleissheim.
[4] Fitzpatrick, T.B., The validity and practicality of sun-reactive skin types I through VI. *Arch Dermatol.* **124** (1988), 869-71.
[5] Sandmann, H., Das solare UV-Messnetz des BfS/UBA. *StrahlenschutzPRAXIS* (2015), 38-40.
[6] Feister, U., et al., UV index forecasts and measurements of health-effective radiation. *J Photochem Photobiol B.* **102** (2011), 55-68.
[7] McKenzie, R.L., et al., Erythemal UV irradiances at Lauder, New Zealand: relationship between horizontal and normal incidence. *Photochem Photobiol.* **66** (1997), 683-9.
[8] Siani, A.M., et al., Occupational exposures to solar ultraviolet radiation of vineyard workers in Tuscany (Italy). *Photochem Photobiol.* **87** (2011), 925-34.
[9] Zaratti, F., et al., Proposal for a modification of the UVI risk scale. *Photochem Photobiol Sci.* **13** (2014), 980-5.

30   *German Medical Data Sciences: Visions and Bridges*
R. Röhrig et al. (Eds.)

doi:10.3233/978-1-61499-808-2-30

Routine Data Analyses to Compare Outpatient Depression Treatment Regimens

Robin SIEGEL[a,1] ,Thomas OSTERMANN[a], Reinhard SCHUSTER[b], Timo EMCKE[c]

[a] *Department for Psychology and Psychotherapy, Witten/Herdecke University, Alfred-Herrhausen-Straße 50, 58448 Witten, Germany*
[b] *Department of Health Economics, Epidemiology and Medical Informatics, University of Lübeck, Katharinenstraße 11, 23554 Lübeck, Germany*
[c] *Department of Prescription Analysis, Association of Statutory Health Insurance Physicians, Bismarckallee 1-6,23812 Bad Segeberg, Germany*
robin.siegel@uni-wh.de, thomas.ostermann@uni-wh.de,
reinhard.schuster@mdk-nord.de, timo.emcke@kvsh.de

Abstract. *Background:* Routine data analyses are becoming increasingly important for health policy decision making. However such databases often vary in data quality, completeness and accessibility. The aim of this study is to describe the quality of a large outpatient healthcare database, the process of data extraction and to give a brief overview of data-structure with focusing on provider-type and disease severity in an example of the treatment of depressive disorders. *Method*: The quality of the database is described and diagnosis rates of depression in outpatient care (ICD-10 diagnoses F32/33) in relation to the provider-type (i.e. general or somatic physician vs. physicians specialized in mental-health vs. psychotherapist) were calculated using Cramers V as a measure for effect size. *Results:* The database consisted of 2,383,672 cases from 2015. Most depressive patients were diagnosed and treated by general or somatic physicians. A clear relationship between the severity of depression and provider-type is shown. In contrast to psychotherapists or physicians specialized in mental-health, general or somatic physicians diagnose a higher rate of unspecified depressive episodes.
Keywords. depression, outpatients, secondary data analysis, provider-type, mental health services

1. Introduction

Decision making in health services research has always been a point of critical discussion between the stakeholders involved. In particular, the planning of resources for epidemiologically relevant diseases like depression is often is discussed controversially and routine data analyses are becoming increasingly important to generate an evidence base.

Due to its high prevalence [1-4] depression is associated with high costs [5-8] and increasingly high numbers of disability days [9]. Therefore it has become important to analyse treatment costs and provider efficiency for depression among the large variety of healthcare providers in inpatient-care and outpatient-care [10].

Analyzing data of a German health insurance company and the German pension fund from 2005 till 2007 Gaebel, Kowitz and Zielasek [11] found that the majority of

---

[1] Corresponding Author: Thomas.Ostermann@uni-wh.de

depressive patients in Germany were treated in outpatient care. Of those patients 71.3 % utilized general medicine services only, while 19.3 % were treated by general practitioners and specialized practitioners (i.e. psychiatrists or psychotherapists) and just 9.4 % were treated by specialized practitioners. Similar results were shown by Boenisch et al. [12] who analyzed data of the Bavaria Association of Statutory Health Insurance Physicians (Association of SHI-Physicians). Only 31.8% of the depressive patients received a threshold treatment, while 13.6 % received a sub-threshold treatment and the majority of 54.9% patients received no depression specific treatment at all.

These studies show the importance of secondary data analysis using databases provided by insurance companies, pension funds and panel physician associations to identify "real-world-problems" such as treatment-adequacy, or the misallocation of resources [13, 14]. However there are limitations and problems using secondary data, such as bias in the database, which can be caused by confounding, missing data, and misclassification [15, 16]. This article aims at describing the quality of the given database described below and the process of data extraction as well as giving a brief overview of the data-structure with focus on provider type and disease severity.

2. Methods

Without special authorization the accounting data present in the Association of SHI-Physicians can only be analyzed for specific statutory purposes and it has to comply with all regulations for person-related data. This paper is based on an internal report necessary for care management.

2.1. Data background

Our presented data covers all patients with invoiced services at the Association of SHI-Physicians of the federal state of Schleswig-Holstein in 2015 (n = 2,383,672). Since statutory health insurance is very common in Germany approximately 86.1 % of the German citizens are covered by Statutory Health Insurance [18].

The quarterly accounting process of the Association of SHI-Physicians requires diagnoses, information about the particular treatment, patient master data, physician groups and a stable id for patients. These routine data allow the compilation of stable research datasets especially for long-term time series analyses and research not easily accessible for primary research. Additional data present for care management (i.e. prescriptions, admission data) can be used for refinement and extension. All datasets are available at least from 2009 till 2016 and stored in separate relational databases (ORACLE, MySQL).

According to the quality criteria from Black and Payne [17] the coverage quality of the database can be assumed as high (level 3 to level 4), with a very high representative population and a nearly complete dataset. However, since there is no possibility to measure the reliability of the diagnostics and treatments the accuracy of the data is somewhat lower (level 1 to level 2).

2.2. Process of Data extraction

This paper is based on accounting data from 2015 (see figure 1) including all cases that visited any physician at least once, but excluding cases with only laboratory services and no physician-contact ($n = 8,442$) invoiced, with missing data for gender ($n = 1,589$) or patients who were younger than 18 ($n = 129,194$) years. The final sample consists of data from $n = 2,252,063$ individuals.

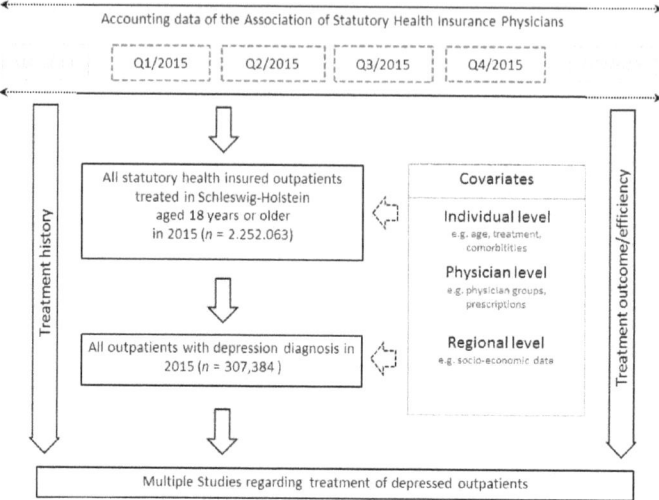

Figure 1. Process of data extraction for current and future studies.

We focused the data extraction on diagnosis of depression and included all corresponding ICD-10 codes F32 and F33 except F33.4 (recurrent depressive disorder, currently in remission). Only secured diagnoses were included in analysis. For calculations psychiatrists, child psychiatrists, specialists in psychosomatic medicine and specialists in neuro-psychiatry were defined as 'physician specialized in mental health' (SP; $n = 270$), while psychological psychotherapists, child and youth psychotherapists as well as physicians exclusively working as psychotherapists were defined as 'psychotherapists' (PT; $n = 690$). All other physicians (i.e. general physicians, specialists for internal medicine) were grouped together as 'general or somatic physicians' (GP; $n = 4425$). Cases treated by two or all three different physician groups (e.g. GP and PT) were accounted half or one third for each group. The same procedure was chosen for different diagnoses, if a patient received more than one different diagnosis above. To test differences in the distribution of diagnoses between the physicians disciplines we used Chi-square tests and calculated Cramer's V as effect sizes and as a measurement for practical significance. The level of statistical significance was defined as $\alpha = 0.05$.

3. Results

In 2015 a total number of 307,384 outpatient patients in Schleswig-Holstein were diagnosed with depression. This corresponds to a 12-month-prevalence of 13.6 %. The average age of this sample was 54.8 years ($SD = 18.0$), 69.7 % of the depression diagnosed patients were female. As shown in table 1 the majority of depressive patients ($n = 262,442$; 85.4 %) were diagnosed by GPs, whereas 10.1% were treated by SPs ($n = 31,088$) and only 4.5 % by PTs ($n = 13,854$). Almost two-third ($n = 194,001$; 65.8 %) of the patients held the diagnosis of other depressive episodes or depressive episode (F3x.8), unspecified as "most severe" diagnosis (F3x.9). Mild (F3x.0;

$n = 16,821$; 5.5 %), moderate (F3x.1; $n = 63,730$; 20.7 %), severe (F3x.2; $n = 21,313$; 6.9 %) and depression with psychotic symptoms (F3x.3; $n = 3,391$; 1.1 %) were diagnosed less often.

Three-quarter of the individuals treated by GPs received a diagnosis of other depressive episodes or depressive episode, unspecified (73.9 %) while only 23.4 % or 6.2 % of the patient treated by SPs or PTs were diagnosed this way. On the other hand most depressions treated by PTs were diagnosed as mild (19.0 %) or moderate (68.8 %) in contrast to 7.0 % (mild) or 46.2 % (moderate) for the SPs and 4.8 % (mild) or 17.5 % (moderate) for the GPs. The highest number of severe depression and depression with psychotic symptoms were diagnosed by SPs.

Table 1. Identified depressions classified by diagnose and disciplines

	F32.8/F32.9 F33.8/F33.9 n (%)	F32.0/F33.0 n (%)	F32.1/F33.1 n (%)	F32.2/F33.2 n (%)	F32.3/F33.3 n (%)	Total n
GP	194001 (73.9 %)	12006 (4.6 %)	39821 (15.2 %)	14016 (5.3 %)	2598 (1.0 %)	262442
SP	7271 (23.4 %)	2189 (7.0 %)	14371 (46.2 %)	6495 (20.9 %)	762 (2.5 %)	31088
PT	857 (6.2 %)	2626 (19.0 %)	9538 (68.8 %)	802 (5.8 %)	31 (0.2 %)	13854
Total	202129 (65.8 %)	16821 (5.5 %)	63730 (20.7 %)	21313 (6.9 %)	3391 (1.1 %)	307384

Chi-square test shows a significant relationship in the distributions of severity between the disciplines ($\chi2$ (8) = 63240; $p < 0.001$) with a moderate effect (Cramer's V = 0.321). Even the comparison of SPs and PTs, without including GPs, shows a moderate effect ($\chi2$ (8) = 5375; $p < 0.001$; Cramer's $V = 0.346$).

4. Discussion

This article provides a short insight on the use of routine data analysis in the field of health services and health policy research. Our results reveal a clear relationship between medical disciplines and diagnosis of depression. The high amount of unspecified depressions diagnosed by GPs could either be due to a high amount of subclinical depressions or due to a lack of certainty and reliability of diagnostics by GPs. This could also explain the calculated 12-month-prevalence of 13.6 %, which is considerably higher than in most German interview-based studies [1, 2, 4]. In accordance with Boenisch et al. [11] most patients were treated by general practitioners. Since this is only a short cross-sectional analysis without information about multiple healthcare utilization, further research on long-term development and treatment of depression is necessary and should include the characteristics of patients utilizing multiple different healthcare suppliers.

5. Conclusion

There are some important conclusions regarding future studies. Due to its high coverage the dataset of the Association of SHI-Physicians has the potential to address and answer socially relevant topics. Apart from our example this might also include the analysis of comorbidities of other psychiatric or somatic illnesses, the extent and cost of treatments regarding the number of psychotherapy sessions or the drugs-description-rate in relation to the diagnosis or discipline. Since the dataset consists of data from 2009 till 2016, long term time-series-analyses about treatment-outcome or the change of treatment regimen might also be possible. In contrast to data of the health insurance companies the data does not cover treatment in inpatient care. Finally, by linking the datasets to regional geo-referenced data (such as inhabitant-physician-rate, income, and unemployment rate) the identification of important socioeconomic factors for treatment utilization on regional level might be a promising field of research.

6. Conflict of Interest

The authors state that they have no conflict of interests.

References

[1] F. Jacobi, M. Höfler, J. Strehle et al., Psychische Störungen in der Allgemeinbevölkerung. Studie zur Gesundheit Erwachsener in Deutschland und ihr Zusatzmodul Psychische Gesundheit (DEGS1-MH), *Nervenarzt* **85** (2014), 77 - 87.

[2] A. Bramesfeld, T. Grobe, F. Schwartz, Who is treated, and how, for depression? An analysis of statutory health insurance data in Germany, *Soc Psychiatry Psychiatr Epidemiol* **42** (2007), 740–746.

[3] J. Alonso, M.C. Angermeyer, S. Bernert et al. Prevalence of mental disorders in Europe: results from the European Study of the Epidemiology of Mental Disorders (ESEMeD) project. *Acta Psychiatr Scand* **109** (2004), 21–27.

[4] M.A. Busch, U.E. Maske, L. Ryl, R. Schlack, U. Hapke, *Bundesgesundheitsblatt* **56** (2013) 733 – 739.

[5] M. Luppa, S. Heinrich, M.C. Angermeyer, H.H. König, S. G. Riedel-Heller, Cost-of-illness studies of depression. A systematic review, *Journal of Affective Disorders* **98** (2007), 29–43.

[6] S. Friemel, S. Bernert, M.C. Angermeyer, H.H. König, The direct costs of depressive disorders in Germany. *Psychiatr Prax* **32** (2005), 113–121.

[7] K. Kleine-Budde, R. Müller, W. Kawohl, A. Bramesfeld, J. Moock, W. Rössler W. The cost of depression - a cost analysis from a large database. *Journal of Affective Disorders* **147** (2013) 137 – 143.

[8] B.G. Druss, R.A. Rosenheck, W.H. Sledge, Health and disability costs of depressive illness an a Major U.S. Corporation. *Am. J. Psychiatr.* **157** (2000), 1274–1278.

[9] T. Grobe, S. Steinmann TK-Gesundheitsreport 2016. Schwerpunktthema: Gesundheit zwischen Beruf und Familie. www.tk.de

[10] A. Bramsfeld, et al., Who is diagnosed as suffering from depression in the German statutory health care system? An analysis of health insurance data. *Eur J Epidemiol* **22** (2007), 397 – 403.

[11] W. Gaebel, S. Kowitz, J. Zielasek, The DGPPN research project on mental healthcare utilization in Germany: inpatient and outpatient treatment of persons with depression by different disciplines. *Eur Arch. Psychiatry Clin Neurosci* **262** (Suppl 2) (2012), 51 – 55.

[12] S. Boenisch, R.D. Kocalevent, H. Matschinger et al., Who receives depression-specific treatment? A secondary data-based analysis of outpatient care received by over 780,000 statutory health-insured individuals diagnosed with depression. *Soc Psychiatry Psychiatr Epidemiol* **47** (2012), 475 – 486.

[13] S. Schneeweiss & J. Avorn, A review of uses of health care utilization databases for epidemiologic research in therapeutics. *J Clin Epidemi* **58** (2005), 323 – 337.

[14] C.R. Crooke, & T.J. Iwashyna, Using existing data to address important clinical questions in critical care. *Crit Care Med* **41** (2013), 886 – 896.

[15] Y. Murakami, Secondary Data Analysis of Epidemiology in Asia, *J Epidemiol* **24** (2014), 345 – 346.

[16] D.D. Terris, D.G. Litaker, S.M. Koroukian, Health state information derived from secondary databases is affected by multiple source of bias, *Journal of Clin Epidemiol* **60** (2007), 734 – 741.

[17] N. Black, & M. Payne, Directory of clinical databases: improving and promoting their use. *Qual Saf Health Care* **12** (2003), 348 – 352.

[18] VdeK - Verband der Ersatzkassen. Daten zum Gesundheitswesen: Versicherte. Verfügbar unter https://www.vdek.com/presse/daten/b_versicherte.html / [23.03.2017]

3. Research Methods

German Medical Data Sciences: Visions and Bridges
R. Röhrig et al. (Eds.)
© 2017 German Association for Medical Informatics, Biometry and Epidemiology (gmds) e.V. and IOS Press.
doi:10.3233/978-1-61499-808-2-37

Standards-Based Procedural Phenotyping: The Arden Syntax on i2b2

Sebastian MATE [a,1], Ixchel CASTELLANOS [b], Thomas GANSLANDT [c],
Hans-Ulrich PROKOSCH [a,c] and Stefan KRAUS [a]

[a] *Medical Informatics, Univ. of Erlangen-Nürnberg, Erlangen, Germany*
[b] *Department of Anesthesiology, University Hospital Erlangen, Erlangen, Germany*
[c] *Center for Medical Information and Communication, University Hospital Erlangen, Erlangen, Germany*

Abstract. Phenotyping, or the identification of patient cohorts, is a recurring challenge in medical informatics. While there are open source tools such as i2b2 that address this problem by providing user-friendly querying interfaces, these platforms lack semantic expressiveness to model complex phenotyping algorithms. The Arden Syntax provides procedural programming language construct, designed specifically for medical decision support and knowledge transfer. In this work, we investigate how language constructs of the Arden Syntax can be used for generic phenotyping. We implemented a prototypical tool to integrate i2b2 with an open source Arden execution environment. To demonstrate the applicability of our approach, we used the tool together with an Arden-based phenotyping algorithm to derive statistics about ICU-acquired hypernatremia. Finally, we discuss how the combination of i2b2's user-friendly cohort pre-selection and Arden's procedural expressiveness could benefit phenotyping.

Keywords. phenotyping, cohort identification, i2b2, Arden Syntax

1. Introduction

The process of identifying patient cohorts based on a set of characterizing patient data elements is commonly referred to as "phenotyping" in the literature. According to the SHARPn project [1], phenotyping is the algorithmic recognition of patients. It includes clinical trials, quality metrics, outcomes research, observational studies, decision support, and other tasks [1]. The search strategy to identify a patient cohort is called "phenotyping algorithm". According to [1], such algorithms consist of complex sets of inclusion and exclusion criteria, coupled using sets of logical operators. Mo et al. [2] have found that "phenotyping algorithms can involve multiple complex logical steps, integrating various operations". These can be Boolean logic, numeric comparator operations, arithmetic functions (e.g. to calculate BMI), aggregative operations (e.g. COUNT, FIRST), negation (negative assertion vs. exclusion/empty set) and temporal relations between events [2]. Ross et al. [3] found that 85% of the eligibility criteria of clinical trials had a significant semantic complexity and 40% relied on temporal data.

The widely used *Informatics for Integrating Biology and the Bedside* (i2b2) [4,5] is a software platform that can be used for basic phenotyping. The system contains

---

[1] Corresponding Author: **Sebastian.Mate@fau.de**

special features such as automatic unit conversion or conceptual subsumption to automatically query for child concepts as found in hierarchically structured terminologies. The query logic relies on Boolean logic, numeric comparison operations, negation and temporal aspects. However, as outlined by Mo et al. [2], the complexity of phenotyping algorithms (like those in eMERGE [6]) can exceed the capabilities of platforms such as i2b2. While the current i2b2 version 1.7 has included support for complex temporal relations, there are still some limitations. For example, i2b2 limits numeric comparators to fixed values (e.g. "$A > 120$") and it is not possible to model relative comparisons (e.g. "$A > B$"). Furthermore, it does not support arithmetic functions, which could be used to compute criteria on-the-fly (e.g. "$BMI = weight / height^2$").

The Arden Syntax for Medical Logic Systems [7] may be a suitable technology to address these shortcomings. It is an HL7 standard that was designed to enable clinical decision support functions in the form of Medical Logic Modules (MLMs), which are typically used to monitor clinical events. It was intended to be user-friendly, enabling even non-experts in computer science to write MLMs. It also features a rich set of operators and a time-stamped data type system that is tailored to medical data.

In this paper, we investigate if i2b2 can be used together with the Arden Syntax to go beyond the functionality of current phenotyping systems. It is our aim to provide a proof of concept and to discuss the assets and drawbacks of this approach.

2. Methods

We created a prototypical Java tool. It contains an integrated MLM editor that uses the RSyntaxTextArea library (https://github.com/bobbylight/RSyntaxTextArea) for which we implemented Arden Syntax highlighting (see Figure 1).

We then developed and integrated a method for translating i2b2 queries into "template" MLMs. By deriving and parsing the i2b2 query XML definitions from the i2b2 database, we create Arden Syntax lists for all i2b2 ontology concepts that were used in the original query. To populate these with data, our tool creates Arden "curly braces" expressions, which contain the SQL statements to retrieve the data records directly from the i2b2 database. It then adds further Arden code, which merges all lists into one central data structure in the form of a list of patient objects, which we called "Patient-Data". Each patient object within "PatientData" provides an attribute for the patient number, as well as one attribute for each original i2b2 query concept. To assist the user with later converting the "template" MLM into a true phenotyping algorithm, a comment is automatically generated and inserted into the MLM to reveal the available attributes of the "PatientData" object (Figure 1, first visible line of code).

Finally, we integrated Arden2ByteCode, a Java-based, open source Arden Syntax environment [8], into our tool. The execution of an MLM in Arden2ByteCode can be triggered from within our program, which also displays the result of the execution.

3. Results

Our implementation allows for post-processing i2b2 query results with Arden Syntax MLMs by applying additional (more restrictive) filtering or computations on patient data, which have been found with the i2b2 system previously. The user has to go through the following steps to use our system:

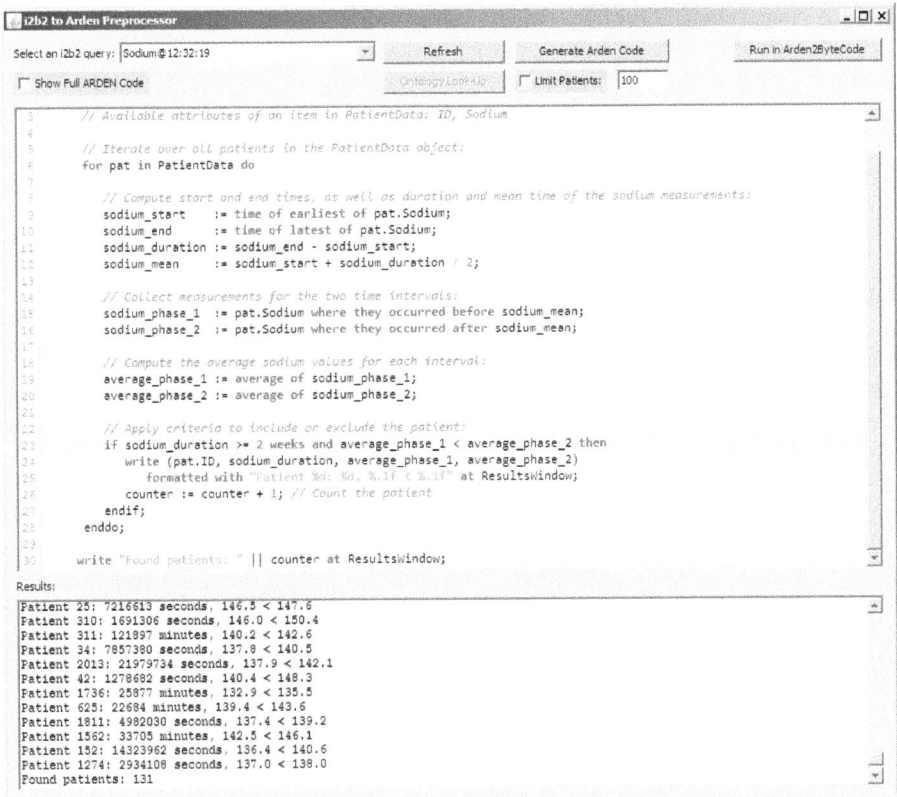

Figure 1. i2b2Arden user interface with a phenotyping algorithm (patient numbers anonymized).

1. The user creates and executes a query within the i2b2 environment. This query includes the clinical data elements of interest, along with their Boolean relations. It may also use other i2b2 features, such as temporal relations and value restrictions.

2. The user opens our tool and selects this i2b2 query. The tool then analyzes the i2b2 query and automatically prepares an MLM template. This transforms the facts data of the i2b2 query's data elements into appropriate Arden Syntax data structures.

3. The user adds further phenotyping logic, based on the Arden Syntax' rich set of around 150 operators, to the MLM. This may include complex temporal logic, operations on values and comparisons between multiple data elements.

To test our prototype in a real environment, we designed and performed a data analysis for the largest 35-bed ICU at our local University Hospital. ICU-acquired hypernatremia (IAH) is a commonly described phenomenon, where sodium blood values increase during hospitalization. Risk factors associated with IAH have been reported, such as male gender and age above 50 [9].

We exported the patient age, gender and sodium measurements since 2015 from our ICU system and uploaded these into an i2b2 project on our i2b2 version 1.7.07 instance. As described above, the first step was to run a query in i2b2. In our example, this initially included only one concept, "*Sodium*". This i2b2 query returned 2,242 patients (the whole database). After creating the MLM template with our tool, we created the phenotyping algorithm, which is shown in Figure 1. The program counts and lists all applicable patients with increasing sodium values. By replacing the "<" comparator in line 23 with ">", the patients with decreasing sodium were found. For 43.8%, the sodium values were increasing. We then repeated the test and modified the initial i2b2 query to include the constraints "*Age > 50 years*" and "*Gender = Male*". After running the Arden Syntax MLM again, we found 48.5% of second group having increasing values, which supports the findings of [9].

4. Discussion

While our phenotyping MLM still needs refinement and further evaluation of the results, it demonstrates that our approach is capable of executing complex procedural phenotyping algorithms, and is able to benefit from the easy-to-use, graphical pre-selection of patient cohorts within i2b2. We plan further investigations on how to design easy-to-use, yet powerful, phenotyping environments. Tools such as i2b2 were not intended to be fully featured data analysis or dedicated phenotyping environments, but rather meant to serve as user-friendly hypothesis generation and validation tools to allow for pre-selecting patient cohorts. Yet, it would still be useful for researchers not having to fall back on low-level technology (such as SQL) or complex statistical software for pursuing complex phenotyping. It is a matter of discussion where to draw the line between user-friendliness and computational power. Future work might focus on integrating our Arden code editor directly into the i2b2 workbench.

Similar approaches are described in the literature. For example, there are various "R" environment integrations for i2b2 (e.g. [10]). These, however, do not allow for "live" editing of program code, in contrast to our approach. There are also other procedural approaches (e.g. [11]), but these do not build upon i2b2 or similar platforms to enable an easy-to-use pre-selection of patient cohorts.

From a technical point of view, computationally equivalent "phenotyping power" could be achieved in any Turing-complete programming language. However, we believe that our example illustrates that the Arden Syntax code might be easier to understand for non-experts in computer science, which was one of the design goals of the Arden Syntax standard [12]. Applying an all-purpose programming language instead may considerably reduce the number of potential users.

Our tool is of prototypical character and there is room for future improvements. It is based on Arden Syntax version 2.5, which is the latest version supported by Arden2Bytecode. Therefore we had to make some concessions: As described above, our tool prepares an MLM to include all concepts from the i2b2 query. This has been implemented by embedding SQL queries to access the i2b2 database. However, as they only return a database record set, we had to post-process these data records to properly align values and their associated time stamps. Otherwise it would not be possible to make use of certain Arden Syntax constructs, such as *time of*. This post-processing requires about 40 lines of additional Arden Syntax code for each concept that has been used in the i2b2 query. Our current workaround is to allow hiding the automatically generated code in our tool via a checkbox (as shown in Figure 1). Therefore support for later versions of the Arden Syntax would considerably facilitate the integration process. In particular, the *as time* operator introduced in version 2.8 would save the additional code required to transform the string representation of a timestamp into the time data type of the Arden Syntax.

Finally, another aspect of later versions of the Arden Syntax is the support for fuzzy logic. The possibility of applying "soft" inclusion and exclusion criteria instead of "hard" Boolean logic could improve current patient identification methods.

5. Acknowledgements

The present work was performed in (partial) fulfillment of the requirements for obtaining the degree "Dr. rer. biol. hum." from the Friedrich-Alexander-Universität Erlangen-Nürnberg (FAU) (SM).

6. Human Subjects Protection

This study is in accordance with the German Bavarian Hospital Law (BayKrg §27). Only anonymized routine care patient data were used, no formal intervention was performed and no additional patient data were collected.

7. Software Availability

The source code and the full demonstration MLM from this paper are available on GitHub (https://github.com/sebmate/i2b2Arden).

References

[1]   Rea S, Pathak J, Savova G, et al., Building a Robust, Scalable and Standards-Driven Infrastructure for Secondary Use of EHR Data: The SHARPn Project, J Biomed Inform 45 (2012), 763–71.
[2]   Mo H, Thompson WK, Rasmussen LV, et al., Desiderata for Computable Representations of Electronic Health Records-Driven Phenotype Algorithms, J Am Med Inform Assoc 22 (2015), 1220–30.
[3]   Ross J, Tu S, Carini S, et al., Analysis of Eligibility Criteria Complexity in Clinical Trials, AMIA Summits Transl Sci Proc (2010), 46–50.
[4]   Kohane IS, Churchill SE, Murphy SN, A Translational Engine at the National Scale: Informatics for Integrating Biology and the Bedside, J Am Med Inform Assoc 19 (2012), 181–5.
[5]   Murphy SN, Weber GM, Mendis ME, et al., Serving the Enterprise and Beyond with Informatics for Integrating Biology and the Bedside (i2b2), J Am Med Inform Assoc 17 (2012), 124–30.
[6]   McCarty CA, Chisholm RL, Chute CG, et al., The eMERGE Network: A Consortium of Biorepositories Linked to Electronic Medical Records Data for Conducting Genomic Studies, BMC Med Genomics 4 (2011), 13.
[7]   Pryor TA, Hripcsak G, The Arden Syntax for Medical Logic Modules, Int J Clin Monit Comput 10 (1993), 215-224.
[8]   Gietzelt M, Goltz U, Grunwald D, et al., Arden2ByteCode: A One-Pass Arden Syntax Compiler for Service-Oriented Decision Support Systems Based on the OSGi Platform, Comput Methods Programs Biomed 106 (2012), 114–25.
[9]   Alansari M, Abdulmomen A, Hussein M, et al., Acquired Hypernatremia in a General Surgical Intensive Care Unit: Incidence and Prognosis, Saudi J Anaesth 10 (2016), 409.
[10]   Segagni D, Ferrazzi F, Larizza C, et al., R Engine Cell: Integrating R Into the i2b2 Software Infrastructure, J Am Med Inform Assoc 18 (2011) 314–7.
[11]   Li D, Endle CM, Murthy S, et al., Modeling and Executing Electronic Health Records Driven Phenotyping Algorithms Using the NQF Quality Data Model and JBoss® Drools Engine, AMIA Annu Symp Proc (2012), 532–41.
[12]   Samwald M, Fehre K, de Bruin J, et al., The Arden Syntax Standard for Clinical Decision Support: Experiences and Directions, J Biomed Infor 45 (2012), 711–8.

42

German Medical Data Sciences: Visions and Bridges
R. Röhrig et al. (Eds.)
© *2017 German Association for Medical Informatics, Biometry and Epidemiology (gmds) e.V. and IOS Press.*
This article is published online with Open Access by IOS Press and distributed under the terms
of the Creative Commons Attribution Non-Commercial License 4.0 (CC BY-NC 4.0).
doi:10.3233/978-1-61499-808-2-42

On-The-Fly Query Translation Between i2b2 and Samply in the German Biobank Node (GBN) Prototypes

Sebastian MATE [a,1,*], Patric VORMSTEIN [b,*], Dennis KADIOGLU [a,c], Raphael W. MAJEED [d], Martin LABLANS [e], Hans-Ulrich PROKOSCH [a,f] and Holger STORF [b]

[a] *Medical Informatics, Univ. of Erlangen-Nürnberg, Erlangen, Germany*
[b] *Medical Informatics Group, University Hospital Frankfurt, Frankfurt, Germany;*
German Cancer Consortium (DKTK), partner site Frankfurt;
and German Cancer Research Center (DKFZ), Heidelberg, Germany
[c] *Institute of Medical Biostatistics, Epidemiology and Informatics, University Medical Center of the Johannes Gutenberg University Mainz, Mainz, Germany*
[d] *German Center for Lung Research, Justus-Liebig-University, Giessen, Germany*
[e] *Medical Informatics in Translational Oncology, German Cancer Research Center (DKFZ), Heidelberg, Germany*
[f] *Center for Medical Information and Communication, Erlangen University Hospital, Erlangen, Germany*

Abstract. Information retrieval is a major challenge in medical informatics. Various research projects have worked on this task in recent years on an institutional level by developing tools to integrate and retrieve information. However, when it comes down to querying such data across institutions, the challenge persists due to the high heterogeneity of data and differences in software systems. The German Biobank Node (GBN) project faced this challenge when trying to interconnect four biobanks to enable distributed queries for biospecimens. All biobanks had already established integrated data repositories, and some of them were already part of research networks. Instead of developing another software platform, GBN decided to form a bridge between these. This paper describes and discusses a core component from the GBN project, the OmniQuery library, which was implemented to enable on-the-fly query translation between heterogeneous research infrastructures.

Keywords. Data harmonization, federated search, biobanking, interoperability

1. Introduction

Medicine is a highly heterogeneous environment, and information integration is a recurring challenge in a medical informatics researcher's day-to-day business. Not only does the information content differ from the medical perspective, one has to deal with a plethora of different data sources. This is a major issue in networked research, where medical data has to be integrated in order to build large-scale data pools to enable the identification of patients with e.g. rare diseases or special types of cancer. In recent years, different approaches to address this problem were developed (an overview can

---

[1] Corresponding Author: **Sebastian.Mate@fau.de**　　[*] These authors contributed equally to this paper.

be found in [1]). However, when different toolsets are used across institutions, the issue of merging and retrieving medical information on a national or international level remains. Furthermore, the willingness of research partners to install additional software and to keep data available in a duplicated fashion is certainly limited, resulting in a need to interconnect already existing platforms.

The German Biobank Node project (GBN) [2], which is part of the *Biobanking and BioMolecular resources Research Infrastructure* (BBMRI) [3], aims to build a network of interconnected biobanks on a national level in Germany. The ultimate goal is to give researchers the ability to search for patients with certain diseases and their associated specimens. The project faced the above-mentioned issues of already exiting, heterogeneous research infrastructures. Aiming not to establish a dedicated GBN platform, the project decided to implement an approach for direct query message translation between the already existing research architectures. By injecting these translated messages into the other system, queries could be executed natively, without implementing an abstraction layer. In this paper, we describe a core component, the OmniQuery library, which enables this on-the-fly query translation between these different research architectures, and discuss the current limitations of our approach.

2. Methods

The GBN prototypes were implemented by four GBN partners and tested with their associated biobanks. Those are the DZL biobank (Giessen University Hospital), the Charité ZeBanC (Berlin), the biobank of the University Cancer Center Frankfurt (UCT Frankfurt) and the biobank of the Comprehensive Cancer Center Erlangen (CCC Erlangen-EMN). In recent years, research teams in Giessen and Erlangen developed i2b2-based data warehouses (DWHs) that are fed with sample data from their biobank systems [4,5]. Similarly, Berlin and Frankfurt established the commercial software CentraXX® (Kairos GmbH), which has been enhanced to serve as local DWHs within the German Cancer Consortium's (DKTK) bridgehead architecture "Samply" [6].

Against this background, GBN decided to support CentraXX® and i2b2 in its prototypes. The challenge was to establish a new hybrid architecture integrating both types of DWH. This required bridging between the already existing two architectures and enabling the translation of queries that were created with the user interface of one platform to the schema and ontology of the other platform. If the query was properly translated, it could be injected into the other architecture without the architecture recognizing that it originated from an external system. By that, it would not have been necessary to modify the original architectures on a large scale.

To meet the goal of executing shared queries (created at a central point within the network) on CentraXX® and i2b2, these have to be distributed to the biobanks at the different sites. To implement the GBN query distribution, we based our two prototypes on components from the Samply system and the "lightweight i2b2 server and client libraries" (li2b2, https://github.com/li2b2), a development from the AKTIN project in Giessen [7]. The Samply components, which were developed by the DKTK and used in Berlin and Frankfurt, allow distributed search among (in this case) CentraXX®-based biobanks. Likewise, the li2b2 components allow interconnecting i2b2-based DWHs.

Given that Samply and li2b2 were already available for query transport, GBN's major challenge was the query translation between CentraXX® and i2b2. To achieve a better understanding of both systems' query capabilities, we conducted a thorough analysis of the two query formalisms used in Samply/CentraXX® and li2b2/i2b2. Both use XML-based query definitions to communicate the medical concepts used in a query, along with their logical relationships ("AND" and "OR"). They also share a similar approach for formulating and executing queries. The inclusion and exclusion criteria for feasibility queries are expressed by medical data elements, which are retrieved from a terminology service. Queries are then formulated by combining multiple data elements with Boolean logic. Data elements may describe the plain existence of a condition (e.g. "male gender") or a more detailed observation (e.g. blood glucose measurements). Furthermore, data elements can be grouped hierarchically on both systems. Depending on the data type of the data elements in a query, a numeric value including a comparator can be attached to the data element, but is also possible to simply check for the plain existence of a data element by omitting the numeric comparison. On both systems, it is also possible to exclude patients from the query result.

Table 1. Comparison between the two different query logics.

Feature	Samply/CentraXX®	li2b2/i2b2
Query Formalism	Full Boolean logic, models SQL formalism	Boolean logic in conjunctive normal form (CNF), models i2b2 formalism
Numeric Comparators	Greater or equal, greater than, equal, less or equal, less than, not equal, between, in (with slightly different naming)	
Check for Existance	"Is Not Null" comparison	Removal of numeric constraint
Non-Existence	"Is Null" comparison	Exclusion of query panel
Metadata	Samply MDR (ISO-11179-based [8])	i2b2 ontology (own model)
Grouping of Data Elements	Mono-hierarchical and catalogs (e.g. for LOINC, ICD-10)	Mono-hierarchical incl. utilization during query runtime (hierarchical subsumption)
Temporal Logic	None	Constrain by fixed dates, complex relative logic (sequence of events)
Other Features	None	Unit conversion, occurs, grouping (financial encounter, modifier)

Despite these similarities, and as outlined in Table 1, there are differences between both platforms, which need to be addressed in order to allow for translating query messages. Both systems express queries in XML syntax, but it is not possible to perform direct XML transformations due to the different types of Boolean logic used. However, this can be overcome by utilizing logic transformations based on rules on logic equivalence. The different naming of numeric comparators can be addressed by replacing the identifiers. Both systems support the "Check for Existence" query feature, which requires a data element to be available for a patient, independently of its value (for catalogs or numeric values). For numeric data elements, compatibility can be achieved by simply removing the numeric value in i2b2 queries or by replacing the comparator with "Is Not Null" in CentraXX® queries. Similarly, the opposite operator "Check for Non-Existence" can be translated in both directions easily. Because both systems utilize their metadata internally during query run-time, it is not necessary to perform syntactic translations related to metadata, except for concept mapping. This can be addressed by providing 1:1 mappings. Similarly, the conceptual subsumption feature of i2b2 can be replicated in CentraXX® by providing 1:n mappings.

3. Results

This analysis enabled us to implement OmniQuery, a Java library, which uses Plain Old Java Objects to hold content and logic of "generic" feasibility queries. Its instantiated objects represent a tree-like structure and are composed out of three main classes. An *OmniQuery* class acts as a root node, which can contain an unlimited number of child nodes, a *LogicNode* class represents logical associations as a child node and a *ConstraintNode* class defines the actual constraints as leaves of the tree structure. Furthermore, enumerations for marking *LogicNodes* and *ConstraintNodes* such as AND, OR, EQUALS, etc. have been integrated. This approach enables performing arbitrary, tree-related algorithms on the data structure and easily manipulating the structure such as changing ancestor and children of a given node. This object structure allows to represent the common features of both Samply and i2b2 queries. To perform the logic transformations, we integrated the open source library AIMA3e (https://github.com/aimacode/aima-java), an implementation based on algorithms from [9], which allows us to normalize any structure from full Boolean logic into conjunctive normal form (CNF, see Table 1). For the purpose of query translation, the OmniQuery Library implements a class for each query formalism, which invokes the transformation of the respective language into the OmniQuery format and vice versa. Those transformation implementations consume an interface provided by OmniQuery so that any other query language can be added to the tool belt of available translators. In the context of the GBN prototypes, we implemented two of these translator classes, *I2B2Translator* and *SamplyTranslator*. Both parse the original query formalism and build an OmniQuery object, which can then be translated into the other syntax by using the other translator. In this process, the translators address the differences that were described above, except for the CNF conversion (which is a feature of the core OmniQuery library).

4. Discussion

The idea to mediate between different data sources is not new, in particular on the "lower" level of databases. One approach is to combine heterogeneous data sources with a virtualization layer, as it has been done e.g. in SALUS [10]. However, attempts to integrate data sources on the "higher" level of heterogeneous software platforms are rare, at least to our knowledge. The EHR4CR system is capable of executing feasibility queries directly on the i2b2 database [11]. It does not, however, utilize the native i2b2 software stack to run these queries. In contrast, and to the best of our knowledge, our approach is the first successful attempt of interconnecting heterogeneous cohort selection platforms directly by utilizing automatic query translation and adhering to the platforms' native interfaces.

The intention behind OmniQuery was to create a generic method to translate queries between arbitrary cohort selection platforms and allow usage of different DWHs. Thus far, the library has only been used in the two GBN prototypes to translate between i2b2 and Samply. While most cohort selection platforms build on a set of features that is very similar to those two systems, OmniQuery is not fully generic. For instance, it is lacking support for advanced features that are not present in one of the systems (such as temporal constraints). In the case of our two prototypes this has not been a problem as it successfully translated queries that met the requirements of the GBN demonstrator in terms of query complexity. Both prototypes were demonstrated to the GBN consortium in February 2017, and they were able to translate and execute queries. The system currently supports querying categorical data elements, such as "gender" or "type of sample", as well as numeric data elements, which is in particular useful for lab values.

The follow-up project German Biobank Alliance will dictate future directions of OmniQuery. However, ongoing efforts in BBMRI are indicating that its platform will also be based on Samply for injecting and distributing queries in the European network. In contrast to this pilot, it is currently planned to use MOLGENIS [12] for local data integration and as a local DWH. We plan to investigate whether OmniQuery could also act as a bridge between Samply and MOLGENIS.

5. Software Availability

The source code of OmniQuery is available on GitHub (https://github.com/German-Biobank-Node/OmniQuery).

6. Acknowledgements

The present work has been funded by the Federal Ministry of Education and Research of Germany within the project *German Biobank Node* (project number 01EY1301). It was performed in (partial) fulfillment of the requirements for obtaining the degree "Dr. rer. biol. hum." from the Friedrich-Alexander-Universität Erlangen-Nürnberg (SM).

References

[1] Xu J, Rasmussen LV, Shaw PL, et al., Review and Evaluation of Electronic Health Records-Driven Phenotype Algorithm Authoring Tools for Clinical and Translational Research, *J Am Med Inform Assoc* 2015, ocv070.

[2] Lablans M, Kadioglu D, Mate S, et al., Strategies for Biobank Networks, *Bundesgesundheitsblatt* **59.3** (2016), 373-378.

[3] van Ommen G-JB, Törnwall O, Bréchot C, et al., BBMRI-ERIC as a Resource for Pharmaceutical and Life Science Industries: The Development of Biobank-Based Expert Centres, *Eur J Med Genet* **23.7** (2015), 893-900.

[4] Majeed RW, Röhrig R., Automated Realtime Data Import for the i2b2 Clinical Data Warehouse: Introducing the HL7 ETL Cell, *Stud Health Technol Inform* **180** (2012), 270-4.

[5] Ganslandt T, Mate S, Helbing K, et al., Unlocking Data for Clinical Research – The German i2b2 Experience, *Appl Clin Inform* **2.1** (2011), 116.

[6] Lablans M, Kadioglu D, Muscholl M, et al., Exploiting Distributed, Heterogeneous and Sensitive Data Stocks While Maintaining the Owner's Data Sovereignty, *Methods Inf Med* **54.4** (2015), 346-352.

[7] Ahlbrandt J, Brammen D, Majeed RW, et al., Balancing the Need for Big Data and Patient Data Privacy - An IT Infrastructure for a Decentralized Emergency Care Research Database, *Stud Health Technol Inform* **205** (2013), 750-754.

[8] Kadioglu D, Weingardt P, Ückert F, et al., Samply.MDR – Ein Open-Source-Metadaten-Repository, *German Medical Science GMS Publishing House* 2016, doi:10.3205/16gmds149.

[9] Russell SJ, Norvig P, Artificial Intelligence, Prentice Hall, 2010.

[10] Sun H, Depraetere K, De Roo J, et al., Semantic Processing of EHR Data for Clinical Research, *J Biomed Inform* **58** (2015), 247-259.

[11] Bache R, Miles S, Taweel A, An Adaptable Architecture for Patient Cohort Identification From Diverse Data Sources, *J Am Med Inform Assoc* **20.e2** (2013), e327-e333.

[12] Swertz MA, Dijkstra M, Adamusiak T, et al., The MOLGENIS Toolkit: Rapid Prototyping of Biosoftware at the Push of a Button. *BMC Bioinformatics* **11.12** (2010), S12.

German Medical Data Sciences: Visions and Bridges
R. Röhrig et al. (Eds.)

doi:10.3233/978-1-61499-808-2-47

Evaluation of the IT Infrastructure of the RESIST Study with the Evidence-Based CIPROS Checklist

Doris LINDOERFER[a,1] and Ulrich MANSMANN[a]

[a] *Institute for Medical Information Processing, Biometry and Epidemiology (IBE),*
Ludwig-Maximilians-Universität München, Munich, Germany

Abstract. Efficient and powerful information systems are substantial to perform medical research projects successfully. Especially, translational medicine poses specific challenges to the corresponding IT infrastructure. The RESIST study is a translational research project in oncology where xenografts inform about patients second-line treatment. DBFORM, an in-house developed system, was used as EDC system. It was enhanced with project specific features. We demonstrate how the CIPROS checklist has the potential to optimize the related requirements engineering process. The CIPROS checklist consists of 72 items, organized within 12 Aspects/Topics and was developed to assess such patient registry software systems. In this paper we use the CIPROS checklist (1) to elucidate the projects requirements and (2) to assess systems features. The application of the CIPROS checklist to fix the RESIST project requirements and system features was successful. The interplay between (1) and (2) helped to accelerate the requirements engineering process and to set up a system suitable to perform the translational research project successful.

Keywords. Information Systems, Software, Translational Medical Research, Registries, Checklist

1. Introduction

Efficient and powerful information systems are core instruments in medical research projects. Specific challenges come from translational medicine which aims to apply a growing understanding of the molecular basis of diseases into clinical practice. This challenges informatics and data with regard to representation of data that is suitable for computational inference (knowledge representation), as well as linking heterogeneous data sets (data integration). Information systems are needed which implement these tasks in the execution of translational clinical trials.

The RESIST study (EudraCT number 2016-003295-46) [1] is a translational research project in which xenografts inform second-line treatment for patients with advanced colorectal carcinoma (aCRC). Ethical vote by the Ludwig-Maximilians-Universität München's internal review board (project-no: 131-16, chairperson: Prof. Dr. Wolfgang Eisenmenger) is available. The trial consists of three parts: 1.) a patient

---

[1] Corresponding Author: Doris Lindoerfer, Dipl.-Inf.; Institute for Medical Information Processing, Biometry and Epidemiology (IBE), Ludwig-Maximilians-Universität München, Marchioninistrasse 15, D-81377 Munich, Germany; Email: lindoerf@ibe.med.uni-muenchen.de.

registry, 2.) a clinical trial where patients are treated with cetuximab until secondary resistance, and 3.) a large collection of avatars carrying probes of individual patients and being treated with alternative substances. In the second phase of the clinical trial, patients are treated with an experimental treatment which has turned out to be predicted as most effective by the patient's AVATARMODELs.

Electronic data capture (EDC) uses an in-house developed system (DBFORM) [2], which is enhanced with features specifically needed for the RESIST study. Since requirements engineering is also essential in the medical domain [3], it is of interest that the extension of the basic DBFORM system is guided by a clear requirements engineering process [4], [5], with results which are compliant with essential aspects of a good EDC system for translational studies.

The CIPROS checklist [6] is an evidence-based assessment tool, which consists of 72 items, organized within 12 Aspects/Topics, developed to assess patient registry software systems. It supports developers to assess requirements for existing systems, to formulate requirements for own systems, and it strengthens the reporting of patient registry software system descriptions. It can be a first step to create standards for patient registry software system assessments.

The objective of this paper is to describe the use of the CIPROS checklist: (1) To elucidate the IT infrastructure needed for the RESIST trial, and (2) to assess the architectural profile of DBFORM. The interplay of both aspects results in a development plan for the IT infrastructure of the RESIST project.

2. Methods

2.1. Evaluation of the RESIST Study Requirements with CIPROS

In order to perform the requirements assessment for the RESIST project we use four categories of answers per CIPROS item: *Yes, needed; yes, nice to have; no;* and *no, but nice to have*. Items which are *yes, nice to have* are more urgent to implement, than the items which are categorized as *no, but nice to have*.

2.2. Evaluation of the DBFORM System Features with CIPROS

Each CIPROS item is checked if it is implemented in DBFORM or not. A rating of the degree of implementation is used: *Yes, implemented in the system*; *partly implemented in the system*; *yes, implemented in special projects*; *partly implemented in special projects*; *configurable in special projects*; *partly configurable in special projects*; and *not available*. Items with the rating *"implemented in special projects"* are not or not yet necessary for the RESIST study.

2.3. Combination of the Both Rating Results

In order to compare both assessments we introduced four categories: yes/yes, (feature is available in DBFORM and is needed for the RESIST study); no/no, (feature is not available in the system and not necessary for the RESIST study); yes/no (feature is available in the system but is not needed for the RESIST study) and no/yes (feature is not implemented in the system, but necessary for the RESIST study). CIPROS items only partly implemented in the DBFORM system or configured easily are regarded as yes. The implementation of only partly implemented items, is either sufficient for the RESIST study, or is not needed in the RESIST study, or is discussed below.

3. Results

3.1. Evaluation of the DBFORM System Features with CIPROS regarding need to perform the Project

The evaluation of the 72 CIPROS items for the DBFORM System regarding the need to perform the project resulted in 37 are yes, needed, 7 are rated as yes, nice to have, 20 are no and 8 are no, but nice to have.

3.2. Evaluation of the DBFORM System Features with CIPROS regarding the existing Implementation

The evaluation of the DBFORM System Features with CIPROS regarding the existing implementation is shown in Figure 1. A total of 24 items out of 72 are implemented in the system, 22 fully and 2 partly. 27 items are implemented in special projects, 22 fully, 2 partly 2 are configurable and 1 is partly configurable. A total of 21 items are not implemented in DBFORM.

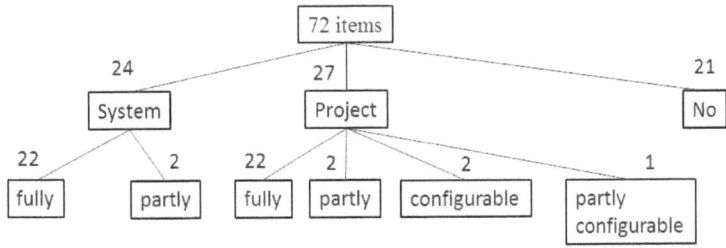

Figure 1. Overall evaluation result of the DBFORM system features with CIPROS.

3.3. Combination of the Both Assessment Results

We combined the results, evaluating the RESIST IT infrastructure and the one evaluation the DBFORM system features (58 out of 72 items got congruent answers: 80.6%). Forty items are available in the system and necessary in the RESIST study. Eighteen items are not available in the system, but also not needed in the RESIST study. Eleven items are available in the DBFORM system but not necessary in the RESIST study. They are irrelevant for the requirements plan. Only three items are not available in the system but needed in the RESIST study.

Item 4.2 "Standardized data are used whenever possible" is not available in the system, but needed in the RESIST study. Using check-boxes based on a vocabulary using international clinical standards will solve this problem. Item 7.4 "Graphical presentation of results" is not yet implemented in the system. At the moment we export the data into the R software [7] where the graphs are produced. Item 10.4 "Source documentation of CRFs in pdf format is possible" is categorized with "yes, nice to have" and will be implemented. The complete evaluation list with the 72 CIPROS items is available by email from the corresponding author of this paper.

4. Discussion

The RESIST trial needs a phenotype database for patient as well as avatar data, and databases for corresponding extensive molecular findings. The following items represent a selection from the 27 project specific items shown in Figure 1.

"Item 2.5, Performance testing" is only partly available in DBFORM. Performance testing is less challenging in the RESIST study because there are only a limited number of users. "Item 3.4, Messaging interface" is implemented in the RESIST study IT infrastructure. "Item 3.13, Integration of biological data" is categorized as "Yes, Project" and DBFORM has to be enhanced to meet the RESIST study requirements. "Item 6.1, Pseudonymous patient identifier", is needed in the RESIST study on several levels. Data protection requirements request different identifiers for the clinical patient data, for the tumor probes and for the AVATARMODEL data, therefore three parallel pseudonymous identifiers for each patient are created.

The CIPROS items "6.2, CRF is divided in parts", "6.7, Multiple choice is used", "6.8, No predefined selection", "6.9, Data validation components", will be implemented in DBFORM and are adapted for the RESIST study. CIPROS items "6.12, Manual data queries", "6.13, Data query flags" and "6.14, Plausibility flags" are not available in DBFORM and are not necessary in the RESIST study. But, they are on the implementation list of DBFORM.

The "Item 9.1, Data protection concept" is established for the RESIST study and "Item 9.2, Double pseudonymization", will be implemented.

CIPROS items "11.1, Compliance with regulations", "11.2, Informed consent", "11.3, Rights on the data", "11.4, Data protection guidelines", "12.1, User manuals" are implemented in the RESIST study. Item "12.2, User training" was considered as not necessary, but will be performed at a later stage. Also item "12.3, User feedback" will be perhaps performed later. Item 12.4, "Online help" would be nice to have and is on the implementation list.

DBFORM is not developed following a design model (item 2.1), but uses elements of design models, dependent of the specific project. DBFORM did not implement an online discussion forum, (item 3.5). Up to now DBFORM has no patient interface (item 3.7) implemented. It has no interface to HIS/CIS, (item 3.12). We gave answer "no" for standardization of CRFs, Data, Metadata and Vocabularies, (items 4.1 – 4.4), because there is no implemented thesaurus, but standardized answers with multiple choice menus are used. There is no XML-Schema for data exchange, (item 4.5). Manual data queries, (item 6.12), are not possible also data query flags, (item 6.13), and plausibility flags, (item 6.14), are not implemented. There is no query builder for researchers, (item 7.1), and report generation, (item 7.2), graphical presentation of results, (item 7.3), and risk analysis, (item 7.5), are not possible. Encrypted data storage at the single-item level, (item 8.4), is not possible, except for user passwords. Multi-client capability, (item 10.2), is not supported, there is no update mechanism, (item 10.3), and source documentation of CRFs in pdf format, (item 10.4), is also not possible.

In our example the evaluation turned out to be successful. We found some new items for DBFORM, which will be implemented in the future.

The complete evaluation can be done in two to four hours dependent on the experience with CIPROS and with the concrete system and project, which is very fast if new requirements can be detected.

5. Conclusion

The CIPROS checklist is developed to assess patient registry software systems. It can be used to specify the requirements for projects as well as to evaluate existing systems to show their features. Combining both assessments shows the degree of conformity and helps to find appropriate systems for real projects. The CIPROS checklist is an instrument to accelerate the requirements engineering process. It helps to specify features for further development of patient registry software systems and it strengthens the reporting about patient registry software systems.

The CIPROS checklist complements existing general requirements specification templates. It accelerates the requirements engineering process of building new systems for patient registries by implementing the already published treasure trove of experiences into the development process of new systems.

Using the CIPROS checklist is no guarantee that all requirements are considered. CIPROS is based on the actually published literature which may not cover very new techniques.

Furthermore, CIPROS is not developed to find requirements for specialized registries with special requirements.

6. Conflict of Interest

The authors state that they have no conflict of interests.

7. Acknowledgement

German Cancer Aid (Deutsche Krebshilfe) for funding the RESIST study.

References

[1] Lindoerfer D, Mansmann U. IT infrastructure of an oncological trial where xenografts inform individual second line treatment decision, *Stud Health Technol Inform.* **235** (2017), 226-230.
[2] Müller TH, Adelhard K. A web-based central diagnostic data repository, *Stud Health Technol Inform.* **90** (2002), 246-250.
[3] Kossmann M. The significance of requirements engineering for the medical domain, *J Med Eng Technol.* **38** (2014), 238-43. doi: 10.3109/03091902.2014.918199.
[4] Bruegge B, Dutoit A. *Object-Oriented Software Engineering Using UML, Patterns, and Java, Third Edition,* Pearson, Harlow, Essex, 2014, 115-165.
[5] Wiegers K, Beatty J. *Software Requirements, Third Edition,* Microsoft Press, Redmont, Washington, 2013, 190-201.
[6] Lindoerfer D, Mansmann U. A Comprehensive Assessment Tool for Patient Registry Software Systems: The CIPROS Checklist, *Methods Inf Med.* **54** (2015), 447-54. doi: 10.3414/ME14-02-0026.
[7] The R Project for Statistical Computing. Available: https://www.r-project.org/ (Accessed: 17 Mar 2017)

German Medical Data Sciences: Visions and Bridges
R. Röhrig et al. (Eds.)
© *2017 German Association for Medical Informatics, Biometry and Epidemiology (gmds) e.V. and IOS Press.*
doi:10.3233/978-1-61499-808-2-52

Analysis of Age and Gender Structures for ICD-10 Diagnoses in Outpatient Treatment Using Shannon's Entropy

Fabian SCHUSTER[a] , Thomas OSTERMANN[b] ,Timo EMCKE[c]
and Reinhard SCHUSTER[1,d,e]
[a] *European University Viadrina Frankfurt (Oder), Germany*
[b] *Witten/Herdecke University, Herdecke, Germany*
[c] *Associations of Statutory Health Insurance Physicians, Bad Segeberg, Germany*
[d] *Medical Advisory Board of the Statutory Health Insurance, Lübeck, Germany*
[e] *Lübeck University, Lübeck, Germany*

Abstract. Introduction: Diagnostic diversity has been in the focus of several studies of health services research. As the fraction of people with statutory health insurance changes with age and gender it is assumed that diagnostic diversity may be influenced by these parameters. Methods: We analyze fractions of patients in Schleswig-Holstein with respect to the chapters of the ICD-10 code in outpatient treatment for quarter 2/2016 with respect to age and gender/sex of the patient. In a first approach we analyzed which diagnose chapters are most relevant in dependence of age and gender. To detect diagnostic diversity, we finally applied Shannon's entropy measure. Due to multimorbidity we used different standardizations. Results: Shannon entropy strongly increases for women after the age of 15, reaching a limit level at the age of 50 years. Between 15 and 70 years we get higher values for women, after 75 years for men. Discussion: This article describes a straight forward pragmatic approach to diagnostic diversity using Shannon's Entropy. From a methodological point of view, the use of Shannon's entropy as a measure for diversity should gain more attraction to researchers of health services research.

Keywords. ICD-10 codes, diagnoses, age structure, gender structure, outpatient treatment, statutory health insurance, Shannon's entropy

1. Introduction

Outpatient treatment due to specific patient groups with related cost effects has gained more and more attention to health policy makers in recent years. Several works have concentrated in the analysis of medical diagnoses in outpatient treatment (Jutel 2009). In particular, diagnostic diversity has been in the focus of several studies (Bell 2014). In particular, Jutel (2009) found that sociodemographic parameters including social class, age and gender might be regarded influencing factors for diagnostic diversity. Thus there is an urgent need to analyze medical diagnoses in this context. One possible way to do so is to analyze secondary data i.e. from large patient registers or insurance data.

The fraction of people with statutory health insurance changes with age and can suspect that on average they have a lower morbidity. Due to reimbursements not all

---

[1] Corresponding Author, Reinhard Schuster, Katharinenstraße 11, 23554 Lübeck, Germany; E-mail: reinhard.schuster@mdk-nord.de

treatments of patients with private insurance are reported to those insurances. There are no valid morbidity data for the comparison of private and statutory health insurances. This complicates or prevents population based considerations. In contrast to hospital treatment there are no main diagnoses defined by the statutory physicians.

The main objective of this paper is to analyze whether there is an influence of gender and age with respect to diagnostic diversity. This supports the development of interdisciplinary treatment concepts for patient subgroups with a focus on multimorbidity.

2. Material and Methods

This article considers all diagnoses for all patients of statutory health insurance in Schleswig-Holstein in quarter 2/2016. We analysed all diseases diagnosed coded in the International Statistical Classification of Diseases and Related Health Problems in its 10th Revision (ICD-10) by physicians treating the patient. Thus this article takes a patient centered point of view.

The first descriptive part analyzes, if the resolution level of chapters (e.g. Chapter IX, Diseases of the circulatory system, I00-I99), ICD-Blocks (e.g. Ischaemic heart diseases, I20-I25) or first three digits of the ICD (e.g. Angina pectoris, I20) influences the results. It also determines which ICD-10 chapter is most central for the treatment of patients with respect to age and gender. Due to multimorbidity patients can have diseases of different chapers, which is also considered as influencing factor.

To detect diagnostic diversity, we applied Shannon's entropy measure (Ostermann et al.). Shannon's entropy is based on a system of mutually exclusive and exhaustive events A_1, A_2, ..., A_n and a set of probabilities $p_1 := p(A_1)$, $p_2 := p(A_2)$,..., $p_n := p(A_n)$. Then, the entropy is given by

$$E(p_1,\ldots,p_n) = -\sum_{k=1}^{n} p_k \log p_k$$

where $0 \cdot \log 0 = 0$ is assumed due to the special limit procedure. The largest value of E is given for the equal distribution of the events A_i with $p_k = \frac{1}{n}; k = 1,2,\ldots,n$, which is easy to proof. A comparison of Shannon's entropy, Lorentz curves with Gini coefficients and deviations from the mean value (F.Schuster et al.) showed similar results with respect to a naturally ordered set (weekdays), here we have no ordered structure with respect to ICD Chapters and prefer Shannon's entropy which is robust against scaling effects which is also used in physics.

3. Results

3.1. Descriptive analysis

For male and female patients under the age of one year only the chapter XVIII (Symptoms, signs and abnormal clinical and laboratory findings, not elsewhere classified) is most central. Between one and 31 years diseases of the respiratory system (chapter X, J00-J99, fig. 1 top left) are most dominant for patients with the exception of boys between 6 and 8 years, for which mental and behavioral disorders (chapter V, F00-F99, fig. 1 top right) are most relevant. For females aged 32 mental and behavioral disorders are at the top. For men between 32 and 53 and woman between 33 and 59 diseases of the musculoskeletal system and connective tissue (Chapter XII, M00-M99, fig.1 bottom left) are in the focus. Above that age diseases of the circulatory system (Chapter IX, I00-I99, fig.1 bottom right) are most common.

Regarding Chapter X (see fig. 1 top left) there is a decreasing importance in the childhood with a new peak around the age of 17. There are slightly increased values for men untill around 40 years, above that age the situation reverses. Above 70 years there are surging values for males.

Untill the age of 15 years there is a male dominance in mental and behavioral disorders (most relevant between 6 and 15 years), after the age of 17 years there is a stable and relevant female dominance (see. fig.1 top right, Chapter V). The part of patients with diseases of the musculoskeletal system and connective tissue (see. fig.1 bottom left, Chapter XII) shows only minor differences untill an age of around 45 years. Afterwards it increases to an upper limit value of 60 % for men and 70 % for women.

The part of patients with diseases of the circulatory system (see fig. 1 bottom right, Chapter XII) is monotonically increasing up to a limit value of 90 % for both men and women with up to 5% higher values for men between 45 and 75 years.

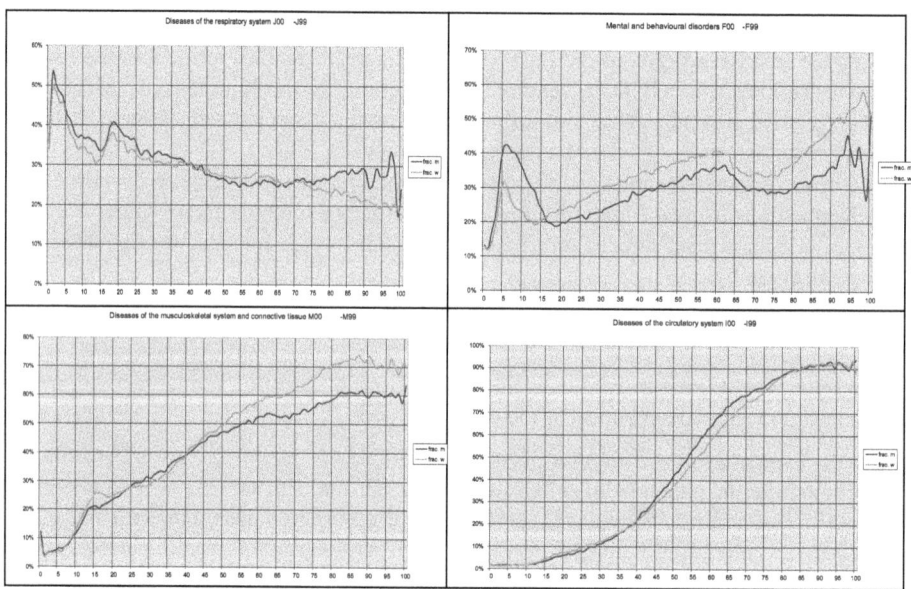

Figure 1. Percentages of diseases with respect to age and gender. Top left: Diseases of the respiratory system (J00-J99, Chapter X) Top right: Mental and behavioral disorders (F00-F99, Chapter V) Bottom left: Diseases of the musculoskeletal system and connective tissue (M00-M99, Chapter XII) Bottom right: Diseases of the circulatory system (I00-I99, Chapter IX) with respect to age and gender

3.2. Shannon Entropy

Shannon entropy strongly increases for women after the age of 15, reaching a limit level at the age of 50 years. Between 15 and 70 years we get higher values for women, after 75 years for men (cf. fig 2).

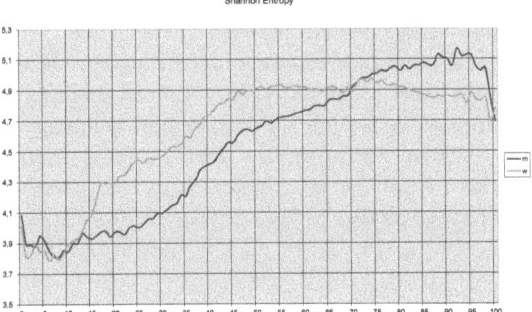

Figure 2. Shannon entropy with respect to age and gender

As mentioned in the methods section there is a multimorbidity effect included in the calculations. We can address this by standardization of the population by means of rescaling to 100 % for each year of birth and gender. Another solution is a patient oriented standardization using a counting value of 1/n if a patient has n diagnoses. Both approaches lead to nearly the same result, cf. fig. 3 left.

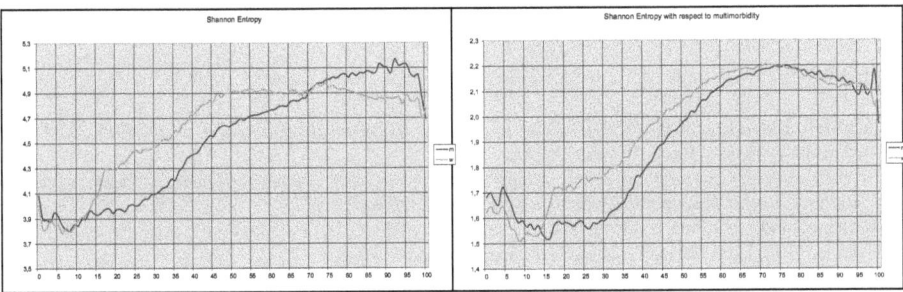

Figure 3. Shannon entropy with respect to age and gender with population standardization (left) and multimorbidity standardization (right)

Finally we consider (cf. fig. 3 right) the Shannon entropy with the respect to the number of diseases (ICD-10 chapters). Above 15 years we have increasing values for women untill an age of 75. Thereafter we get moderately decreasing values for both genders.

4. Discussion

The analysis of secondary data is a promising approach for health care policy makers and stakeholders. This article describes a straight forward pragmatic approach to diagnostic diversity using Shannon's Entropy from a sample of patients of statutory health insurance in Schleswig-Holstein in quarter 2/2016.

This approach has already been used in the analysis of inpatient data (Erben 2000, Ostermann & Schuster 2015). This article applies this approach to outpatient data, which might be a limiting factor, many outpatient procedures lack a definitive diagnosis and thus unspecified diagnoses may be overrepresented (Siegel 2017).

From a methodological point of view, Shannon's entropy is sensitive to rare events, which makes it one of the most reliable diversity indices (Leinster & Cobbold (2012). Another study found similarities to Gini's Coefficient of inequality (Schuster 2017). In conclusion the use of Shannon's entropy as a measure for diversity should gain more attraction to researchers of health services research to learn more about this measure, which still needs to be rediscovered.

5. Conflict of Interest

The authors state that they have no conflict of interests.

6. Acknowledgement

This article is dedicated to Christoph Erben who died in March 2017 and encouraged us to use Shannon's entropy as a marker of diversity.

References

[1] A.V.Bell, Diagnostic diversity: *The role of social class in diagnostic experiences of infertility.* Sociology of health & illness, **36(4)**, 516-530, 2014.

[2] W.H.Courtenay, *Constructions of masculinity and their influence on mens well-being: A theory of gender and heal,* Social Science and Medicine, **50**, 1385-1401, 2000.

[3] K.Deaux, and M.LaFrance, M. Gender, In G. Lindzey (Ed.), *The Handbook of Social Psychology, 4th edition,* Vol. I (pp. 788-827), New York, Random House, 1998.

[4] N.Ebner, G.Fischer *Psychiatrie.* In: Rieder A.,Lohoff B. (Hrsg), Gender Medizin – geschlechts-spezifische Aspekte für die klinische Praxis. Springer-Verlag, Wien-New York, 77-111, 2004.

[5] T.Emcke, Th. Ostermann, M. Heidbreder, R.Schuster, *Comparison of Different Implementations of a Process Limiting Pharmaceutical Expenditures Required by German Law,* HealthInf, 2017.

[6] C.M.Erben, *The concept of entropy as a possibility for gathering mass data for nominal scaled data in health status reporting.* Stud Health Technol Inform 2000; **77:**118-9, 2000.

[7] A.Jutel, *Sociology of diagnosis: a preliminary review.* Sociol Health Illn. Mar, **31(2):**278-99, 2009.

[8] P.J.Offner, E.E.Moore, W.L.Biffl, *Male gender is a risk factor for major infections after surgery,* Arch Surg; **134:** 935-938, 1999.

[9] Th.Ostermann, R.Schuster, R., *An Informationtheoretical Approach to Classify Hospitals with Respect to Their Diagnostic Diversity using Shannon's entropy,* HealthInf, 2015.

[10] R.Schuster, T.Emcke, E.v.Arnstedt, M.Heidbreder, *Morbidity Related Groups (MRG) for epidemiological analysis in outpatient treatment,* IOS Press 783-787, 2016.

[11] F.Schuster, Th. Ostermann, R. Schuster and T. Emcke: *Deviations in Birth Rates with Respect to the Day of the Week and the Month for a 100 Year Period Regarding Social and Medical Aspects in Explaining Models.* Proceedings of the 10th International Joint Conference on Biomedical Engineering Systems and Technologies (BIOSTEC), Vol. **5:** HEALTHINF, 41-47, 2017.

[12] M.Sieverding: *Sind Frauen weniger gesund als Männer? Überprüfung einer verbreiteten Annahme anhand neuerer Befunde,* Kölner Zeitschrift für Soziologie und Sozialpsychologie, **50**, 471-489, 1998.

[13] M.Sieverding, G.Weidner, B. von Volkmann, B., *Cardiovascular reactivity in a simulated job interview: The role of gender role self-concept,* International Journal of Behavioral Medicine, **12**, 1-10, 2005.

[14] L.M. Verbrugge, *Females and illness: Recent trends in sex differences in the United States,* Journal of Health and Social Behavior, **17**, 387-403, 1976.

[15] C.Vögele, A.Jarvis and K.Cheeseman, *Anger suppression, reactivity, and hypertension risk: Gender makes a difference,* Annals of Behavioral Medicine, **19**, 61-69, 1997.

German Medical Data Sciences: Visions and Bridges
R. Röhrig et al. (Eds.)
© 2017 German Association for Medical Informatics, Biometry and Epidemiology (gmds) e.V. and IOS Press.
This article is published online with Open Access by IOS Press and distributed under the terms
of the Creative Commons Attribution Non-Commercial License 4.0 (CC BY-NC 4.0).
doi:10.3233/978-1-61499-808-2-57

Markov Model of the Outpatient Classification System Morbidity Related Groups (MRG)

Timo EMCKE[a,1], Thomas OSTERMANN[b] and Reinhard SCHUSTER[c,d]

[a] *Association of SHI Physicians, Bad Segeberg, Germany*
[b] *Witten/Herdecke University, Herdecke, Germany*
[c] *Medical Advisory Board of SHI in Northern Germany, Lübeck, Germany*
[d] *Lübeck University, Lübeck, Germany*
timo.emcke@kvsh.de, thomas.ostermann@uni-wh.de, reinhard.schuster@mdk-nord.de

Abstract. *Background* Benchmarking and guidance of outpatient physicians in Germany are almost always based on one year data. This also holds true for morbidity related groups, a classification system applied in northern Germany since 2017. A study of the markov properties of prescription based grouping algorithms is reported here. *Results* There is a strongly connected graph for almost all components and the resulting markov chain has a unique stationary solution. *Conclusions* Target values based on the status quo of prescription behavior can provide stable guidelines for outpatient physicians. Every set of partitions converging like MRG should be considered for controlling measures.

Keywords. markov process, outpatient care, morbidity related groups, big data, benchmarking

1. Introduction

Modern health care systems have to ensure the quality and equity of treatment while controlling costs and distribution of funds. Controlling measures are essential instruments necessary for the administration of today. While actual values are available in health care databases (e.g. accounting/prescription data), standards for the determination and analysis of target values and benchmarks are at an early stage. Originating in probability theory this paper shows that under certain conditions a policy maker doesn't need to know the process's full history. Targets and forecasts can be based solely on the present state without losing model accuracy.

In 2017 statutory health insurances and the associated physicians in the German federal state of Schleswig-Holstein launched expenditure controlling of outpatient prescriptions by morbidity related groups (MRG) [3,8]. Quarterly the underlying grouping algorithm assigns outpatients to a group based on drug classes (Anatomical Therapeutic Chemical Classification System). Prescription budgets and consultation materials are the end result used by policy makers and auditors. The question is, how stable those MRG, the dependencies among them and the observable changes from one quarter to the next are. Is a one year foundation of data sufficient for controlling prescription behavior?

---

[1] Corresponding author, Timo Emcke, Bismarckallee 1-6, 23795 Bad Segeberg, Germany; E-mail: timo.emcke@kvsh.de

2. Methods

The analysis is based on detailed prescription data of the statutory health insurance in Schleswig-Holstein from Q4/2015-Q3/2016 used for physician budget calculations. Each outpatient treated in one of the quarters has been classified (n = 7,708,711 ≈ 1.93M classifications of patients per quarter). For the sake of simplification only the grouping of patients in adjacent quarters are analyzed (n = 3,039,580 ≈ 0.76M per quarter).

This dataset has a countable state space (15 ATC main groups [defined by first character of the ATC code] or 238 MRGs based on the first three characters of ATC) and discrete time (quarters) for each individual. We analyze if a first degree markov model (DTMC) [4, 7] of the transition probabilities from one quarter to the next is balanced. This would mean that grouping predictions for the next future quarter can be made based solely on the current one.

3. Results

The majority of patients is in main group C of the ATC (cardiovascular system). Followed by groups A (alimentary tract and metabolism) and N (nervous system) (figure 1)

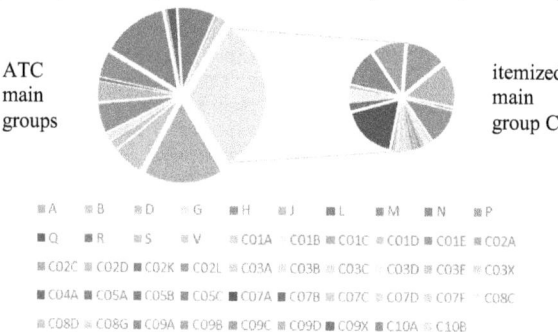

Figure 1. Outpatient shares based on first level of ATC (main group C itemized)

Looking at the 2,279,685 possible transitions between quarters (three per patient) one gets the following result for the 15 main groups of ATC (table 1).

Table 1. Quarterly transitions between ATC main groups

	A	B	C	D	G	H	J	L	M	N	P	Q	R	S	V
A	213487	7782	40123	3185	2149	5605	5525	846	8113	15480	317	3183	9562	1126	13288
B	8596	84703	20092	862	1011	1684	1487	394	2400	6937	68	1962	3207	223	883
C	41560	18105	472733	5830	3843	10238	10488	599	13272	21012	295	3788	13492	1177	1157
D	3701	848	5994	21150	742	1593	2090	158	1518	2217	228	2356	3237	781	210
G	2123	848	3942	694	113498	677	1331	278	709	1903	42	389	897	108	77
H	5775	1614	10026	1497	736	62307	3883	371	3253	4078	210	603	3469	560	216
J	5353	1278	9785	1941	1313	3605	11814	277	2501	3343	303	961	4890	865	160
L	941	392	608	209	350	375	360	37217	916	720	58	563	227	30	63
M	8588	2016	13633	1551	784	3308	2792	879	51270	7000	306	940	3832	514	188
N	16491	6559	21707	2137	1982	3905	3631	746	7462	316988	183	3355	6509	578	782
P	364	55	309	222	29	219	353	58	325	174	1807	116	604	100	18
Q	3612	2093	4218	2259	510	609	1106	601	1011	3715	96	35041	1810	400	470
R	9788	2731	13272	2813	934	3386	5216	224	3562	6120	514	1792	122793	1514	1054
S	1131	191	1267	601	103	514	923	41	461	586	90	983	1616	60716	55
V	13420	808	1155	215	90	200	156	46	181	756	19	420	1055	46	17688

About 71.2 % of the population studied (1,623,212) remains in the same main group. Considering the third level of ATC (239 different MRG) about 62.7 % of patients (1,428,805) keep their classification in the next quarter. Visualizing the most important edges/components illustrates the central relevance of group C (figure 2).

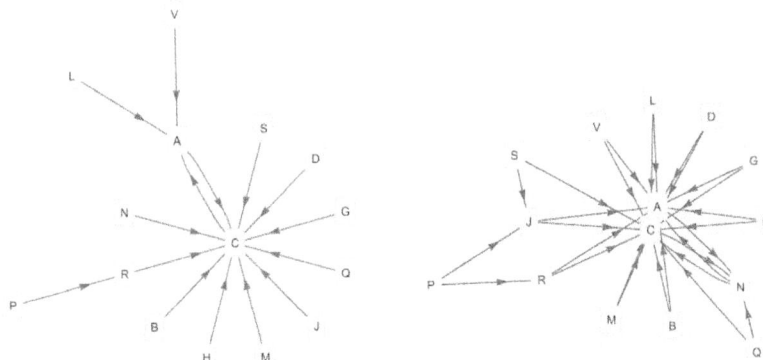

Figure 2: Top 2 (left) and top 3 transitions (right) between ATC main groups excl. self loops

Adding transition probabilities to this simplified representation of main effects shows that some other (intermediate) main groups are also worth considering (e.g. A, R, J and N) (figure 3).

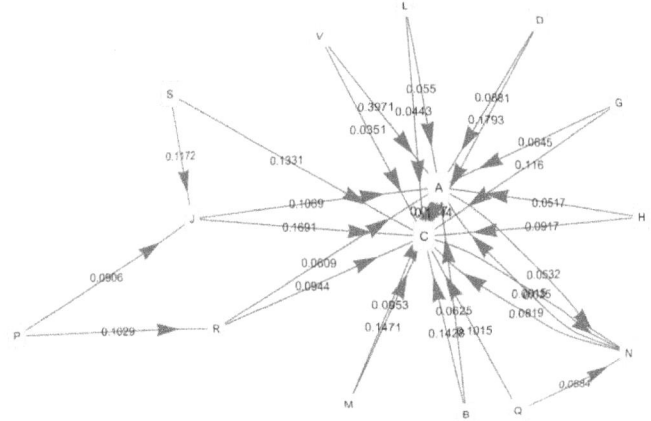

Figure 3: Transitions probabilities of Top 3 transitions excl. loops

If we look at all 235 MRG and exclude four groups only covering 0.1 % of patients with prescriptions, we get a strongly connected graph. The tool used for determination of the subset of relevant edges was *Mathematica* 10.3.1 by Wolfram Research. The inclusion of patients with no drug prescriptions (e.g. patients missing in the subsequent periods because of their death) would result in a strongly connected graph for all components.

The adjacency matrix of a strongly connected graph is irreducible [6, 9]. All components of powers of the adjacency matrix are positive and thereby the markov chain is aperiodic. Hence and due to fact that the number of states is finite we get a unique stationary solution [1, 6]. The rate of convergence is determined by the quotient of the first ($\lambda_1=1$) and the second (λ_2) of decreasingly ordered eigenvalues [5].

Table 2. Unique stationary distribution of the markov process of the 15 ATC main groups

	A	B	C	D	G	H	J	L	M	N	P	Q	R	S	V
A	0.6252	0.0256	0.1244	0.0106	0.0063	0.019	0.0238	0.0021	0.0292	0.0532	0.001	0.0101	0.0277	0.0029	0.0387
B	0.0625	0.6298	0.1428	0.0078	0.0064	0.0136	0.014	0.002	0.0175	0.0564	0.000	0.0179	0.0225	0.0018	0.0045
C	0.0617	0.0301	0.7655	0.0104	0.006	0.0163	0.0184	0.0008	0.023	0.035	0.000	0.0067	0.0214	0.0022	0.0017
D	0.0881	0.0276	0.1793	0.2971	0.0129	0.0476	0.0797	0.0025	0.0619	0.0751	0.007	0.0338	0.0697	0.0147	0.0028
G	0.0645	0.0292	0.116	0.0154	0.5929	0.0176	0.0267	0.0013	0.0263	0.0606	0.001	0.0121	0.0299	0.0037	0.0026
H	0.0517	0.0148	0.0917	0.0153	0.0048	0.6655	0.0402	0.0022	0.0317	0.0386	0.002	0.0052	0.0302	0.0046	0.0012
J	0.1069	0.0263	0.1691	0.0405	0.0127	0.069	0.26	0.0022	0.0865	0.0879	0.007	0.0155	0.0971	0.0172	0.0021
L	0.055	0.0204	0.0443	0.0069	0.0036	0.0188	0.0143	0.7108	0.0328	0.043	0.004	0.0229	0.0175	0.0029	0.0025
M	0.0953	0.0268	0.1471	0.0232	0.008	0.0381	0.0612	0.0041	0.4379	0.0892	0.003	0.0107	0.0458	0.0073	0.0019
N	0.0615	0.027	0.0819	0.0106	0.0069	0.0178	0.023	0.0018	0.0303	0.6922	0.000	0.0141	0.0263	0.0029	0.0027
P	0.073	0.0158	0.0674	0.0471	0.0081	0.0476	0.0906	0.0082	0.0677	0.0489	0.388	0.0166	0.1029	0.0166	0.0015
Q	0.0753	0.0513	0.1015	0.081	0.008	0.0151	0.0259	0.0059	0.0244	0.0884	0.002	0.5216	0.0351	0.0053	0.0091
R	0.0609	0.0216	0.0944	0.0192	0.0062	0.0246	0.0425	0.0014	0.0315	0.0495	0.004	0.01	0.6235	0.0077	0.0028
S	0.0906	0.023	0.1331	0.0571	0.0127	0.0583	0.1172	0.0016	0.0669	0.073	0.009	0.0205	0.1088	0.2258	0.0023
V	0.3971	0.0201	0.0351	0.0033	0.0022	0.0049	0.005	0.001	0.0059	0.0235	0.000	0.012	0.014	0.0008	0.4748

The starting and the stationary distribution (table 2) of the transition probabilities are very similar. All transition matrices from one to any subsequent quarter are nearly the same and thereby the transition process has markov property. The stability of the iterations is to some extent a local property because external factors may slowly change the transition matrix and the normalized eigenvector to largest eigenvalue.
This holds true for the ATC main group scenario as well as the detailed MRG classification.

4. Discussion

Our results reveal that the patient classification algorithm used for MRG produces stable groups. Nevertheless outpatient care in Germany and therefore our results are dominated by patients older than 45 years. The majority of patients in the second half of life have diseases of the circulatory system (figure 4).

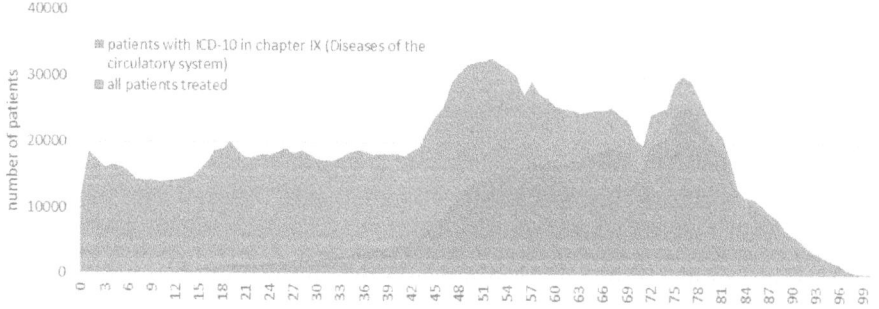

Figure 4. Shares of patients in Schleswig-Holstein (Q4/2015-Q3/2016) with diseases of the circulatory system

To a certain extent this explains the central relevance of the classifications related to the main group C (cardiovascular system) and the overall balance of the grouping. It can be assumed that the transitions and the statistical properties in younger populations differ. The intermediate main groups shown in figure 2 provide first indications.

The exclusion of patients with prescription gaps longer than one quarter might destabilize the system of transitions. Especially patients dying, recovering or falling ill can be important for equilibrium solutions.

Additionally, a grouping (of patients) can be based on certain ICD-10 codes [2] from accounting data (e.g. F32 [depressions] and F45 [somatoform disorders]) (figure 5).

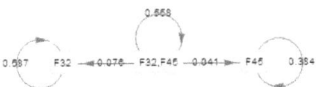

Figure 5: Example transitions (incl. probabilities and self loops) between certain mental and behavioural disorders

An algorithm based on prescription and diagnostic data might provide better groups.

5. Conclusion

For practical purposes the health care system applies target values based on todays status quo without taking past developments into account (e.g. MRG). Checking for markov properties can be a valuable tool for validation and adjustment of the underlying grouping and pooling algorithms.

Good guidelines motivate and enable better allocation of resources.

6. Conflict of Interest

The authors state that they have no conflict of interests.

References

[1] A. Berman, J.R. Plemmons, *Nonnegative Matrices in the Mathematical Sciences*, SIAM, 1994.
[2] T. Ostermann and R. Schuster, *An Informationtheoretical Approach to Classify Hospitals with Respect to Their Diagnostic Diversity using Shannon's Entropy*. Proceedings of the International Conference on Health Informatics (HealthInf) 325-329, 2015.
[3] T. Emcke, Th. Ostermann, M. Heidbreder, R. Schuster, *Comparison of Different Implementations of a Process Limiting Pharmaceutical Expenditures Required by German Law*, Proceedings of the 10th International Joint Conference on Biomedical Engineering and Technologies (BIOSTEC), Vol. **5**: HealthInf, 35-40, 2017.
[4] A.A. Markov, *Extension of the limit theorems of probability theory to a sum of variables connected in a chain*. Reprinted in Appendix B of: R. Howard. Dynamic Probabilistic Systems, volume **1**: Markov Chains. John Wiley and Sons, 1971.
[5] S.P. Meyn and R.L. Tweedie, *Markov Chains and Stochastic Stability*. London: Springer, 1993.
[6] E. Nummelin, *General irreducible Markov chains and non-negative operators*. Cambridge University Press, 1984, 2004.
[7] E. Seneta, *Non-negative matrices and Markov chains*. 2nd rev. ed., 1981, XVI, 288 p., Softcover Springer Series in Statistics, 2nd rev. ed. XVI, 1981.
[8] R. Schuster, T. Emcke, E.v. Arnstedt, M. Heidbreder, *Morbidity Related Groups (MRG) for epidemiological analysis in outpatient treatment*, IOS Press 783-787, 2016
[9] H. Wielandt, *Unzerlegbare, nicht negative Matrizen*, Mathematische Zeitschrift, **52** (1): 642-648, 1950.

4. IT Infrastructure for Biomedical Research/Data Integration Centers

German Medical Data Sciences: Visions and Bridges
R. Röhrig et al. (Eds.)
© *2017 German Association for Medical Informatics, Biometry and Epidemiology (gmds) e.V. and IOS Press.*
This article is published online with Open Access by IOS Press and distributed under the terms
of the Creative Commons Attribution Non-Commercial License 4.0 (CC BY-NC 4.0).
doi:10.3233/978-1-61499-808-2-65

IT Infrastructure for Biomedical Research in North-West Germany

Insa SEEGER[a,1], Atinkut ZELEKE[a], Michael FREITAG[b] and Rainer RÖHRIG[a]

[a] *Medical Informatics, Carl von Ossietzky University Oldenburg, Germany*
[b] *General Medicine, Carl von Ossietzky University Oldenburg, Germany*

Abstract. The efficient use of routine data for biomedical research presupposes an IT infrastructure designed for health care facilities. The objective of this study was to analyse which IT infrastructure is used in hospitals and by general practitioners' (GP) practices in the region Oldenburg-Bremen and to examine how well this supports research projects. To this end, IT managers and GPs were interviewed. The usage of hospital information systems (HIS) and data warehouse systems (DWS) in hospitals is of major importance for the study. Over 90 % use DWS for administration, 42 % for clinical research. None of the hospitals implemented consent for the use of routine data for research. Only a third of the GPs have participated in studies. The GPs' offices based EHR systems in use offer virtually no support for research projects. The study results demonstrate that technical and organisational measures are required for the further usage of routine data in the region.

Keywords. hospital information system, CIO, general practitioners, electronic health records, medical informatics

1. Introduction

"Real world data" of daily routine data are the most important sources for health system research. The usage of routine data within medical research extends from the support of clinical studies to epidemiological studies, up to studies of research in health services depending on the secondary analysis of data [1, 2]. For example, routine data are suitable to assess compliance of the use of antibiotics (inpatient, outpatient) and the reason for decisions [3–5].

Medical data gathered in electronic health records (EHR) offer potential for future medical research. There are initiatives on a European level to link the distributed and heterogeneous data resources and make efficient secondary use of hospital EHR data to support clinical research studies [6]. But to evaluate collected routine data for research, a powerful IT infrastructure is necessary. Because of the frequent use of hospital information systems data is more often available in an electronic form, yet the data quality or the access to this data for research is insufficient [2]. Apart from research in hospitals, research with routinely collected data by general practitioners is an underused resource [7]. To link research and patient-centered care, the funding concept "medical informatics" of the German Federal Ministry for Education and Research (BMBF) supports innovative IT solutions [8].

---

[1] Corresponding author: insa.seeger@uni-oldenburg.de

Until now, the region Oldenburg-Bremen has been only little experienced with medical research. With the establishment of the medical faculty at the University of Oldenburg the increasing number of students and graduates need a good IT infrastructure for research.

The objective of this study was to prepare an analysis of the current status of the IT infrastructure to support research and establish new business areas in the region.

The following questions should be answered:

1. Which IT infrastructures are employed in hospitals and GP's practices?
2. How is the access to the existing electronic data regulated?
3. To what extent can the existing IT infrastructure support research projects in the present facilities?

2. Methods

After the approbation of the ethical committee we conducted two descriptive surveys: Firstly, we interviewed hospitals in north-west Germany, and secondly, we surveyed resident GPs who were interested in education and research at the faculty of Medicine and Health Sciences of the Carl von Ossietzky University in Oldenburg. Both aspects were important to describe the region, so they were combined in the study.

From 33 hospitals in the region of Oldenburg-Bremen, 25 hospitals were chosen, both rural and urban, furthermore hospitals of differing care levels and funding models. We knew from previous projects, that the remaining eight hospitals were not interested in research or did not provide any information.

In the period between August and December 2016, interview requests were sent to CIOs of 25 selected hospitals. If an interest in the study was expressed in an initial telephone request, further information and the questionnaire were sent by email. A semi-structured method served as a framework for data acquisition and evaluation. The questions were developed according to the functionality described in the literature [2, 9–12] and the development of the medical informatics funding concept initiated by the BMBF [8]. The CIOs were asked for what purpose they use the data warehouse and how the access rights are regulated; whether an electronic patient record is available; what other IT software is used for patient care; and whether patients agree to the usage of their data for research during data collection.

Subsequently a pre-test was conducted with a CIO, some changes to the questionnaire were made following his replies. The data collection for the hospital IT infrastructure included personal and telephone interviews as well as the opportunity to complete and return the questionnaire.

The network of teaching and research practices of the Faculty of Medicine and Health Sciences includes 181 general and 135 specialist practices in north-west Germany. To access potential participating GPs and to create a picture of their IT infrastructure, emails with online questionnaires were sent to 316 GPs in the network. This part of the study took place in spring 2017 over a period of four weeks. The online survey of GPs included mainly closed yes/no questions about the IT infrastructure during their medical service, also about their participation in studies in general and possible participation in clinical studies by the University of Oldenburg. The pre-test was conducted by three GPs. The survey was executed by means of the SoSci Survey software package. Both surveys were analysed with SPSS 23®.

3. Results

Data from twelve CIOs (response rate 48 %) and 64 practitioners (response rate 20 %) were included in the analysis. The results are indicated in table 1 and table 2.

Table 1. Answers of the Chief Information Officers of 12 hospitals

Answers CIOs	n	% of 12
Electronic Medical Record in use	8	67 %
Internal electronic transmission of medical findings	12	100 %
External electronic transmission of medical findings	5	42 %
Software implemented to improve drug safety	3	25 %
Data warehouse in use	11	92 %
for administration/operational purposes	11	92 %
for archiving in clinical trials	5	42 %
Heads of clinical department have access to data warehouse for research purposes	2	17 %
Use and access rules for clinical research implemented	7	58 %
Established graduated consent management for data usage	7	58 %
Implemented consent for the use of routine data for research	0	0 %

Table 2. Answers of the 64 general practitioners

Answers practitioners	n	% of 64
Participation in studies (last three years)	**33**	**21 %**
epidemical studies	9	22 %
observation studies with other principals	9	22 %
application monitoring	8	20 %
drug trials	8	20 %
Sponsors of the studies		
university institutes	13	45 %
pharmaceutical companies	8	28 %
Medical information system (for general practitioner offices)	**64**	**100 %**
Medistar (CompuGroup, Germany)	13	20 %
x.concept (Medatixx, Germany)	11	17 %
Turbomed (CompuGroup, Germany)	9	14 %
Other (16 other systems with four or less installations)	31	49 %
Existing medical information system support for carrying out studies	1	5 %
Interest to take part in clinical or health system research in collaboration with the University of Oldenburg	52	81 %

4. Discussion

One third of all the hospitals in the north western region took part in the survey. It can be assumed that the non-responding hospitals have a lower interest in research and the implementation rates are over-estimated.

Over 90 % of the CIOs surveyed in hospitals use a DWS in addition to a hospital information system. However, in a great majority of cases the full functionality of the DWS is not fully used, for example only two chief physicians are allowed to use the DWS for research. In a European study of the developmental status of electronic information systems German hospitals ranked in the lower third - far behind the Benelux and Scandinavian countries; only 60 % of the 201 surveyed hospitals use electronic patient record [13]. The difference in the distribution of DWS and processes for an informed consent for data usage for biomedical research indicates that building an infrastructure for biomedical research is not only a big technical but also a big organisational challenge. There are some technical improvements necessary and possible, but the required human and technical resources are the leading problems [2, 9, 10]. In our survey, the DWS is used mainly for medical controlling and financial purposes and thus serves the management in business. According to a study of the role of IT in German hospitals, user access to the IT resources in hospitals is defined (up to 90 %) by the management board [14]. Apart from the lack of clarity in the legal position regarding data usage, the costs for additional IT or the lack of interest in research could be causative. To use the data collected by the HIS for research purposes, the implementation of a HIS-based recruiting support could be useful, however a most complete documentation is required for this [15]. Furthermore, hospitals must set up guidelines for data protection, access, and data standardisation.

The results of the GP study show that more than half of the surveyed GPs use the medical information systems Medistar, x.concept and Turbomed. A study by Schmiemann et al. also showed these three medical information systems to be the most commonly used systems in the Bremen/Lower Saxony region. [16].

There were relatively few studies (33 %) carried out by GPs involved in this study. A survey of 408 German GPs in 2010 revealed that 53 % of those surveyed had experience of observation studies and 69 % were generally prepared to participate in studies [17]. Over 80 % of our participants indicate willingness for research; however, the survey results show that the practice software does not support the execution of studies. Through the establishment of research networks as they have existed for many years in the United Kingdom [18], individual solutions can be developed for study implementation because of the inter-professional collaboration of practice owners and scientists. An example is the usage of open and free data management systems. In the field of health system research there is no alternative to the expansion of multiple use of care data. In doing so it cannot be restricted to secondary routine or social data, but rather include the primary treatment documentation [19].

In our study we only questioned GPs in a close networking with the University of Oldenburg. This can be an indicator of greater interest in research compared to other GPs. There are many IT systems with functions usable for biomedical research. But there is still a technical and an immense organisational challenge to implement an IT infrastructure to use routine data for biomedical research. The IT infrastructure in medical practices was found not suitable for clinical research. The health facilities must set up guidelines for data protection, access, and data standardisation to encourage biomedical research.

Acknowledgements and Conflict of Interests

This study was funded by Stiftung Bremer Wertpapierbörse. The authors thank E. Gildehaus & J. Lotz for supporting the design of the study and B. Whelan and S. Gacek for copy editing. All authors state that there are no conflicts of interest.

References

[1] Trinczek B, Kopcke F, Leusch T, et al.: Design and multicentric implementation of a generic software architecture for patient recruitment systems re-using existing HIS tools and routine patient data. Appl Clin Inform 2014; 5(1): 264–83.

[2] Prokosch H-U, Ganslandt T: Perspectives for Medical Informatics. Methods Inf Med 2009.

[3] Hartmann B, Junger A, Brammen D, Röhrig R, Klasen J, Quinzio L, Benson M, Hempelmann G: Review of antibiotic drug use in a surgical ICU: management with a patient data management system for additional outcome analysis in patients staying more than 24 hours. Clin Ther 2004 Jun; 26(6): 915–24.

[4] Vercheval C, Gillet M, Maes N, et al.: Quality of documentation on antibiotic therapy in medical records: evaluation of combined interventions in a teaching hospital by repeated point prevalence survey. Eur J Clin Microbiol Infect Dis 2016; 35(9): 1495–500.

[5] Liu P, Ohl C, Johnson J, Williamson J, Beardsley J, Luther V: Frequency of empiric antibiotic de-escalation in an acute care hospital with an established Antimicrobial Stewardship Program. BMC Infect Dis 2016; 16(1): 751.

[6] Moor G de, Sundgren M, Kalra D, et al.: Using electronic health records for clinical research: the case of the EHR4CR project. J Biomed Inform 2015; 53: 162–73.

[7] Lusignan S de, Hague N, VanVlymen J, Kumarapeli P: Routinely-collected general practice data are complex, but with systematic processing can be used for quality improvement and research. jhi 2006; 14(1): 59–66.

[8] Bundesministerium für Bildung und Forschung: Förderkonzept Medizininformatik: Daten vernetzen - Gesundheitsversorgung verbessern. http://www.gesundheitsforschung-bmbf.de/de/medizininformatik.php. (last accessed on 9 March 2017).

[9] Williams R, Kontopantelis E, Buchan I, Peek N: Clinical code set engineering for reusing EHR data for research: A review. J Biomed Inform 2017; 70: 1–13.

[10] Martin-Sanchez FJ, Aguiar-Pulido V, Lopez-Campos GH, Peek N, Sacchi L: Secondary Use and Analysis of Big Data Collected for Patient Care. Contribution from the IMIA Working Group on Data Mining and Big Data Analytics. Yearb Med Inform 2017; 26(1).

[11] Bauer, C R K D, Ganslandt T, Baum B, et al.: Integrated Data Repository Toolkit (IDRT). A Suite of Programs to Facilitate Health Analytics on Heterogeneous Medical Data. Methods Inf Med 2016; 55(2): 125–35.

[12] TMF - Technologie- und Methodenplattform für die vernetzte medizinische Forschung e.V. (ed.): IT-Infrastrukturen in der patientenorientierten Forschung: Aktueller Stand und Handlungsbedarf 2015. Berlin: Akademische Verlagsgesellschaft AKA GmbH 2015.

[13] Sabes-Figuera R, Maghiros I, Abadie F: European hospital survey. JRC scientific and policy reports; 26355. Luxembourg: Publ. Off. of the Europ. Union 2013. doi:10.2791/55646.

[14] Böckmann B, Elbel G-K, Radunz O: Die Rolle der IT im Krankenhaus: IT als strategischer Partner der Unternehmensleitung [2012 Nov 1; cited 2017 Mar 8]. Available: https://www2.deloitte.com/

[15] Kopcke F, Trinczek B, Majeed RW, et al.: Evaluation of data completeness in the electronic health record for the purpose of patient recruitment into clinical trials: a retrospective analysis of element presence. BMC Med Inform Decis Mak 2013; 13: 37.

[16] Schmiemann G, Schneider-Rathert W, Gierschmann A, Kersting M: Arztinformationssysteme in Hausarztpraxen - zwischen Pflicht und Kür. Zeitschrift für Allgemeinmedizin (ZFA) 2012; 88(3): 127–32.

[17] Peters-Klimm F, Hermann K, Gagyor I, Haasenritter J, Bleidorn J: Erfahrungen und Einstellungen zu Klinischen Studien in der Hausarztpraxis: Ergebnisse einer Befragung von deutschen Hausärzten. Gesundheitswesen 2013; 75(5): 321–7.

[18] Sullivan F, Butler C, Cupples M, Kinmonth A-L: Primary care research networks in the United Kingdom. BMJ 2007; 334(7603): 1093–4.

[19] Müller-Mielitz S, Lux Thomas (eds.): E-Health-Ökonomie. Wiesbaden: Springer Gabler 2017.

German Medical Data Sciences: Visions and Bridges
R. Röhrig et al. (Eds.)
© *2017 German Association for Medical Informatics, Biometry and Epidemiology (gmds) e.V. and IOS Press.*

doi:10.3233/978-1-61499-808-2-70

Data Collection of Medication – Impact of Autocompletion in eCRFs on Efficiency and Data Quality

Tolga P. NAZIYOK[a,1], Corinna FEEKEN[a], Atinkut A. ZELEKE[a],
Michael DÖRKS[b] and Rainer RÖHRIG[a]
[a] *Dep. Medical Informatics,*
[b] *Dep. Outpatient care and Pharmacoepidemiology,*
Carl von Ossietzky University Oldenburg, Germany

Abstract. Objective: Openclinica Input Completion (OIC) was developed to increase the efficiency to enter drugs in eCRF in OpenClinica®. The aim of the study was to evaluate the impact on efficiency and data quality as well as usability. **Methods:** 20 participants were asked to input 15 drugs with the new tool and by hand. **Results:** The mean input time got decreased from 16:12m to 3:59m. 31 of 300 (10%) of manual entered medication data sets had one or more errors versus 10 of 300 (3,3%) data sets entered with OIC. **Conclusion:** OIC was able to increase efficiency and data quality. We conclude that new additions to the graphical user interface in electronical Case-Report-Form (eCRF) systems should be validated before usage in research projects.

Keywords. Data Collection, Organizational Efficiency, Data Accuracy, eCRF, Usability

1. Introduction

The quality of clinical research is directly dependent on the quality of the data it had acquired at the time of data collection and management [1]. Electronic data capture such as electronics case report form (eCRF) has in recent years been increasingly used in clinical research to improve the data quality and shorten the study period [2-4].The data entry errors in clinical research are common and if the error is large enough to affect the investigators' conclusions, it can have a risk to the level of changing the standard of care of thousands of patients. Researchers indicated that up to 26% of errors can be caused by mistakes in data entry and misinterpretation of the result in the original document [5] and source-to-database error rates are highly dependent on the amount of structured data collection in the clinical setting [4]. The use of customized form for data entry found to increase the accuracy and efficiency of data recorders [6]. However; little is known on the use of specific functionalities of eCRF-systems such as autocomplete and its effect on the efficiency and quality of the data.

In a recent clinical study, the pharmacotherapy of autistic patients was documented. In order to be able to evaluate the data, a clear coding is needed; in this case the ATC (Anatomical Therapeutic Chemical Classification System) code was used to extract the

---

1 Corresponding Author: tolga.philipp.naziyok@uni-oldenburg.de

active substance apart from the different brands of each drug. To assist their study we developed an extension tool for the *OpenClinica®* study management system, which enables a user to search for drug names and map them automatically to various attributes such as the ATC code. In this study we aim to evaluate the effect on efficiency (time) and data quality of said extension tool. Moreover, the usability was assessed accordingly.

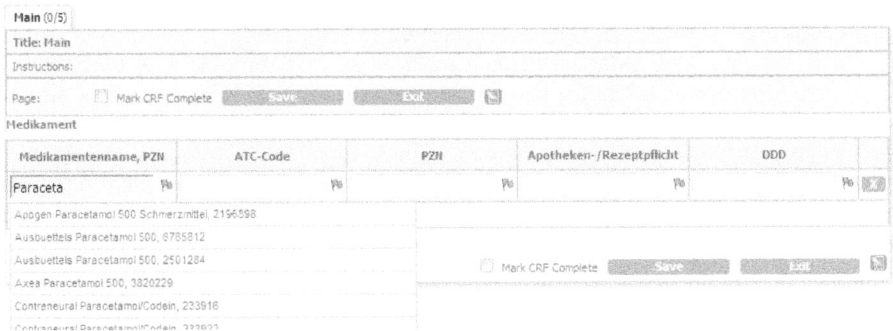

Figure 1: The *OpenClinica®* eCRF to input medications and other parameters. It shows how the user inputs a medication name and is presented with a list of matching medications. The eCRF without the OIC feature looks identical, but offers no autocomplete.

2. Study Setting

The data entry is done in *OpenClinica®*, the system for which OIC (Openclinica Input Completion) was designed for. *OpenClinica®* is the worldwide first commercial open source software for clinical trials and has become one of the most distributed systems for them. In *OpenClinica®* you input your data via electronic Case Report Forms (eCRF) as seen in figure 1.

OIC enhances the regular CRF with an autocomplete functionality that is triggered the moment a user enters more than 4 signs into the drug name row. It looks similar to the autocomplete from google, but it is comprehensive and therefore longer. It contains the full retailer name and the PZN (Pharmazentralnummer) a unique identifier given for each drug, aid or other pharmacy product in Germany. After selecting an item from the list, the ATC-Code, PZN, prescription status and the Defined Daily Dose (DDD) are filled in automatically. The autocomplete is populated from a database that was built on the basis of WIdO's (Wissenschaftliches Institut der AOK) table, which we were allowed to use, of nearly 140,000 drugs and their associated properties. It was developed with JavaScript and PHP.

3. Methods

After the approval of the ethical committee of the Universität Oldenburg (vote no: 2017-008) 20 individuals were recruited to perform a data entry of various drugs. The recruitment was done without any emphasis on previous knowledge or skill, the only requirement was that none of the participants have used OIC before. They were asked to input 15 specific drugs and search for additional parameters. A pharmacist, who has used OIC before, was tasked to choose the 15 drugs with the requirement to include some that are difficult to search or to type. The participants have to input them two times: One time using the manual approach by searching the correct Information in a table and a second time using OIC. They were randomized into two groups: One group does the manual entry first and semi-automatic afterwards (M/A), the second group the other way around (A/M). Before the test, each participant singed the participant information and consent, and they got a brief instruction of what to do and how to do it for the respective variant. The time was measured for each pass.

After the data entry, each participant received an invitation for a usability-survey via e-mail. First, it was asked the participant about his medical experience. The second page consisted of the 10 questions to evaluate the System Usability Scale (SUS) [7]. On the last page we gave them the opportunity to leave a comment of any kind regarding the study.

Data collection errors was detected and classified into seven groups by two independent researchers (authors). An explorative data analysis was performed for the required time and the count of entries with one or more errors for one medication. The 95% confidence intervals were determined by a bootstrap method (1000 samples). If no event occurred {n=0 Events of N Cases}, the confidence intervals were simulated with an additional case with an event {n=1 /(N+1)}.

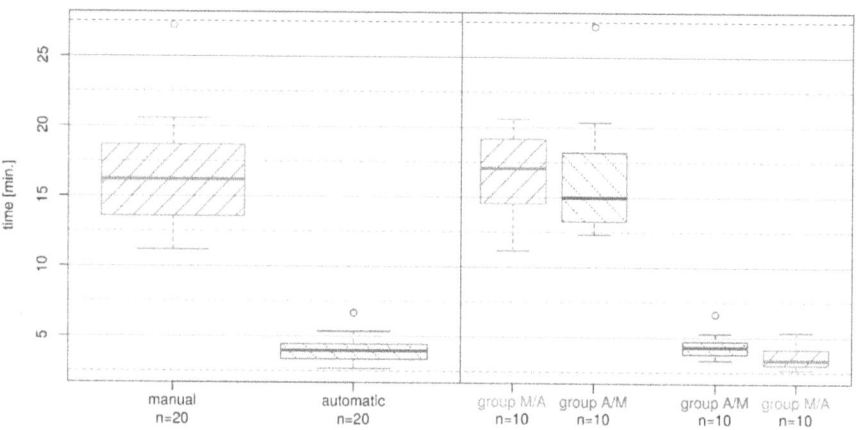

Figure 2: The time differences between both variants. Left are both variants compared directly, on the right, the variants are also grouped according to the corresponding sequence.

4. Results

The effects on efficiency are shown in Figure 2 via boxplots. The left graph shows a median time reduction of 16:12m to 3:59m (75% reduction) between the old and the new variant. The right graph clusters both variants into their respective groups. The group M/A scored 17:04m, 3:23m (-80%) and group A/M 4:18m, 14:59m (-71%) as median times for the respective first and second run. The right graph also reveals a learning effect in the form of reduced input times of 4:18m to 3:23m (-21%) for M/A and 17:04m to 14:59m (-12%) for A/M, regarding their second run.

Table 1: 300 drugs were entered into two different systems. For each type of error, the amount, total and percentage, as well as the 95% confidence interval (CI) is displayed (n=1/(N+1) for each type with n=0).

	Manual			Autocomplete		
Type	n	%	95%-CI	n	%	95%-CI
Wrong drug	1	0.33%	0 - 1 %	0	0.00%	0 - 1 %
Wrong dose	6	2.00%	0.7 - 3.7 %	1	0.33%	0 - 1 %
Wrong administration	5	1.67%	0.3- 3.3 %	3	1.00%	0 - 2.3 %
Supplement missing	2	0.67%	0 - 1.7 %	1	0.33%	0 - 1 %
Confusion of data fields	14	4.67%	2.3 - 7.3 %	0	0.00%	0 - 1 %
Wrong manufacturer	3	1.00%	0 - 2.3 %	4	1.33%	0.3 - 2.7 %
Missing Data	0	0.00%	0 - 1 %	1	0.33%	0 - 1 %
Total Errors	31	10.33%	7-14 %	10	3.33%	1.3-5.7 %

The results on data quality are presented in table 1. There was no correlation found between input speed and error rate.

18 participants, eight with medical background and ten without answered the SUS questionnaire. In average the score was 90.8, those with medical background ranked it slightly lower (89.4) and those without medical background higher (92.0). The results are shown in table 2.

Table 2: This table shows the mean results for the SUS questionnaire answered by 18 participants. Subgroups are analyzed for groups with and without medical background. 1 means "strong disagree" and 5 means "strong agree".

SUS Question	Medical Background	Others	Both
1. I think that I would like to use this system frequently	4.50	4.25	4.39
2. I found the system unnecessarily complex.	1.20	1.25	1.22
3. I think that I would need the support of a technical person to be able to use this system.	1.40	1.13	1.28
4. I found the various functions in this system were well integrated.	4.50	4.00	4.28
5. I thought there was too much inconsistency in this system.	1.40	1.50	1.44
6. I would imagine that most people would learn to use this system very quickly.	4.70	4.88	4.78
7. I felt very confident using the system.	4.50	4.38	4.44
8. I found the system very cumbersome to use.	1.10	1.13	1.11
9. I thought the system was easy to use.	4.80	4.50	4.67
10. I needed to learn a lot of things before I could get going with this system.	1.10	1.25	1.17

5. Discussion

OIC is able to complete the task without problems and does so, as expected, with less work time (about 4 times faster) and is therefore validated. It would be interesting to find out in which degree typing time was saved and in what degree decision time. Our study setup was not prepared to measure this, but a follow up study might be able to.

As in [2], the errors found were either a misinterpretation or an error in the entry itself. Almost half of the manual errors happened because of a confusion of data fields (14 times), for example by copy-pasting the data in the wrong data field. This kind of error never happened in the automatic approach, since that would require editing of the data after the autocomplete took place. It is important to note, that in the real work environment the users would rearrange the table and thus may be able to work faster and/or with less errors made, but for the study the original table was maintained. The other manual mistakes resulted from a faulty search, for example, similar medicine was selected from the table because the exact entry was not immediately found. This work confirms that there is not only a difference between paper and eCRF on data quality [2-5], there is also an important influence by the design and functionality of the graphical user interface of eCRF. This is in accordance with studies to clinical information systems [8].

In terms of usability, OIC seems to do well with a mean SUS score of 90.8. However, the score could be distorted because the point of comparison was entering it by hand, which is a long and tedious task. In addition, the comments provide constructive suggestions to improve the program even further. Another follow up study could have the inclusion criteria to include specialists like documentarists and study nurses. These individuals might have more in depth feedback or might use such system differently and provide different results.

6. Conclusion

We successfully implemented an enhancement tool (OIC) for *OpenClinica*® to support the input of drug names and their associated values by autocomplete. The evaluation study carried out shows benefits on efficiency and data quality. In conclusion, new functionalities in eCRF-systems should be validated before usage in research projects.

Acknowledgements and Conflict of interest

The authors thank all participants and the ASD-net study team. The authors have no conflict of interest.

References

[1] Gaddale, Jagadeeswara Rao. "Clinical data acquisition standards harmonization importance and benefits in clinical data management." *Perspectives in clinical research* 6.4 (2015): 179.
[2] Kuchinke, Wolfgang, et al. "Heterogeneity prevails: the state of clinical trial data management in Europe-results of a survey of ECRIN centres." *Trials* 11.1 (2010): 79.
[3] El Emam, Khaled, et al. "The use of electronic data capture tools in clinical trials: Web-survey of 259 Canadian trials." *Journal of medical Internet research* 11.1 (2009): e8.
[4] Nahm, Meredith L., Carl F. Pieper, and Maureen M. Cunningham. "Quantifying data quality for clinical trials using electronic data capture." *PloS one* 3.8 (2008): e3049.
[5] Goldberg, Saveli, Andrzej Niemierko, and Alexander Turchin. "Analysis of data errors in clinical research databases." *AMIA*. 2008.
[6] Stein, Benjamin, and Joseph L. Kannry. "Comparison of Three Methods of Entering Clinical Information in a Prototype Triage System." *AMIA Annual Symposium Proceedings*. Vol. 2003. American Medical Informatics Association, 2003.
[7] Brooke, John. "SUS-A quick and dirty usability scale." *Usability evaluation in industry* 189.194 (1996): 4-7.
[8] Ahlbrandt, Janko et. al.: *Small cause - big effect: improvement in interface design results in improved data quality - a multicenter crossover study*". Stud Health Technol Inform. 2012: 180: 393-7.

© 2017 German Association for Medical Informatics, Biometry and Epidemiology (gmds) e.V. and IOS Press.
This article is published online with Open Access by IOS Press and distributed under the terms
of the Creative Commons Attribution Non-Commercial License 4.0 (CC BY-NC 4.0).
doi:10.3233/978-1-61499-808-2-75

A Decentralized IT Architecture for Locating and Negotiating Access to Biobank Samples

Rumyana PROYNOVA [a,1], Diogo ALEXANDRE [a], Martin LABLANS, [a] David VAN ENCKEVORT[b], Sebastian MATE[c], Niina EKLUND[d], Kaisa SILANDER[d], Michael HUMMEL[e], Petr HOLUB[f] and Frank ÜCKERT[a]

[a] German Cancer Research Center, Heidelberg.&BBMRI.de
[b] Universitair Medisch Centrum Groningen, Groningen & BBMRI.nl
[c] Friedrich Alexander Universität, Erlangen-Nürnberg & BBMRI.de
[d] Terveyden Ja Hyvinvoinnin Laitos, Helsinki & BBMRI.fi
[e] Charité, Berlin & BBMRI.de
[f] BBMRI-ERIC, Graz

Abstract. There is a need among researchers for the easy discoverability of biobank samples. Currently, there is no uniform way for finding samples and negotiate access. Instead, researchers have to communicate with each biobank separately. We present the architecture for the BBMRI-CS IT platform, whose goal is to facilitate sample location and access. We chose a decentral approach, which allows for strong data protection and provides the high flexibility needed in the highly heterogeneous landscape of European biobanks. This is the first implementation of a decentral search in the biobank field. With the addition of a Negotiator component, it also allows for easy communication and a follow-through of the lengthy approval process for accessing samples.

Keywords. Biological specimen banks, Information storage and retrieval, Decentral search, European research infrastructure

1. Introduction

Biobanks are an essential part of the research infrastructure in the life sciences. They offer access to human biological samples, as well as the associated epidemiological, clinical, biological, genealogical and molecular information, which is critical for researchers who work on the major challenges that medical science is facing today.

The European biobank landscape is highly heterogeneous. Each biobank uses its own process for sample requests. Researchers have to first locate candidate biobanks, then, if the needed samples are available, negotiate access with each biobank separately. Biobanks desire more external cooperation, but find that few requests reach them.

BBMRI-ERIC is a distributed research infrastructure of biobanks and biomedical resources [1]. One of its aims is to provide the Common Service IT (CS-IT) platform, which supports researchers in locating samples and gaining access to them, providing a

---

[1] Corresponding Author: Rumyana Proynova, Medical Informatics in Translational Oncology, German Cancer Research Center, Im Neuenheimer Feld 580, 69120 Heidelberg, Germany. r.proynova@dkfz.de.

unified search process, while being flexible enough to account for the differences between biobanks. It allows for focused searches on the sample level, cutting down on the inefficiencies inherent in sending and processing queries to biobanks which might or might not have the desired material.

In work with stakeholders, Lablans [2] identified the major requirements:

- **Technical heterogeneity.** The system should be able to represent sample data from different source systems without the need for manual reentry.
- **Semantic interoperability.** The system has to make the sample descriptions from different organizations comparable to each other.
- **Minimal effort.** Participating in the system should require minimal effort.
- **Data minimization.** The system should avoid saving sample data outside of the biobank where possible.
- **Data sovereignty.** The biobanker should control which data leaves the biobank, and there should be no pressure to justify a decision to deny access.

2. State of the art

Several platforms already facilitate to some degree sample access to biobanks. They all offer partial solution of the access problem, but cannot function as a comprehensive solution on the European level.

Some biobanks provide a sample search on the Internet, for example the Auria biobank [3]. This type of system best represents the dataset of one biobank, and grants perfect data sovereignty, but is not interoperable with other biobanks and requires the researcher to actively seek out a biobank.

A more interconnected approach is seen in biobank registries such as the German biobank registry [4]. The registry approach requires the biobanker to preemptively provide data, which hurts the requirements of minimal effort, data minimization and sovereignty. Its minimal dataset only allows a search with low precision and recall. For situations where this is sufficient, the registry-based approach offers an attractive option for low-friction data access. Centralized search systems such as CRIP [5] work on a similar principle and have similar advantages and disadvantages.

All these options are focused on discovering potentially collaborating biobanks. To our knowledge, none of them supports the subsequent negotiation process.

3. Concept

The BBMRI CS-IT platform allows for the connection of large numbers of biobanks. Its architecture follows the principles of the "decentral search" [6] developed in the German Cancer Consortium [7]. Its main advantage is that the information never leaves the biobank uncontrolled, allowing the biobanks to retain data sovereignty and implement privacy protection, unlike the central solutions discussed in the previous section. Figure 1 shows a diagram of the architecture.

To address the problem of semantic interoperability, BBMRI-ERIC supports a set of data models. The central one is the BBMRI-ERIC core terminology, which encompasses a minimal list of data elements, related to the MIABIS dataset [8, 8]. It is extended by optional purpose-specific data models. The core terminology and the extension data models are defined as data dictionaries contained in a *Metadata repository* (MDR) based on the ISO/IEC 11179 standard [9].

When a biobank joins the platform, its data has to be harmonized. BBMRI-ERIC provides a suite of *Mapping & ETL* tools, with which the biobanker maps the source data structure to one or more of the data dictionaries supported by the platform. After the mapping of the metadata, the data itself is uploaded into a *local data silo*. Unlike the source systems, it contains harmonized data. The biobank also installs a *Connector*. It can execute queries against the dataset in the data silo, but does not actively send information to the outside.

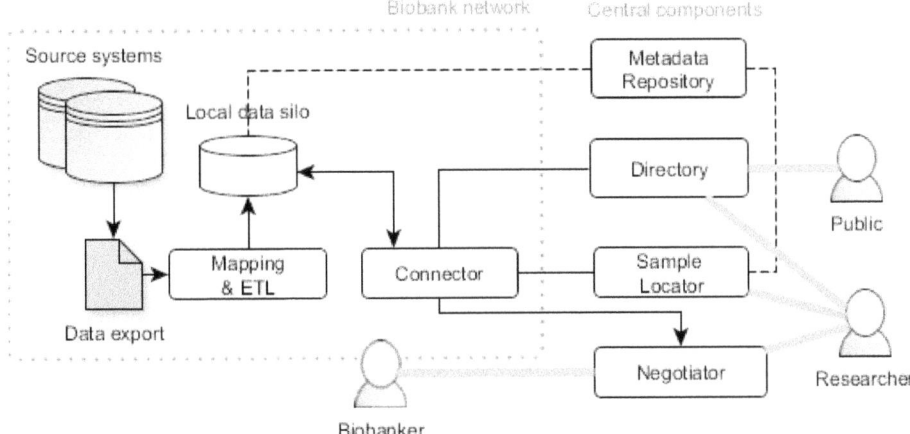

Figure 1. Architecture of the BBMRI-ERIC CS-IT platform

When a researcher needs samples, he or she first interacts with the *Sample Locator* component, which offers an interface for the construction of search queries based on the data elements provided by the MDR. The next step is to enrich the request by composing a short description in the *Negotiator*. The connectors fetch the query from the Sample Locator and execute it locally. If the data silo has matching samples, the Connector notifies the biobanker that a request is waiting. At that point, nobody outside of the biobank knows which biobanks matched the query.

The biobanker visits the Negotiator and uses the freetext description and the query criteria to determine if his or her biobank can actually provide the desired samples. As the request can be underdefined, the Negotiator allows the biobanker to ask for clarification and guide the researcher in improving the query criteria to better match his or her research question. When a biobank is confident that it can provide the samples, the biobanker can start a confidential conversation with the researcher to discuss the logistical, organizational and legal details.

This process offers high data protection, but may become cumbersome to the users. Its complexity is only needed when sample access is desired. Sometimes researchers or members of the public need non-sensitive information only, and the overhead of the sample request process is not necessary. For this use case, the platform also incorporates the *Directory [10]*. This is a registry-based service, offering low-detail information not violating the donors' privacy. It has a search interface that delivers immediate search results. For the convenience of biobankers, they can update their biobank's information in the Directory through the Connector.

4. Implementation

The implementation of the BBMRI-ERIC CS-IT platform follows an agile approach, stepwise releasing the components in a way that the system can be used to some extent even before the planned scope has been completed. All components are released as free and open source software.

At the time of this writing, the Directory is in active use and contains the data of over 1000 biobanks. The Negotiator is in a rollout phase, and in use by a small number of piloting biobanks, allowing for negotiation after a Directory search. The MDR is completed and contains two datasets: a first version of the BBMRI core terminology, and a colon cancer data dictionary as a first example of an extension data dictionary.

The connector, the local data silo, and ETL tools for a user-friendly mapping process are under active development. The public release is planned in fall 2017.

The Sample Locator is not yet implemented. It is expected to be released in 2018. Until then, users can locate biobanks with candidate samples by using the Directory, and proceed from here to negotiation.

5. Discussion

The architecture presented here meets the five major requirements elicited from stakeholders. Transferring the source data into a data silo using a unified structure solves the problem of technical interoperability. The MDR-driven approach with a core dataset and extensions is a scalable approach to the semantic interoperability problem. As both the data silo and the connector remain within the biobank, the principles of data sovereignty and data minimization are upheld – information is only transmitted with regard to a request, following approval of a biobanker.

The effort needed to setup the system is not trivial, but we argue that it is still small in comparison to the gains from participation. The highest additional effort for the biobank is the one-time process of mapping the source data to the provided data dictionaries. The ETL tools are usable by domain experts without IT background. So while the goal of minimal effort is not completely reached, it is still at a very good level and allows for realistic system adoption.

The decentral search approach is not as convenient for the requester as the immediate serving of search results familiar from other domains. We chose this solution as a response to the need for confidentiality and data protection inherent in biological sample data, since even non-identifying information such as a diagnosis is subject to some confidentiality under current social and legal norms. The non-sensitive data about biobanks and their samples can be found in the Directory, which offers a conventional search with immediate results.

The Negotiator is a novel component, which has not been employed in previous search systems. It lets humans take over the communication after the search has discovered which potential communication partners have relevant samples. This adds flexibility to the system, allowing it to support a large variety of collaboration models, and making it robust to imperfect search queries and missing data sources.

System success is highly dependent on gaining acceptance from biobanks and ensuring high data quality. To achieve this, we are engaged in dialogue with selected biobanks and BBMRI's national nodes since the earliest project phases. We rely on their feedback for creating a system which they are willing and capable of using.

6. Conclusion

In this paper, we present an architecture for a platform which allows researchers to locate and request samples from biobanks. It is an implementation of a decentral search approach, enriched by a Negotiator component which supports a flexible approval and collaboration process between biobankers and researchers.

Some components of the future system are already released and are well-received among users. Close work with stakeholders ensures that the remaining components will also meet the users' needs and allows us to overcome the challenges inherent in the creation of a system of this scale.

7. Conflict of Interest

The authors state that they have no conflict of interest.

8. Acknowledgements

We thank Saher Maqsood, Maximilian Ataian, Paul Weingardt, Polina Litvak, Jonattan Jetten, Fleur Kelpin and Mark de Haan for their work on implementing the platform. The work is part of the ADOPT BBMRI-ERIC project, funded by the EC, topic H2020-INFRADEV-3-2015, Grant Agreement Nr 676550.

References

[1]   BBMRI-ERIC. What is BBMRI-ERIC?: BBMRI-ERIC [cited 2017 March 14]
[2]   Lablans M. Die dezentrale Suche für die medizinische Verbundforschung. Doctoral thesis, Mathematisch-Naturwissenschaftliche Fakultät, Universität Münster 2015.
[3]   Auria Biobank Catalog [cited 2017 March 14] Available from: URL: https://www.auriabiopankki.fi/katalogi/.
[4]   Deutsches Biobankregister [cited 2017 March 14] Available from: URL: http://dbr.biobanken.de/de/web/guest/bdb/.
[5]   Schroder C, Heidtke KR, Zacherl N, Zatloukal K, Taupitz J. Safeguarding donors' personal rights and biobank autonomy in biobank networks: the CRIP privacy regime. Cell Tissue Bank 2011; 12(3): 233–40
      [https://doi.org/10.1007/s10561-010-9190-8][PMID: 20632213]
[6]   Lablans M, Kadioglu D, Mate S, Leb I, Prokosch H-U, Uckert F. Strategies for biobank networks. Classification of different approaches for locating samples and an outlook on the future within the BBMRI-ERIC. Bundesgesundheitsblatt Gesundheitsforschung Gesundheitsschutz 2016; 59(3): 373–8
      [https://doi.org/10.1007/s00103-015-2299-y][PMID: 26753865]
[7]   Lablans M, Kadioglu D, Muscholl M, Uckert F. Exploiting Distributed, Heterogeneous and Sensitive Data Stocks while Maintaining the Owner's Data Sovereignty. Methods Inf Med 2015; 54(4): 346–52
      [https://doi.org/10.3414/ME14-01-0137][PMID: 26196653]
[8]   Norlin L, Fransson MN, Eriksson M, et al. A Minimum Data Set for Sharing Biobank Samples, Information, and Data: MIABIS. Biopreserv Biobank 2012; 10(4): 343–8
      [https://doi.org/10.1089/bio.2012.0003][PMID: 24849882]
[9]   ISO/IEC. ISO/IEC 11179, Information Technology -- Metadata registries (MDR); 2015 2015 Nov 5 [cited 2017 March 16]
[10] van Enckevort D, Reihs R, Swertz M, et al. BBMRI-ERIC directory: Metadata and aggregate data about biobanks and other bioresources 2016.

German Medical Data Sciences: Visions and Bridges
R. Röhrig et al. (Eds.)
© *2017 German Association for Medical Informatics, Biometry and Epidemiology (gmds) e.V. and IOS Press.*
doi:10.3233/978-1-61499-808-2-80

Semi-Automatic Terminology Generation for Information Extraction from German Chest X-Ray Reports

Jonathan KREBS[a,1], Hamo COROVIC[b], Georg DIETRICH[a], Max ERTL[c], Georg
FETTE[c], Mathias KASPAR[c], Markus KRUG[a], Stefan STOERK[c], Frank PUPPE[a]

[a] *Würzburg University, Chair of Computer Science 6; Germany*
[b] *Bamberg Hospital, Department of Radiology, Germany*
[c] *Würzburg University and University Hospital, CHFC, Germany*

Abstract. Extraction of structured data from textual reports is an important sub-task for building medical data warehouses for research and care. Many medical and most radiology reports are written in a telegraphic style with a concatenation of noun phrases describing the presence or absence of findings. Therefore a lexico-syntactical approach is promising, where key terms and their relations are recognized and mapped on a predefined standard terminology (ontology). We propose a two-phase algorithm for terminology matching: In the first pass, a local terminology for recognition is derived as close as possible to the terms used in the radiology reports. In the second pass, the local terminology is mapped to a standard terminology. In this paper, we report on an algorithm for the first step of semi-automatic generation of the local terminology and evaluate the algorithm with radiology reports of chest X-ray examinations from Würzburg university hospital. With an effort of about 20 hours work of a radiologist as domain expert and 10 hours for meetings, a local terminology with about 250 attributes and various value patterns was built. In an evaluation with 100 randomly chosen reports it achieved an F1-Score of about 95% for information extraction.

Keywords. Information Extraction, Terminology Generation, Data Warehouse, Radiology Reports.

1. Introduction

Developing information extraction (IE) applications from medical text documents, like reports and discharge letters, is a laborious task and requires adapting IE-tools to the structure and terminology (ontology) of the respective domain. Although standard terminologies like ICD, SNOMED, LOINC, RadLex etc. exist, those terms are often not easy to match to the terms used in text documents, written or dictated by physicians. In addition, IE of languages other than English faces many challenges [1], e.g. the standard terminologies may be partially or not at all translated. As for RadLex, a translation into German is announced for 2017 by the German X-ray Society (Deutsche Röntgengesellschaft)[2]. Although the German X-ray Society offers templates for struc-

---

[1] Corresponding Author, Jonathan Krebs, Würzburg University, Institute for Informatics, Am Hubland, 97074 Würzburg, Germany; E-mail: jonathan.krebs@uni-wuerzburg.de.

[2] http://www.befundung.drg.de/de-DE/2910/deutsches-radlex (visited 18.3.2017)

tured reporting[3], they are often not used by physicians, since dictating is a faster way for documentation. For the same reason, physicians often dictate noun phrases in a telegraphic style instead of using grammatically correct sentences. Similar observations can be made in other domains like sonography, pathology etc.

Our goal is to support the process of building an IE terminology from a sample of reports, since this is the most time consuming part in the development of IE applications. Examples of IE systems from German reports include radiology reports [2], German Patient Records [3], transthoracic echocardiography reports [4], and lung function tests [5]. Building large terminologies usable in an IE pipeline is very time-consuming. Such pipelines are often implemented using natural language processing frameworks that offer many useful components, e.g. GATE[4] and UIMA[5]. Some well-known systems for clinical information extraction are HITEx ([6]; based on GATE) and Apache cTAKES ([7]; based on UIMA). We used a special IE pipeline similar to [4] based on UIMA consisting of the following main steps for reports:

1. Anonymization (if necessary).
2. Segmentation of documents in sections and section classification (if necessary).
3. For each section, information extraction with section specific terminologies:
   3.1. Segmentation.
   3.2. Shallow parsing.
   3.3. Extraction of clinical concepts (attribute-value-pairs) with IE terminology.
   3.4. Special processors for detecting negations, time dependencies etc.
   3.5. Disambiguation of clinical concepts using context information.
   3.6. Postprocessing operations e.g. for information aggregation.

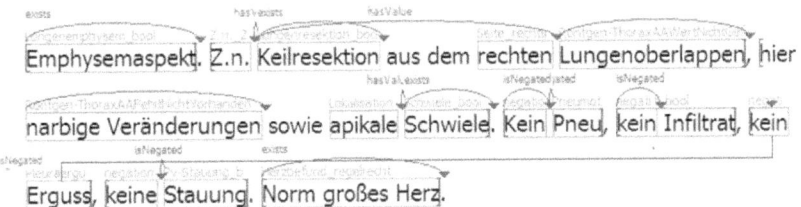

Figure 1. Example for a chest X-ray report (in German) with inferred annotations.

2. Methods

Our goal is not to develop a new IE-algorithm, but a semi-automatic terminology generation algorithm with a set of reports as input and a list of attribute-value pairs with synonyms and regular expressions as output. This knowledge is used by the IE pipeline described above to generate annotations as attribute-value pairs (see Fig. 1).

The first step is anonymization using a two-pass algorithm eliminating known named entities and using heuristics to detect names, addresses, phone-numbers etc. Since many phrases are stereotypical, the second step is to segment a report in phrases and aggregate phrases from different reports into one document without phrase duplication. This step uses mainly punctuation marks as separators with special treatment of

---

[3] http://www.befundung.drg.de/de-DE/2909/befundvorlagen (visited 18.3.2017)
[4] https://gate.ac.uk/
[5] https://uima.apache.org/

abbreviations, enumerations (like 4. in Fig. 2), and numbers. The main part of the terminology generation algorithm operates on the aggregated document (see Fig. 2).

1.	Herz normal groß ((152)).
2.	Kein Infiltrat ((141)).
3.	Aortensklerose ((103)).
4.	Normaler Herz-, Mediastinal- und Lungenbefund ((49)).
5.	Aortenelongation ((43)).
6.	Aorta elongiert und sklerosiert ((2)).
7.	Postoperative Veränderungen und Minderbelüftungen im linken Mittelfeld ((1)).

Figure 2. Excerpt of an aggregated document with some frequent (1-5) and some rare phrases (6-7) from 3000 chest X-ray reports (in German). The numbers in double parentheses represent the frequency of the phrases in the original reports.

After anonymization and segmentation the main steps of the semi-automatic terminology generation algorithm are:
1. Candidate terminology generation.
    1.1. Extract nouns from phrases and aggregate them by stemming and edit distance.
    1.2. Suggest an attribute type (e.g. Boolean, choice or number) for each noun.
    1.3. Filter nouns which are unlikely to be an attribute.
    1.4. Expand nouns occurring within enumerations (like 4 in Fig. 2).
    1.5. Display all relevant nouns with additional information in a terminology table.
2. Candidate terminology validation and elaboration (manual step by domain specialist, usably by making simple entries in the generated terminology table).
    2.1. Mark irrelevant nouns
    2.2. Group equivalent nouns.
    2.3. Add synonyms and regular expressions for relevant nouns.
    2.4. Check and modify the types of the attributes if necessary.
    2.5. Mark values for laterality, location, degree of severity, etc. for each attribute
    2.6. Define value templates for categories, e.g. for laterality: right, left, both sides.
3. Terminology update: The program processes the notes of step 2 and generates an updated terminology table. Steps 2 and 3 may be iterated several times.
4. Terminology application: The table is translated into a data structure suitable for the IE, loaded into the tool ATHEN[6] (Annotation and Text Highlighting Environment) and applied. ATHEN highlights all extracted entities, see Figure 1.
5. Reference standard definition: The domain specialist defines a reference standard of correct relations in ATHEN de novo or based on the suggestions of the IE when applying the terminology.
6. Evaluation with previously unseen documents. If necessary, steps 2-6 are repeated.

3. Results

We measured both, the precision and recall of the IE result and the time spent by the physician for terminology development. The physician (HC) spent about 20 hours of work mainly by editing and correcting documents in MS-Excel generated by the terminology extraction algorithm described above. He spent additional 10 hours for meet-

---

[6] https://gitlab2.informatik.uni-wuerzburg.de/kallimachos/Athen

ings with the computer science group (including the time spent for the evaluation). The computing time on a standard workstation took just a few minutes for steps 1 and 4.

The terminology was built based on a training corpus of 3000 chest X-ray reports from Würzburg university hospital. Its final version consists of 258 attributes with the following value categories: negation, laterality (right, left, both sides; relevant for 137 of the 258 attributes), location (38 possible values; relevant for 47 attributes), degree of severity (5 values; relevant for 131 attributes), condition-after ("Zustand nach"; relevant for 67 attributes), and progression note (3 values; relevant for 73 attributes).

With this terminology fed into the IE pipeline we performed an evaluation with 100 randomly chosen chest X-ray documents that were not already included in the training set. The manually defined reference standard contained 735 attribute-value pairs for the 352 segments (roughly half of them were negated) within the 100 documents. Each value category for an attribute (existence/negation, laterality, location, severity, condition-after, progression) was counted separately, if the report mentioned a value for the attribute in the respective category. In addition, since secondary findings are often mentioned in chest X-ray reports, we annotated the core attributes (i.e., the clinically most important attributes) and measured their performance separately. Further on, we measured the recognition rate restricted on the positive findings (not counting negations). The results are shown in Table 1 with an F1 value of 95.1% for all attributes. The core attributes had a precision of 100% in the evaluation sample and an F1 value of 98.9%. If only non-negated, i.e. pathological, attributes are considered, F1 values drop from 95.1% to 90.8% for all attributes and remain constant for the core attributes, since negations are recognized quite well and non-pathological statements have a lower variance than the non-core pathological statements. The accuracy on document level (number of documents with all attribute-value extractions correct) is 70%.

Table 1. Evaluation results with 100 previously unseen chest X-ray documents (TP = True Positive, FP = False Positive, FN = False Negative) on attribute level (# = number of attributes)

Types of attributes included	#	TP	FP	FN	Precision	Recall	F1
All attributes	258	735	4	65	99.4%	91.1%	95.1%
All attributes without negation	258	278	3	53	98.8%	83.9%	90.8%
Core attributes	119	351	0	8	100%	97.8%	98.9%
Core attributes without negation	119	130	0	3	100%	97.7%	98.9%

An error analysis for the 4 FP and 69 FN attributes in Table 1 revealed the following error categories (with frequencies):

- Missing regular expressions for an existing attribute or value: 25
- Segmentation errors: 23
- Missing attributes or values: 12
- Misspellings in report: 4
- Other: 5

Missing regular expressions are the most common error type. In general, it requires little effort for correction. Although it is difficult to cover all variations for a specific attribute, a few iterations would reduce the quantity of this error type considerably. A similar argument holds for missing attributes or values. Segmentation errors are more difficult to correct. Abbreviations ending with "." were a frequent source of error if they finish their segment needing a special disambiguation. Other segmentation errors occurred if an attribute-value was listed in a different segment than the attribute itself.

4. Discussion

From a practical point of view, the results of this rather efficient approach to building hospital specific information extraction models for particular reports are good enough for use in a data warehouse, since in particular the core attributes were found with high precision and recall. The evaluation results are comparable to those of other publication (e.g. [2-6]), but were achieved with a much lower manual effort by the domain expert. To the best of our knowledge, the effort for knowledge engineering is not reported in these and other respective publications. We did not investigate machine learning approaches offering also a potential reduction of manual work. Our approach supports such IE-approaches as well, since they need a gold standard to generalize from and the approach presented is useful to reduce the effort of defining or adapting the gold standard for a particular domain.

5. Summary and future Work

An efficient method for building an IE terminology for a specific domain was presented. The next step is to map this local terminology to a standard terminology like Radlex, if it is translated in German. We plan to apply this method for other domains (e.g. MRT, CT, etc.) in order to populate a data warehouse with structured information from unstructured reports. Further on we will investigate how well such local terminologies can be transferred from one hospital to another with manual adaptions and/or machine learning techniques and assess the efforts required therefore.

6. Conflict of Interest

The authors state that they have no conflict of interests.

References

[1] J. Starlinger, M. Kittner, O. Blankenstein, U. Leser. How to Improve Information Extraction from German Medical Notes, it - Information Technology 58 (10/2016).

[2] C. Bretschneider, S. Zillner, M. Hammon. Identifying pathological findings in german radiology reports using a syntacto-semantic parsing approach.In: Proc. Workshop on Biomedical Natural Language Processing. 2013. p. 27–35. http://www.aclweb.org/anthology/W13-1904.

[3] H.-U. Krieger, C. Spurk, H. Uszkoreit, F. Xu, Y. Zhang, F. Mueller, and T. Tolxdorff. Information extraction from german patient records via hybrid parsing and relation extraction strategies. In LREC, pages 2043-2048, 2014.

[4] M. Toepfer, H. Corovic, G. Fette, P. Kluegl, S. Stoerk, and F. Puppe. Fine-grained information extraction from german transthoracic echocardiography reports. BMC medical informatics and decision making, 15(1):1, 2015.

[5] M. Toepfer, D. Schmidt, G. Dietrich, M. Ertl, G. Fette, M. Kaspar, S. Störk, F. Puppe, Extraktion von Lungenfunktionsparametern aus Arztbriefen, GMDS Jahrestagung 2015,

[6] Q. Zeng , S. Goryachev, S. Weiss, M. Sordo, S. Murphy, R. Lazarus. Extracting principal diagnosis, comorbidity and smoking status for asthma research: evaluation of a natural language processing system. BMC Med Inf Decis Making. 2006;6:30.

[7] G. Savova, J. Masanz, P. Ogren, J. Zheng, S. Sohn, K. Kipper-Schuler et al. Mayo clinical Text Analysis and Knowledge Extraction System (cTAKES): architecture, component evaluation and applications. J Am Med Inform Assoc. 2010;17(5):507–13. 938.

German Medical Data Sciences: Visions and Bridges
R. Röhrig et al. (Eds.)
85
doi:10.3233/978-1-61499-808-2-85

Implementing a Data Management Platform for Longitudinal Health Research

Jan-Patrick WEIß[a,1], Ursula HÜBNER[a], Jens RAUCH[a], Jens HÜSERS[a],
Frank TEUTEBERG[b], Moritz ESDAR[a], Jan-David LIEBE[a]

[a] *Health Informatics Research Group, Osnabrück University AS, Germany*
[b] *Research Group Accounting & Information Systems, University Osnabrück, Germany*

Abstract. Health IT adoption research is rooted in Rogers' Diffusion of Innovation theory, which is based on longitudinal analyses. However, many studies in this field use cross-sectional designs. The aim of this study therefore was to design and implement a system to (i) consolidate survey data sets originating from different years (ii) integrate additional secondary data and (iii) query and statistically analyse these longitudinal data. Our system design comprises a 5-tier-architecture that embraces tiers for data capture, data representation, logics, presentation and integration. In order to historicize data properly and to separate data storage from data analytics a data vault schema was implemented. This approach allows the flexible integration of heterogeneous data sets and the selection of comparable items. Data analysis is prepared by compiling data in data marts and performed by R and related tools. IT Report Healthcare data from 2011, 2013 and 2017 could be loaded, analysed and combined with secondary longitudinal data.

Keywords. Survey data, longitudinal analyses, health IT adoption research

1. Introduction

Health IT adoption research is rooted in the work about the adoption and diffusion of innovation and draws on Rogers' Diffusion of Innovation (DOI) theory [1]. Health IT adoption studies often make use of surveying techniques to obtain the necessary information about IT adoption rates from samples of healthcare organisations and hereby, design their work as cross-sectional studies [2]. However, cross-sectional studies are only snapshots in time and therefore not suitable to study trends as the DOI theory requests. At the same time, longitudinal studies, which are more appropriate to answer these questions, demand more resources and are therefore underrepresented in the health IT adoption research [2,3]. IT Report Healthcare is a regularly conducted survey with a focus on measuring IT adoption in Germany, but also in Austria [4], the Netherlands and Switzerland that was developed in accordance with the OECD eHealth benchmark. IT Report Healthcare surveys like most other repetitive surveys, which capture information in a highly agile environment, face the same kind of issues: 1) new IT developments, 2) changing context, e.g. regulations, 3) changes of the statistical unit, e.g. merging of organisations, 4) availability of new data sources, 5) new research questions that are evolving from previous research findings. Thus, there is the need to

---

[1] Corresponding Author, Jan-Patrick Weiß, Osnabrück University of AS, Health Informatics Research Group, PO Box 1940, 49009 Osnabrück, Germany; E-Mail: j.p.weiss@hs-osnabrueck.de

encapsulate data from each point of time, to easily identify comparable items and to link only these data across time. It is the overall goal of the project to develop, implement and continuously improve an integrated platform for the management, analysis and visualisation of research data in IT adoption studies, but also in health services research. This part of the project focusses on the overall architecture and data management for longitudinal research. The aim of this study therefore was to design and implement a system built on open source components to (i) consolidate different items of one survey which was conducted in different years into one database, (ii) integrate additional secondary data sources and (iii) query and statistically analyse data over multiple years for longitudinal analyses.

2. State of the art

Data warehouse systems face the challenge of integrating several isolated information repositories into one single logical repository [5]. A literature and internet search, which was performed prior to the developments, resulted in no publications of a system that fulfilled the requirements as stated above. There were a few approaches to design and implement data warehouse systems for using survey-based data [6,7]. These approaches have a fixed concept in which the survey file formats, the survey structure and the user requirements stay the same and therefore are not flexible enough for iterative and agile research processes. IT adoption studies [8] often do not refer to any issues of data management but focus on data analytics primarily.

3. Concept

In order to meet these requirements, a hybrid approach for designing and implementing the system was chosen [9]. We combined a supply driven approach [5], in which we identified and analysed the data available, with a demand driven approach [10], in which we determined the requested information from users according to previous IT adoptions studies [11,12].

Our system design comprises a 5-tier-architecture that embraces a *data capture tier*, a *data tier*, a *logic tier* and a *presentation tier* (Fig. 1). They are connected via a fifth tier, the *data integration bus*. The *data capture tier* describes instruments from which the relevant data originates. The *data tier* is represented by a data warehouse for data consolidation and storage consisting of three layers: in the *source layer,* each of the data sources provided by the *data capture tier* is mirrored as a relational database table to ensure compliance with the defined data schema and data constraints. All extraction, transformation and loading (ETL) processes are implemented and executed through the *data integration bus.*

Primary data from different survey datasets and secondary data (e.g. hospital quality reports) are loaded into a consolidated form within the *core layer*. The core layer within the data tier constitutes the centre of data management and lays the foundation for flexible and longitudinal analyses. This is achieved via a schema that is based on the data vault model [13]. This schema is uncoupled from the model of the source layer to ensure flexibility. The data vault schema consists of three types of tables (hub, link, satellite). A hub represents a real-world or abstract object (e.g. survey item, site, quality indicator), which can be uniquely identified by its natural key. Each hub object receives a technical primary key and load timestamp for historicizing within the ETL process.

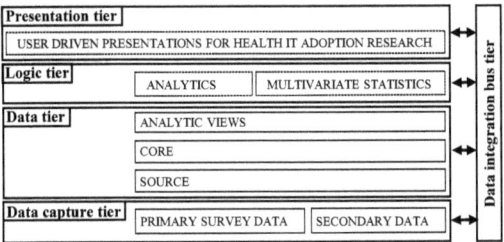

Figure 1. Overview of the system architecture

Links model the relationships between hubs (e.g. item – response, survey – site, site – response – quality indicator). A satellite contains attributes of one hub or one link. To historicize multiple temporal versions of attribute values its primary key is the foreign key of one hub/link with a timestamp. By separating natural keys (e.g. item codes, site ID) and the relationships between them from their attributes, a data schema is created that can, in comparison to the classical relational model [14], historicize various objects from different years and is able to combine these various objects in a flexible way, and to provide data for different, frequently changing query requirements.

Data marts, which constitute the analytics view layer in the data tier, provide optimised views with automatic aggregated data for predefined analyses. To perform more complex calculations, the data is loaded into further tools of the *logic tier* and the relevant results are stored back in additional data marts. This exchange service is represented via the *data integration bus*. In the *presentation tier* the data is displayed for standardised regular reports or for further research.

In contrast to other approaches, this concept does not focus on the integration of some specific types of data for certain use cases (e.g. clinical data [15], patient data [16]) but rather aims at the scalability through the data vault model approach for persistent, historicized storage of multiple surveys from different years.

4. Implementations

Pentaho Data Integration 7 served as the central *data integration bus* for all ETL jobs. Primary survey data were extracted from LimeSurvey 2.54.3 or legacy SPSS survey files from previous years. Secondary data was extracted from publicly available data sources (hospital quality reports, demographic hospital data). All data sources were loaded into relational database tables into the source layer (PostgreSQL 9.6 on Ubuntu Server 16.04). Then the data sources were transformed to one unified, consolidated, physical data vault schema (Fig. 2).

The data warehouse contains surveys of IT Report Healthcare from 2011, 2013 and 2017 (2011: 339 datasets, 203 items: 2013: 259 datasets, 521 items; 2017: 283 datasets, 226 items), historical demographic data of German hospitals from 2003 to 2014 (2883 datasets, 63 attributes) and hospital quality reports from 2012 to 2014 (381 quality indicators). In the design process, synonymously named items are mapped onto one item entity and stored in the hub *h_item*. Descriptive properties from the data sources, from which these items originated, are historicized in the satellites. Data marts were created to provide aggregated data e.g. denormalised demographic data of survey re-spondents or item frequency tables for longitudinal analysis. Data marts were accessed by the statistical software R 3.3.2 for data analysis and visualisation. Same survey items over the years 2011, 2013 and 2017 are provided by one data mart as frequency tables and were then further processed and visualised in R using the package *ggplot2* 2.2.1 [17] (Fig. 3).

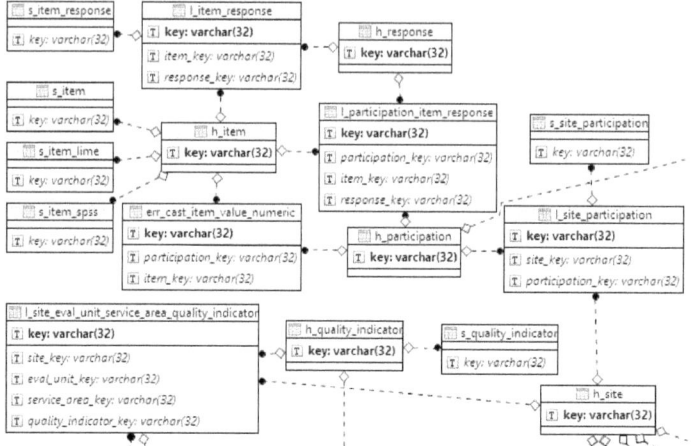

Figure 2. Excerpt of the deployed data vault model centered on the survey structure

5. Lessons learned

The proposed system for collecting, processing, storing and analysing data is composed of separate components, which are connected by ETL jobs. Each component can be replaced without affecting the rest of the system – except for the need of designing new ETL jobs. All tools used are open source and freely accessible. All relevant datasets could be loaded into the source layer. Using the proposed data vault model changes in the structure of the data source will lead to no changes in the structure of the model. Existing data can thus be easily extended by adding additional satellites, hubs or links.

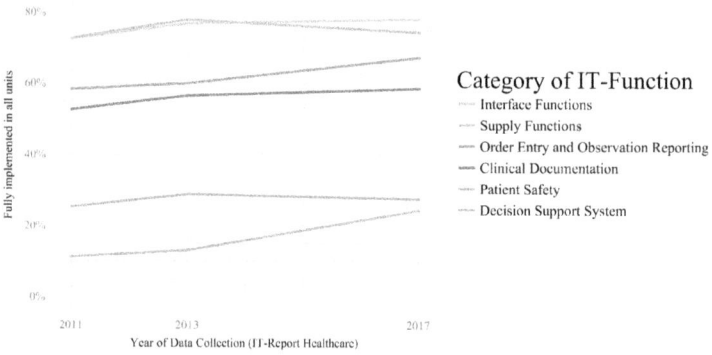

Figure 3. Display of IT adoption rates of six types IT applications for the years 2011, 2013 and 2017

6. Conclusion

We designed and implemented a system that improves data management for longitudinal analyses via the data vault model approach for persistent, historicized storage of datasets. It thus allows for agile, longitudinal analyses of heterogeneous datasets and lays the foundation of more rigorous and theory oriented studies of health IT adoption.

7. Conflict of Interest

The authors state that they have no conflict of interests.

Acknowledgment

This study is funded by Lower Saxony Germany (grants: ZN 3103, ZN 3062).

References

[1] Rogers EM. Diffusion of innovations. 5th ed. New York, London, Toronto, Sydney: Free Press, 2003.
[2] Agarwal R, Gao G, DesRoches C, Jha AK. Research Commentary —The Digital Transformation of Healthcare: Current Status and the Road Ahead. Inf. Syst. Res. **21** (2010), 796–809.
[3] Jones SS, Rudin RS, Perry T, Shekelle PG. Health information technology: an updated systematic review with a focus on meaningful use. Ann. Intern. Med. **160** (2014) 48–54.
[4] Hüsers J, Hübner U, Esdar M, Ammenwerth E, Hackl WO, Naumann L, Liebe JD. Innovative Power of Health Care Organisations Affects IT Adoption: A bi-National Health IT Benchmark Comparing Austria and Germany. J Med Syst. **41** (2017), 33. DOI:10.1007/s10916-016-0671-6.
[5] Inmon WH. Building the data warehouse. 4th ed. Indianapolis Ind.: Wiley, 2005.
[6] Seah BK, Ezam Selan N. Design and Implementation of Data Warehouse with Data Model using Survey-based Services Data. In: INTECH 2014. Piscataway, NJ: IEEE; (2014), 58–64.
[7] Yost M, Nealon J. Using a dimensional data warehouse to standardize survey and census metadata. National Agricultural Statistics Service, U.S. Department of Agriculture, 1999.
[8] Buntin MB, Burke MF, Hoaglin MC, Blumenthal D. The benefits of health information technology: a review of the recent literature shows predominantly positive results. Health aff. **30** (2011), 464–71.
[9] Romero O, Abelló A. A Survey of Multidimensional Modeling Methodologies. IJDWM **5** (2009), 1–23.
[10] Kimball R, Ross M. The data warehouse toolkit: The complete guide to dimensional modeling. 2nd ed. New York: Wiley, 2002.
[11] Liebe J, Hüsers J, Hübner U. Investigating the roots of successful IT adoption processes - an empirical study exploring the shared awareness-knowledge of Directors of Nursing and Chief Information Officers. BMC Med. Inform. Decis. Mak. **16** (2016), 10.
[12] Liebe JD, Hübner U, Straede MC, Thye J. Developing a Workflow Composite Score to Measure Clinical Information Logistics. Methods Inf. Med. **54** (2015), 424–33.
[13] Golfarelli M, Graziani S, Rizzi S. Starry Vault: Automating Multidimensional Modeling from Data Vaults. In: Pokorný J, Ivanović M, Thalheim B, Šaloun P, editors. Advances in Databases and Information Systems. Lecture Notes in Comput. Sci. Cham: Springer Int. Publishing; (2016), 137–51.
[14] Codd EF. A relational model of data for large shared data banks. Commun. ACM **13** (1970), 377–87.
[15] Gui H, Zheng R, Ma C, Fan H, Xu L. An Architecture for Healthcare Big Data Management and Analysis. In: Yin X et al. editors. HIS 2016, Shanghai, China, November 5-7, 2016, Proceedings. Lecture Notes in Comput. Sci. Vol 10038. Cham, s.l.: Springer International Publishing; (2016), 154–60.
[16] Kaspar M, Fette G, Ertl M, Dietrich G, Nagler N, Störk S, et al. Extraktion und Transfer patientenbezogener Daten aus klinischen Informationssystemen in Studiendatenbanken – effektive Unterstützung klinisch-epidemiologischer Forschung durch ein Data Warehouse: GMS Publishing House, 2015.
[17] Wickham H, Chang W. ggplot2: Create Elegant Data Visualisations Using the Grammar of Graphics, 2016.

German Medical Data Sciences: Visions and Bridges
R. Röhrig et al. (Eds.)

doi:10.3233/978-1-61499-808-2-90

A Customizable Importer for the Clinical Data Warehouses PaDaWaN and I2B2

Georg FETTE[a,b,1], Mathias KASPAR[b], Georg DIETRICH[a], Maximilian ERTL[b],
Jonathan KREBS[a], Stefan STOERK[b], Frank PUPPE[a]

[a] *Würzburg University, Chair of Computer Science 6*
[b] *University Hospital of Würzburg, Comprehensive Heart Failure Center*

Abstract. In recent years, clinical data warehouses (CDW) storing routine patient data have become more and more popular to support scientific work in the medical domain. Although CDW systems provide interfaces to import new data, these interfaces have to be used by processing tools that are often not included in the systems themselves. In order to establish an extraction-transformation-load (ETL) workflow, already existing components have to be taken or new components have to be developed to perform the load part of the ETL. We present a customizable importer for the two CDW systems PaDaWaN and I2B2, which is able to import the most common import formats (plain text, CSV and XML files). In order to be run, the importer only needs a configuration file with the user credentials for the target CDW and a list of XML import configuration files, which determine how already exported data is indented to be imported. The importer is provided as a Java program, which has no further software requirements.

Keywords. data warehouse, ETL

1. Introduction

PaDaWaN [1] and I2B2 [2] are clinical data warehouse (CDW) systems, which store their data in an entity attribute value (EAV) model [3]. Both systems can be loaded via a web interface or data can be directly written into the respective database tables. However, further tools are required that read data from a data source (and optionally transform the data as desired) and send it to an import interface in order to get the data into the CDW.

The goal is to provide an import tool for PaDaWaN as well as I2B2, which is able to import the most common import data formats: plain text for unstructured data, e.g. discharge letters and reports; CSV for structured data, e.g. coded diagnoses or laboratory values; XML for semi structured data, like PMDs (see below), which are the majority of document types at university hospital of Würzburg. The import tool should be easy to configure, easy to integrate into arbitrary ETL workflows, and should not require additional software.

---

[1] Corresponding author: Georg Fette, University Hospital of Würzburg, DZHI, Am Schwarzenberg 15, 97078 Würzburg, Germany; E-Mail: georg.fette@uni-wuerzburg.de

2. State of the art

IDRT [4] contains an import and mapping tool that can be used to import catalog and fact data into I2B2. The IDRT tool can be either used as a stand-alone desktop application or it can be used as a component in the ETL suite Talend Open Studio[2]. When IDRT is to be integrated in other ETL environments this is not yet possible out of the box. Also IDRT is not able to process arbitrary XML import files. As the IDRT tool is only able to import into the I2B2 data model we chose to create a new importer tool that has a more abstract data model interface and is easier to integrate into arbitrary ETL tools.

3. Methods

The abstract data model of PaDaWaN, which is quite similar to I2B2, is depicted in Figure 1. It consists of a catalog of attributes (concepts; in I2B2 terminology) and a large set of facts (observation facts). Each fact is linked to a catalog attribute (concept) and is attached to a mandatory patient (patient) and, optionally a patient case (encounter) and/or a reference (instance).

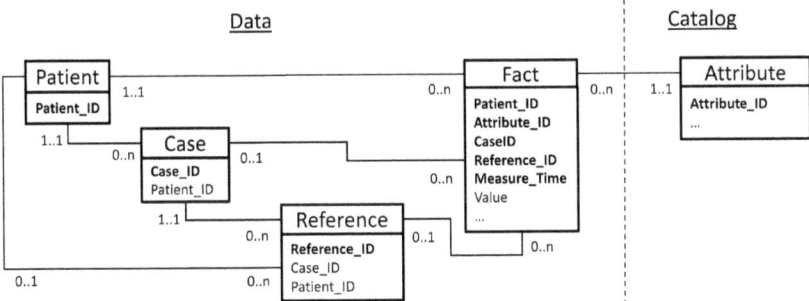

Figure 1: Abstract data model of PaDaWaN and I2B2

Due to the similar data models, a common Java interface for both PaDaWaN and I2B2 was created. The interface unites the shared properties of both systems, currently still neglecting some specific details of I2B2 [5] (e.g. PaDaWaN stores only the facts' measurement timestamps, whereas I2B2 supports start-end-intervals). Using this interface adapter implementations for PaDaWaN, as well as for I2B2 were created. The importer can be configured into which target system to import into. The importer is realized as a set of configurable Java classes for each data format (plain text, CSV, XML), which are altogether provided as a .jar-file. In order to be run, the program needs a configuration file specifying the import target system (CDW type, Server URL, database name) and the corresponding user login credentials. Furthermore, the importer needs the path to a file system directory containing import configurations (ICs), which define what data and how this data has to be imported. Both import parameters are provided to the .jar-file when started via command line parameters.

An IC is an XML file, providing all necessary information for the import process for one data source. An IC specifies a file system directory from which the importer imports all contained files. All further configuration is dependent on the data type of the exported data:

---

[2] *https://www.talend.com/products/talend-open-studio/*

Plain text files: The text content of each file from a given folder is imported as a single textual fact. The fact's metadata (e.g. patient ID) has to be extracted from the file's filename. The IC has to include regular expressions, which provide the identification of the needed metadata within the filename (e.g. Figure 2).

Tabular files: All files in a given folder are comma-separated value (CSV) files, which all have to have the same format. The IC configuration has to contain the syntactical format specification (e.g. delimiter, encoding, escape characters, etc.) and the semantic format specification. Via the tabular files importer the following data can be imported:

- *Catalog data*: The catalog for a specific CDW domain can be imported from a tabular file. The IC has to determine which columns in the CSV file shall be interpreted as the name, the catalog attribute ID, the data type, the unit or further information that is needed for the creation of catalog entries.

- *Fact data*: For the import of fact data from a CSV file the IC has to specify which columns contain the catalog attribute ID, values, measuring time stamps of each fact, etc. (e.g. Figure 2).

- *Import-metadata*: To ease the import of some data sources, patient-, case- and document-metadata can be imported into dedicated import-metadata database tables. These tables can be used when the importer is importing data lacking necessary information, e.g. only case IDs are provided instead of patient IDs. The importer can obtain the corresponding patient IDs from the import-metadata. Another example is in case the source data only contains fact measurement time stamps and no corresponding case IDs. The lacking case ID for a given fact measurement timestamp can be calculated by taking the temporally nearest case from the import-metadata tables.

- *Age*: The stored age for each case is the patient's age at the beginning of the respective case. For this calculation, the patient's date of birth from the import-metadata tables is used.

- *Authorization data*: PaDaWaN possesses an authorization concept managing users, groups, memberships of users to groups and accessibilities to catalog attributes for each group. All information belonging to those domains can be also be imported via the tabular files importer.

XML files: All files in a given folder have to be XML files with the same XML schema. The IC specifies a list of tuples (XML tag, XML attribute1, XML attribute2), which are searched for when the importer traverses the XML during import. For each tag, which is contained in the list of tuples, a fact is created with the catalog attribute identifier given by the XML attribute1 and the fact value given by the XML attribute2. Additional fact metadata (e.g. measure timestamp, patient identifier, etc.) have to be extracted from the filename of the XML file, as it is done for plain text files.

```
<ImportConfig>
    <DataCSV Project="Diagnose" Dir="DiagExport" AttrIDColumn="DKEY1"
        ValueColumn="DITXT" CaseIDColumn="PFALNR"
        MeasureTimestampColumn="DIADTZT" MeasureTimestampFormat="yyyyMMddhhmmss"
        Encoding="UTF8" />
    <DataText Project="Arztbriefe" Dir="BriefExport" AttrID="Brieftext" DocIDRegex="^(\d+)_.*"
        Encoding="UTF8" />
</ImportConfig>
```

Figure 2: Example of an import configuration including a CSV data source and a plain text data source

When run, the importer logs potential errors or warnings that occurred during the import process into a designated table of the target database. After a successful import of an import file, this success is also logged, storing the filename and the file modification timestamp of the respective file. When repeatedly running the importer with the same ICs on the same data source folders the importer can be configured to use the database logs to prevent unnecessary processing of already processed files. Using this mode, the import folders can be re-used for iterative (e.g. daily) export of data deltas without the need for cleaning those folders before every update cycle.

4. Implementation

The presented customizable importer is currently deployed and in use in the CDW projects at the university hospitals of Würzburg and Ulm. Within the CDW project Würzburg the majority of data domains that are loaded into the CDW are processed using the presented customizable importer. The domains processed by the importer at the current stage of the project are (grouped by data format) **CSV**: laboratory reports, diagnoses (ICD10), disease-related groups (DRG), procedures (OPS), age, sex, admission and discharge time stamp, hospital ward; **XML**: echocardiography reports, sonography reports, anamnesis and physical examination reports, electrocardiogram reports, coronary angiography reports, X-ray reports; **Plain text**: discharge letters.
A small fraction of the data domains (e.g. medication) still require additional transformations, therefore their import is performed by Java programs, which are individually created for those data domain.
At the CDW project in Ulm, which is currently still in the prototype phase, the importer processes the domains: **CSV**: diagnoses, laboratory reports, age, sex, admission and discharge time; **Plain text**: discharge letters.

5. Lessons learned

The use of the customizable importer improved the rollout speed at the Würzburg CDW project for the integration of new domains into the CDW, especially for the XML data domains. The XML data domains originate from so-called Parametrized Medical Documents (PMD), which are exported from the local SAP system in a generic XML format. PMDs are hierarchical structured documents comparable to CDAs (Clinical Document Architecture) [6]. At the university hospital of Würzburg, there exist hundreds of PMD domains [7], which represent a big fraction of the total data stock in the local hospital information system. The import process for those domains can now be configured via ICs instead of having to write Java code. Although in both CDW projects where the importer is used (Würzburg, Ulm) the technicians configuring the ICs are also programmers, the configuration of ICs is preferred to writing Java code. The training period for new workers in the ETL process becomes shorter because no programming IDEs have to be installed and configured and no code framework has to be learned. As part of the future development, the importer could be equipped with a user interface and an IC generation wizard like it is the case in IDRT [4] or in the CSV import wizard of Microsoft Excel.
By using the customizable importer and its import configurations the import process is logically separated from processes belonging to another technological level (e.g. database transactions, file access, program logic, etc.). This separation improves the documentability of the loading part of the ETL process. Other people in the CDW

project, e.g. working on quality assurance, can more easily review the import process because all import logic is concentrated in the single folder with IC-files.

The presented importer serves solely for the loading of data and not for any transformations of processed data. For transformations, an additional ETL software has to be used. In the CDW project at the university hospital of Würzburg the importer is included in an additional Java program that controls the ETL process [1]. As the customizable importer only needs text file configurations, an integration in another ETL environment should be easy to accomplish.

The abstraction from the concrete target CDW keeps the importer independent from the CDW system used. When choosing to exchange the underlying software (e.g. switching from I2B2 to PaDaWaN or vice versa) the existing ICs can be re-used without any further adjustments. Other CDW systems could be added to the framework by creating an appropriate adapter implementation for the abstract model (assuming the data model matches the abstract model depicted above). Due to the similar EAV models of PaDaWaN and I2B2 the unification under the same interface did not pose major problems. Other possible CDW data models like FHIR QI-Core[3], OMOP CMD[4] or PCORnet CDM[5] are more complex and would need a more sophisticated abstract model before a unification under a common interface could be achieved.

6. Conclusion

A customizable importer for the two DW systems PaDaWaN and I2B2 was presented which is able to import data in the most common data formats (plain text, CSV and XML). In order to run the importer only needs a configuration file with the credentials of the target DW system and a list of XML import configurations, thus making the importer easy to integrate into ETL workflows.

7. Conflict of Interest

No conflicts of Interest

References

[1] G. Fette, M. Ertl, G. Dietrich, et al., An improved data workflow for a medical data warehouse, *European Journal of Epidemiology* **32** (2016), Health-exploring complexity: an interdisciplinary systems approach HEC2016, 54.
[2] S. Murphy, G. Weber, M. Mendis, et al., Serving the Enterprise and beyond with Informatics for Integrating Biology and the Bedside (i2b2), *J Am Med Inform Assoc.* **17 (2)** (2010), 124-130.
[3] V. Dinu, P. Nadkarni, Guidelines for the effective use of entity-attribute-value modeling for biomedical databases, *Int J Med Inform.* **76 (11-12)** (2007), 769-779.
[4] C. Bauer, T. Ganslandt, B. Baum, et al., The Integrated Data Repository Toolkit (IDRT): accelerating translational research infrastructures, *Journal of Clinical Bioinformatics.* **5 (Suppl. 1)** (2015), S6.
[5] L. Liman, Vergleich und Integration der Data Warehouse Architekturen PaDaWaN und i2b2, *Master thesis (german)* (2017)
[6] R. Dolin, L. Alschuler, C. Beebe, et al., The HL7 Clinical Document Architecture, *J Am Med Inform Assoc.* **8 (6)** (2001), 552-569.
[7] M. Ertl, Erfassung von klinischen Untersuchungsdaten und Transfer in ein Data Warehouse, *Master thesis (german)* (2011).

---

[3] http://hl7.org/fhir/us/qicore
[4] https://www.ohdsi.org/data-standardization/the-common-data-model/
[5] http://www.pcornet.org/pcornet-common-data-model/

German Medical Data Sciences: Visions and Bridges
R. Röhrig et al. (Eds.)
© 2017 German Association for Medical Informatics, Biometry and Epidemiology (gmds) e.V. and IOS Press.
This article is published online with Open Access by IOS Press and distributed under the terms
of the Creative Commons Attribution Non-Commercial License 4.0 (CC BY-NC 4.0).
doi:10.3233/978-1-61499-808-2-95

Automated Transformation of CDISC ODM to OpenClinica

Sophia GESSNER[a,1], Michael STORCK[a], Stefan HEGSELMANN[a], Martin DUGAS[a]
and Iñaki SOTO-REY[a]
[a]Institute of Medical Informatics, University of Münster, Germany

Abstract. Due to the increasing use of electronic data capture systems for clinical research, the interest in saving resources by automatically generating and reusing case report forms in clinical studies is growing. OpenClinica, an open-source electronic data capture system enables the reuse of metadata in its own Excel import template, hampering the reuse of metadata defined in other standard formats. One of these standard formats is the Operational Data Model for metadata, administrative and clinical data in clinical studies. This work suggests a mapping from Operational Data Model to OpenClinica and describes the implementation of a converter to automatically generate OpenClinica conform case report forms based upon metadata in the Operational Data Model.

Keywords. Data Collection, Access to Information, Health Information Systems, Metadata, Surveys and Questionnaires.

1. Introduction

Nowadays, medical research data is predominantly documented in electronic data capture (EDC) systems [1]. The benefits of EDC systems when compared to paper-based data collection, such as facilitated data management and reduced data collection costs, have been discussed previously [2–4]. OpenClinica (OC), an open source EDC system, used in over 3000 clinical studies [5], represents an example for an EDC system. A crucial task, setting up an EDC based study is the generation of electronic case report forms (eCRFs). They contain the metadata for the collected data, i.e. item names, data types, measurement units, questions and answer options.

In OC, eCRFs can be defined in an Excel template to import them into the system [6]. To fill the eCRFs with clinical data, researchers may enter data directly via the user interface. Additionally, OC allows uploading existing clinical data via a REST interface, as long as it is stored in CDISC Operational Data Model (ODM), a platform-independent format for exchanging and storing metadata, administrative and clinical data [6, 7]. In order to further process or share data, OC provides various export formats, including formats used by statistical evaluation tools and ODM.

There is a discrepancy in OCs support for ODM. While clinical data can be imported as ODM files, metadata cannot. The only way to generate eCRFs is to upload metadata via an OC Excel template, hampering the reuse of pre-defined metadata in

---

[1] Sophia Geßner, Institute of Medical Informatics, Albert-Schweitzer-Campus 1, 48149 Münster, Germany; E-mail: Sophia.Gessner@uni-muenster.de.

standard formats. The demand for reuse of metadata in order to save time establishing eCRFs and even routine documentation forms is growing [8].

A research infrastructure, called Portal of Medical Data Models (MDM) [9], an open-access repository for medical forms, offers more than 10.000 medical forms in ODM for reuse in medical research.

The objective of this work is to provide an automated transformation of given metadata from ODM to the OC Excel import template.

2. Methods

Based upon the current version of ODM, 1.3.2, a mapping from ODM to the OC Excel spreadsheet template, v3.9, was defined.

In order to provide the possibility of an automated transformation of ODM's metadata into the Excel template, an ODMtoOpenClinica converter was developed using Java programming language. To validate the ODM files against the ODM 1.3.2 schema, a previously implemented ODM validator [10] was used and improved. To transform elements from the XML structure of ODM to Java objects, a Java library developed by the University of Münster, was used [11]. In order to adhere to OC's restrictions concerning the structure and naming of metadata, OC specific validations and adaptions were developed. The converter was integrated into the Portal of MDM. Furthermore the converter can directly be accessed via web interface or an API [12].

A test set of 10 ODM files with intentionally generated exceptional cases, such as multiple form definitions, missing ODM elements and files, covering all data types and range checks available in ODM, were converted. Additionally 30 random samples were downloaded from the Portal of MDM, converted with ODMtoOpenClinica and examined in OC. Errors leading to invalid OC CRFs were identified and corrected. For errors that could not be resolved due to incompatibility between ODM and OC CRF, a log file is generated and provided to the user.

3. Results

Elements of the ODM XML tree structure, relevant for the mapping to the corresponding columns of the OC template, are presented in Figure 1. The root XML element of an ODM file is named ODM. Its child element Study contains the study's metadata information as GlobalVariables with study name and description, BasicDefinitions for the definition of measurement units and MetaDataVersion elements. Further elements serve as references, such as ItemRef elements, linking elements within and across ODM files. To simplify the presentation of the mapping, ODM, GlobalVariables and reference elements have been omitted in Figure 1.

The OC template consists of five Excel sheets that specify the metadata necessary to set up a study form in OC:
- CRF, capturing information like the name and version of the CRF
- Sections, indicating the layout and organization of items
- Groups, grouping items logically together
- Items, defining all variables and their attributes
- Instructions, briefing users generating forms

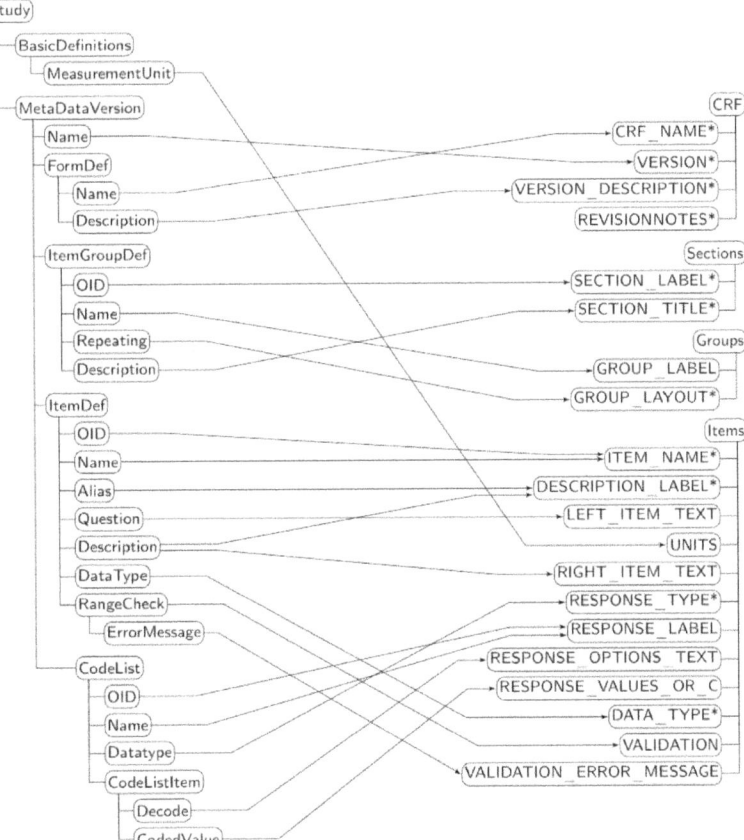

Figure 1. Mapping from ODM to the OC Excel template. (*=required fields in OC)

Figure 1 presents the excerpt of the ODM structure on the left side, linked via arrows to the corresponding elements of the OC template on the right side.

The converter implements the mapping to enable the automated transformation of ODM files into instantly applicable OC eCRFs. While ODM allows the definition of metadata for a whole study with multiple study events and various forms, the OC template is designated to represent a single form in a study. An ODM file containing multiple forms is transformed into multiple Excel files indicating FormDefNames and StudyEventDefNames as filenames.

Reference elements may indicate order numbers on items. If specified, items are sorted ascending, enumerated and transferred to QUESTION_NUMBERS, otherwise the order of items is derived from their positions in ODM. Mandatory items, also defined in ItemRefs, are mapped to the REQUIRED field in OC. The various DataTypes and their mapping are presented in Table 1.

ODM supports multilingual forms, by permitting multiple TranslatedText elements for ItemDefQuestions. Since OC only allows one language to be uploaded in one CRF, the converter checks the ODM for an indicated language code and chooses items in the language available. If no code is transmitted, English TranslatedTexts are used to generate the CRF, otherwise texts in German or the default language serve as backup.

Table 1. Mapping of ODM Item and CodeList DataTypes and their corresponding elements in OC. Further DataTypes, not presented in the table, provided by ODM are mapped to the OC DATA_TYPE "ST" and the OC RESPONSE_TYPE "Text". (ST=any character string, INT=whole numbers, REAL=decimal numbers, PDATE=partial date, either MMM-YYYY or YYYY, Textarea=multi-line box, Text=one-line box)

ODM DataType	OC DATA_TYPE	OC RESPONSE_TYPE
text/string	ST	Textarea
integer	INT	Text
float	REAL	Text
date	DATE	Text
time	ST	Text
boolean	INT	Single-Select (Yes, No)
partialDate	PDATE	Text

Certain OC specific requirements demanded preprocessing of elements. The DESCRIPTION_LABEL gives further information about an item, resembling the information contained in the Description attribute of items in ODM. As the Alias attribute in ODM gives the possibility to indicate further synonyms of the items, this information is also adopted into the DESCRIPTION_LABEL field. Since the REVISION_NOTES field in OC is mandatory, we followed OCs instructions to fill it with the note "This is a brand new form.". With every converted file, a record of all modifications is provided to the user via supplementary csv files, called "conversionNotes". The modifications are classified by their severity level concerning the resulting OC file: NOTICE, for minor changes to generate valid OC files, WARNING for metadata alternating changes and CRITICAL, for modifications that require manual post processing of the OC template after conversion.

Some elements of the OC template, such as subtitles, instructions or layout information, could not be filled in, since the information is not available in ODM. These elements are additional information and not obligatory in OC. RESPONSE_LAYOUT is left blank, displaying items in OC vertically.

4. Discussion

This work presents a solution to the limited possibilities of reuse of eCRFs in a widely used open-source EDC system. By creating a mapping from ODM, the implementation of a converter enabling the automated transformation of ODM files to OC compliant Excel sheets, became feasible.

The integration of ODMtoOpenClinica into the Portal of MDM enables the reuse of more than 10.000 medical forms from clinical trials, routine documentation, standard instruments and common data elements, available in ODM, paving the way for multicentric standardized structured documentation. Medical concepts of items in the Portal of MDM are semantically annotated with Unified Medical Language System codes. This information is transferred to OC, leading to a better semantic interoperability of clinical data. Nevertheless, it might be a valuable feature extension for OC to enable semantic annotation of medical concepts in a separate field.

By generating one Excel file per ODM form, the converter flattens the hierarchy of the original structures. Still, an ODM file may contain further information about the study, such as study title and study events. This information could not be included in the OC template, so the manual input and editing of the study title and definition of study events in OC is inevitable. A newer version of the OC's Excel import template should include Study information, which would enhance its interoperability with ODM.

The efficiency improvement in the set-up of studies as well as the conversion of ODM files issued from other EDC systems should be evaluated.

5. Conclusion

The proposed mapping between ODM and OC enabled the development of a converter for ODM forms into OC compliant forms. By integrating the converter into the Portal of MDM, more than 10.000 medical forms including 6.750 from clinical trials can easily be imported to OC and used for data collection.

Acknowledgements and Conflict of Interest

This work was supported by German Research Foundation (Deutsche Forschungs-gemeinschaft, DFG grant DU 352/11-1). We would like to thank Maurice Heine for his contribution to this project. The authors state that they have no conflict of interests.

References

[1]   K.A. Kessel, S.E. Combs, Review of Developments in Electronic, Clinical Data Collection, and Documentation Systems over the Last Decade - Are We Ready for Big Data in Routine Health Care?, *Frontiers in oncology* **6** (2016) 75.
[2]   I. Pavlovic, T. Kern, D. Miklavcic, Comparison of paper-based and electronic data collection process in clinical trials: costs simulation study, *Contemporary clinical trials* **30** (2009) 300–316.
[3]   P.V. Staziaki, P. Kim, H.V. Vadvala, B.B. Ghoshhajra, Medical Registry Data Collection Efficiency: A Crossover Study Comparing Web-Based Electronic Data Capture and a Standard Spreadsheet, *Journal of medical Internet research* **18** (2016) e141.
[4]   I.C. Olsen, E.A. Haavardsholm, E. Moholt, T.K. Kvien, E. Lie, NOR-DMARD data management: implementation of data capture from electronic health records, *Clinical and experimental rheumatology* **32** (2014) S-158-62.
[5]   OpenClinica - Electronic data capture for clinical research, https://www.openclinica.com/, accessed 8 February 2017.
[6]   OpenClinica Reference Guide, https://docs.openclinica.com/3.1/study-setup/build-study/create-case-report-forms-crfs, accessed 8 February 2017.
[7]   CDISC - Clinical Data Interchange Standards Consortium, Operational Data Model (ODM) - XML, 2016, https://www.cdisc.org/standards/foundational/odm, accessed 21 November 2016.
[8]   M. Dugas, K.-H. Jöckel, T. Friede, O. Gefeller, M. Kieser, M. Marschollek, E. Ammenwerth, R. Röhrig, P. Knaup-Gregori, H.-U. Prokosch, Memorandum "Open Metadata". Open Access to Documentation Forms and Item Catalogs in Healthcare, *Methods of Information in Medicine* **54** (2015) 376–378.
[9]   Metadata Repository for Medical Forms, https://medical-data-models.org/, accessed 29 May 2017.
[10] M. Storck, R. Krumm, M. Dugas, ODMSummary: A Tool for Automatic Structured Comparison of Multiple Medical Forms Based on Semantic Annotation with the Unified Medical Language System, *PloS one* **11** (2016) e0164569.
[11] I. Soto-Rey, M. Dugas, M. Storck, Implementation of an ODM and HL7 Compliant Electronic Patient-Reported Outcome System, *Studies in health technology and informatics* **228** (2016) 421–425.
[12] ODMToolbox, https://odmtoolbox.uni-muenster.de/, accessed 29 May 2017.

100

German Medical Data Sciences: Visions and Bridges
R. Röhrig et al. (Eds.)
© *2017 German Association for Medical Informatics, Biometry and Epidemiology (gmds) e.V. and IOS Press.*
This article is published online with Open Access by IOS Press and distributed under the terms
of the Creative Commons Attribution Non-Commercial License 4.0 (CC BY-NC 4.0).
doi:10.3233/978-1-61499-808-2-100

Proof-of-Concept Integration of Heterogeneous Biobank IT Infrastructures into a Hybrid Biobanking Network

Sebastian MATE [a,1], Dennis KADIOGLU [a,b], Raphael W. MAJEED [c],
Mark R. STÖHR [c], Michael FOLZ [d], Patric VORMSTEIN [d,e], Holger STORF [d,e],
Daniel P. BRUCKER [e,f], Dietmar KEUNE [g], Norman ZERBE [h], Michael HUMMEL [h,i],
Karsten SENGHAS [j], Hans-Ulrich PROKOSCH [a] and Martin LABLANS [j]

[a] *Medical Informatics, Univ. of Erlangen-Nürnberg, Erlangen, Germany*
[b] *Institute of Medical Biostatistics, Epidemiology and Informatics, University Medical Center of the Johannes Gutenberg University Mainz, Mainz, Germany*
[c] *UGMLC, German Center for Lung Research (DZL), Justus-Liebig-University, Giessen, Germany*
[d] *Medical Informatics Group, University Hospital Frankfurt, Frankfurt, Germany*
[e] *German Cancer Consortium (DKTK), partner site Frankfurt; and German Cancer Research Center (DKFZ), Heidelberg, Germany*
[f] *University Cancer Center (UCT) Frankfurt, University Hospital Frankfurt, Frankfurt, Germany*
[g] *Clinical Cancer Registry, Charité Comprehensive Cancer Center, Berlin, Germany*
[h] *Institute of Pathology, Charité - Universitätsmedizin Berlin, Berlin, Germany; and Central Biobank Charité (ZeBanC), Berlin, Germany*
[i] *German Biobank Node*
[j] *Medical Informatics in Translational Oncology, German Cancer Research Center (DKFZ), Heidelberg, Germany*

Abstract. Cross-institutional biobank networks hold the promise of supporting medicine by enabling the exchange of associated samples for research purposes. Various initiatives, such as BBMRI-ERIC and German Biobank Node (GBN), aim to interconnect biobanks for enabling the compilation of joint biomaterial collections. However, building software platforms to facilitate such collaboration is challenging due to the heterogeneity of existing biobank IT infrastructures and the necessary efforts for installing and maintaining additional software components. As a remedy, this paper presents the concept of a hybrid network for interconnecting already existing software components commonly found in biobanks and a proof-of-concept implementation of two prototypes involving four biobanks of the German Biobank Node. Here we demonstrate the successful bridging of two IT systems found in many German biobanks – Samply and i2b2.

Keywords. Translational medical research, biobank network, federated queries, cohort identification, German Biobank Node

---

[1] Corresponding Author: Sebastian Mate, Wetterkreuz 13, 91058 Erlangen-Tennenlohe, Germany; E-mail: Sebastian.Mate@fau.de.

1. Introduction

Biobanks play a pivotal role in facilitating biomedical research in the era of personalized medicine. As research infrastructures, they effectively support the discovery and validation of molecular disease mechanisms and biomarker detection, which will ultimately lead to deep insights into disease pathogenesis and allow the development of innovative treatment options. Such new knowledge can be incorporated into the assessment and stratification of risk factors, new diagnostic methods, pharmacogenomics, and drug development [1]. However, access to samples and associated clinical data of suitable quality is still one of the major challenges (see e.g. [2]). Since almost all diseases are composed of highly diverse molecular subgroups, it becomes more and more difficult, even for large biobanks, to provide sufficient samples and data of a certain molecular subgroup to provide statistical rigor to a study [3,4]. Researchers increasingly require large and sufficiently characterized data sets to uncover the subtle statistical associations between phenotypes and diseases. As stated in [5], "biobanking is required to change strategic focus from a sample dominated perspective to a data-centric strategy." Thus, it is desirable to merge data from multiple biobanks for further analysis [6].

BBMRI-ERIC is a European research infrastructure aiming to interconnect high quality biobanks all over Europe via a federation of national nodes. The planned software platform will enable researchers to identify samples by running queries across participating biobanks. The German Biobank Node (GBN) has been established as one of the BBMRI-ERIC national nodes [7]. In the first funding phase of GBN, it was the goal to design and evaluate the concept of an architecture for integrating biobanks with different local data warehouse (DWH) implementations into one network, and allowing queries from a single consistent user interface. The aim of this paper is to describe the development and lessons learned from two prototypical cross-biobank query implementations within a hybrid IT infrastructure.

2. Methods

The motivation within GBN was to develop a platform that is easily adoptable for the majority of biobanks. Hence, we intended to base our approach on technology that is already available in many biobanks. To this end, we analyzed the status quo at the five GBN-coordinated centralized biobanks (cBMBs) as well as the six biobanks of the BMBF-funded German Centers for Health Research (Deutsche Zentren der Gesundheitsforschung, DZGs), and the m4 Biobank Alliance in Munich, which were considered to be representative for German biobanks in terms of IT infrastructures. We recognized that only a few already had the infrastructure to identify samples or patient cohorts. Some of these were based on the commercial software CentraXX® provided by Kairos GmbH. Many of these CentraXX®-based biobanks, such as the Charité ZeBanC in Berlin and the University Cancer Center's biobank at UCT Frankfurt also participated in the research network of the German Cancer Consortium (DKTK), for which they established "bridgeheads", a combination of CentraXX® and the open-source software Samply [8]. Other sites implemented local research DWHs based on i2b2 [9], e.g. the DZL biobank at Giessen University Hospital and the one at the Comprehensive Cancer Center in Erlangen (CCC Erlangen-EMN). Starting from this initial analysis of available tools, we developed two prototypical GBN architectures. Finally, we evaluated both architectures at the above-mentioned four biobanks.

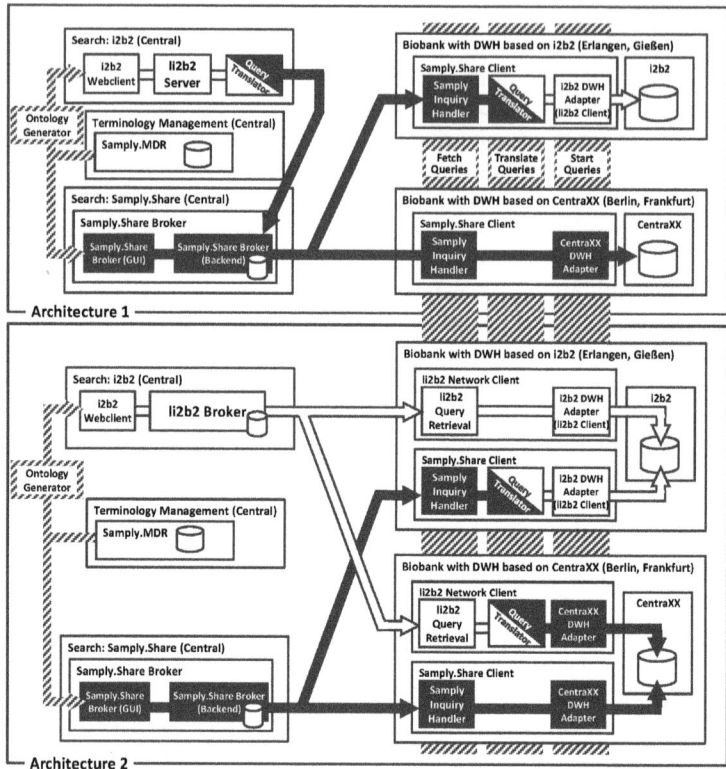

Figure 1. The two prototypical architectures that have been developed within GBN.

3. Results

The pilot was based on data stored in CentraXX® and i2b2, due to their availability at the selected sites. Two prototypical GBN architectures (as shown in Figure 1) have been developed. To enable networking with the i2b2 sites, we utilize li2b2 (https://github.com/li2b2) and not the better-known SHRINE [10], which uses a query push mechanism that is incompatible with firewalls usually installed at university hospitals. The central components, which are used for central terminology management and for issuing queries, are depicted on the left, local biobank components on the right side. i2b2/li2b2-related components and messages are shown in white, Samply/CentraXX®-based ones in black. The main difference between the architectures is that in architecture 1, outgoing queries are managed in a single queue (the *Samply.Share Broker*), whereas in architecture 2, a second queue (the *li2b2 Broker*) exists. Architecture 2 is in fact based on two networks that are not interconnected. This is also apparent on the right side, where for the second architecture, two clients are utilized – one for each technology (*li2b2 Network Client* and *Samply.Share Client*). As indicated by the three vertical stripes in the figure, the clients perform two to three tasks. The first one is to fetch new queries from a broker (*Samply Inquiry Handler* and *li2b2 Query Retrieval*). If necessary, a *Query Translator*, based on the *OmniQuery library* transforms the query into the syntax of the other platform, on the fly. Additionally, a mapping between the common GBN data elements from the central *Samply.MDR* to the respective local ones had to be implemented. The *Samply.Share Client* uses a mapping table, whereas the *li2b2 Network Client* uses an XSL transformation to replace concept identifiers. Finally, *DWH Adapters* issue the query to the DWH (i2b2 or CentraXX®), which reports the patient count back to the initial search component after execution.

We demonstrated both approaches to the GBN consortium in February 2017. We were able to successfully generate queries with both search clients (*i2b2 Webclient, Samply.Share Broker GUI*), automatically distribute them across our hybrid Samply/li2b2 network and execute them on the DWHs based on CentraXX® and i2b2. We currently support querying for patient phenotypes and sample characteristics (e.g. gender, type of sample). Furthermore, numeric data elements, such as laboratory measurements, can be constrained by comparator and value. As a result, the network returns the aggregated patient count for each site.

4. Discussion

The current literature presents different examples for integrating diverse data sources with information regarding biospecimens and their respective donors. These can be implemented at a single institution [11-13], in networks of institutions with identical local DWHs uploaded into central repositories [14], or they can remain in federated systems [8]. In contrast to central repositories, federated networks enable sites to retain more control of their data [15,16]. For example, the Breast Cancer Campaign Tissue Bank is a collaboration of four individual biobanks in the UK, and a platform has been developed to address the challenges of running a distributed network [17].

Our approach integrates already available local components into a federated network, thereby avoiding the establishment of new IT systems. For biobanks without existing local DWHs, this can be addressed by IT tools that have been developed recently (e.g. [18]). Our approach is also open for the integration of further platforms by implementing additional query translators.

To the best of our knowledge, our proof-of-concept is the first successful attempt to connect different DWH and federated search technologies into a single hybrid network. Architecture 1 grants biobanks a high degree of flexibility in their choice of a DWH. In our example, Frankfurt and Berlin employed their existing DKTK "bridgeheads", while Giessen and Erlangen set up an installation based on i2b2. On top of that, architecture 2 allows entire networks that had already settled on different federated search technologies to be interconnected, enabling inter-consortia queries.

However, our prototype also revealed inevitable limitations of hybrid networks. First, they introduce more complexity, as they require additional components to translate between different technologies. A certain degree of resources and technical expertise is required to design, develop, deploy, maintain and troubleshoot these additional components, especially since DWHs operate in secure clinical environments. Second, combining several technologies in consistent and comprehensible user interfaces requires determining and settling on their "lowest common denominator" in terms of features. For example, our prototype removed support for both i2b2's temporal relations in queries (as they are unsupported in CentraXX®' SQL-based query syntax) and Samply's fine-grained access control and privacy-preserving "decentral search" paradigm [8] (as i2b2 only supports *queries* and not Samply *inquiries*).

In conclusion, the high degree of flexibility of hybrid networks comes at a cost of increased complexity and reduced functionality. Obviously, biobank networks should build on a harmonized architecture and interoperable software whenever possible. Our proof-of-concept provides an important contribution by demonstrating that biobank databases and even whole existing networks can be federated across technological boundaries, such as different DWHs or query paradigms.

5. Acknowledgements

The present work has been funded by the Federal Ministry of Education and Research of Germany within the project *German Biobank Node* (project number 01EY1301). It was performed in (partial) fulfillment of the requirements for obtaining the degree "Dr. rer. biol. hum." from the Friedrich-Alexander-Universität Erlangen-Nürnberg (SM).

References

[1] Olson JE, Bielinski SJ, Ryu E, *et al.,* Biobanks and Personalized Medicine, *Clin Genet* **86** (2014), 50.
[2] Mabile L, Dalgleish R, Thorisson GA, *et al.,* Quantifying the Use of Bioresources for Promoting their Sharing in Scientific Research, *Gigascience* **2.1** (2013), 7.
[3] Laffert von M, Penzel R, Schirmacher P, *et al.,* Multicenter ALK Testing in Non–Small-Cell Lung Cancer: Results of a Round Robin Test, *J Thorac Oncol* **9.10** (2014), 1464–1469.
[4] Quinlan PR, Mistry G, Bullbeck H, *et al.,* A Data Standard for Sourcing Fit-for-Purpose Biological Samples in an Integrated Virtual Network of Biobanks, *Biopreserv Biobank* **12** (2014), 184–91.
[5] Quinlan PR, Gardner S, Groves M, *et al.,* A Data-Centric Strategy for Modern Biobanking, *Adv Exp Med Biol* **864** (2015), 165–169.
[6] Pang C, Hendriksen D, Dijkstra M, *et al.,* BiobankConnect: Software to Rapidly Connect Data Elements for Pooled Analysis Across Biobanks Using Ontological and Lexical Indexing, *J Am Med Inform Assoc* **22.1** (2015), 65–75.
[7] Hummel M, Rufenach C, Biomaterial Banks Are Crucial to Developing Genetically-Based Prevention Concepts, *Bundesgesundheitsblatt* **58** (2014), 127–130.
[8] Lablans M, Kadioglu D, Muscholl M, *et al.,* Exploiting Distributed, Heterogeneous and Sensitive Data Stocks While Maintaining the Owner's Data Sovereignty, *Methods Inf Med* **54.4** (2015), 346–352.
[9] Murphy SN, Weber GM, Mendis ME, *et al.,* Serving the Enterprise and Beyond with Informatics for Integrating Biology and the Bedside (i2b2), *J Am Med Inform Assoc* **17** (2010), 124–130.
[10] McMurry AJ, Murphy SN, MacFadden D, *et al.,* SHRINE: Enabling Nationally Scalable Multi-Site Disease Studies, *PLoS ONE* **8.3** (2013), e55811.
[11] Gainer VS, Cagan A, Castro VM, *et al.,* The Biobank Portal for Partners Personalized Medicine: A Query Tool for Working with Consented Biobank Samples, Genotypes, and Phenotypes Using i2b2, *JPM* **6.1** (2016), 11.
[12] McIntosh LD, Sharma MK, *et al.,* caTissue Suite to OpenSpecimen: Developing an Extensible, Open Source, Web-Based Biobanking Management System. *J Biomed Inform* **57** (2015), 456–464.
[13] Eminaga O, Özgür E, Semjonow A, *et al.,* Linkage of Data From Diverse Data Sources (LDS): A Data Combination Model Provides Clinical Data of Corresponding Specimens in Biobanking Information System, *J Med Syst* **37.5** (2013), 9975.
[14] Oberländer M, Linnebacher M, König A, *et al.,* The "North German Tumor Bank of Colorectal Cancer": Status Report After the First 2 Years of Support by the German Cancer Aid Foundation, *Langenbecks Arch Surg* **398.2** (2013), 251-258.
[15] Lablans M, Bartholomäus S, Ückert F, Providing Trust and Interoperability to Federate Distributed Biobanks. *Stud Health Technol Inform* 169 (2011), 644–648.
[16] Lablans M, Kadioglu D, Mate S, et al., Strategies for Biobank Networks, *Bundesgesundheitsblatt* **59.3** (2016), 373-378.
[17] Quinlan PR, Groves M, Jordan LB, *et al.,* The Informatics Challenges Facing Biobanks: A Perspective from a United Kingdom Biobanking Network, *Biopreserv Biobank* **13** (2015), 363–370.
[18] Bauer CRKD, Ganslandt T, Baum B, *et al.,* Integrated Data Repository Toolkit (IDRT). *Methods Inf Med* **55** (2016), 125–135.

5. Health Care Information Systems

German Medical Data Sciences: Visions and Bridges
R. Röhrig et al. (Eds.)
107
© *2017 German Association for Medical Informatics, Biometry and Epidemiology (gmds) e.V. and IOS Press.*
This article is published online with Open Access by IOS Press and distributed under the terms
of the Creative Commons Attribution Non-Commercial License 4.0 (CC BY-NC 4.0).
doi:10.3233/978-1-61499-808-2-107

Alarm Fatigue: Causes and Effects

Marc WILKEN[a,1,2], Dirk HÜSKE-KRAUS[b,2], Andreas KLAUSEN[a],
Christian KOCH[c], Wolfgang SCHLAUCH[d] and Rainer RÖHRIG[a]

[a] *Carl von Ossietzky University, Oldenburg, Germany*
[b] *Philips Medizin Systeme Böblingen GmbH, Böblingen, Germany*
[c] *Justus-Liebig-University, Giessen, Germany*
[d] *Bitsea GmbH, Hennef, Germany*

Abstract. The term "Alarm fatigue" is commonly used to describe the effect which a high number of alarms can have on caregivers: Frequent alarms, many of which are avoidable, can lead to inadequate responses, severely impacting patient safety. In the first step of a long-term effort to address this problem, both the direct and indirect impact of alarms, as well as possible causes of unnecessary alarms were focused. Models of these causes and impacts were developed using a scoping review which included guided interviews with experts from medical informatics, clinicians and medical device manufacturers. These models can provide the methodical grounds for the definition of targeted interventions and the assessment of their effects.

Keywords. Alarm fatigue; Clinical Alarms; Clinical Alarms: organization and administration; Sociotechnical System; Critical Care; Patient Safety

1. Introduction

Physiological monitoring offers more and more data for the surveillance of patients' vital signs. With this, a corresponding increase in clinical and technical alarms can be observed. Almost inevitably, this also results in a growing number of alarms which do not require any action by the caregiver, i.e. non-actionable alarms. But even alarms which do require an action can be avoidable. Improper electrode placement, for instance, can lead to technical alarms which require a reaction (replacement of the electrode) but are preventable nonetheless. In the remainder, we will refer to both non-actionable and avoidable alarms together as "unnecessary alarms". In this study, we focused on Intensive Care Units (ICUs), but similar problems exist in all care areas where patients are being monitored [1; 2]. Of the 150 to 350 alarms per day and patient [3-5] as many as 80 % to 95 % are non-actionable (or "false": the used definitions vary) [6-8]. The workload from managing hundreds of alarms per work shift, including the mental stress from evaluation and prioritization of many alarm conditions in parallel, is often regarded as the main contributing factor for a fatigue in healthcare workers called "Alarm fatigue" [9]. We argue that Alarm fatigue should not be seen as a condition of an individual healthcare worker, but rather as a state of the sociotechnical system ICU where caregivers exposed to too many unnecessary alarms become more likely to react inadequately to alarms. The term "cry-wolf effect" has become common to denote the

---

[1] Corresponding Author, Marc.Wilken@uni-oldenburg.de [2] Shared First author

psychologically plausible – though rarely demonstrated in empirical settings (but see [10]) – mechanism by which high rates of false alarms lead to inadequate responses. While in the US the Emergency Care Research Institute lists "alarm hazards" in the top three of the "Health Technology Hazards" for several years responses [11-13], and while the FDA Manufacturer and User Facility Device Experience (MAUDE) database reports 566 "alarm-related deaths" between 2005 and 2010 [14], outside the US the awareness of the problem and regulatory attempts to improve the situation appear to be sparse.

Quite a few publications focus on advice to reduce unnecessary alarms [10; 15], mostly based on concrete improvement projects, but a comprehensive model of the causes and the effects of these alarms is still a desideratum.

The aim of this study was to develop such models since they are a necessary precondition for the development of a systematic approach to reduce unnecessary alarms.

2. Methods

We conducted a scoping review including a MEDLINE search and guided interviews with clinicians, experts from the field of medical informatics and medical device manufacturers, as described by Arksey and O'Malley [16]. We followed the six stages model for scoping reviews. We divided the study concerning two different goals. First, it was necessary to get an understanding of the underlying causes of unnecessary alarms on ICUs. Second, we used the same method, to elicit input to investigate the effects of unnecessary alarms on ICUs. We grouped the causes of avoidable alarms in a 6M-Ishikawa diagram, with the categories slightly adapted to better match the ICU setting. A potential cause was identified if it was mentioned as such during the focus group sessions or in the literature. However, we did not find explicit mentions of causality very often. More frequently, the literature rather recommends activities to mitigate the problem of unnecessary alarms by addressing a particular topic. We included these "inferred" topics into the model if they were regarded as plausible by focus group members. For the effect model, we used a causal map [18] showing all effects mentioned in the literature. Causal links which were suggested by at least two articles were included in the model, as was a self-evident one ("unnecessary workload" leading to "inefficiencies"). The resulting models were reviewed by the experts.

3. Results

Many publications report experiences from concrete improvement projects [4; 8], sometimes with a stepwise approach so that practice changes and outcome metrics can be correlated [14]. We did not find any publication to relate the baseline status of assumed causes to a general model of possible causes. Other publications give practice recommendations, drawing on past experiences, [19] but they also do not link their suggestions to any causal model. The scoping review shows that a comprehensive overview of all possible causes of unnecessary alarms is missing. The causal contributors to unnecessary alarms identified in the scoping review are shown in Figure 1. This figure has a low granularity with the terminal nodes still covering rather diverse phenomena. Figure 2 shows the identified direct and mediated possible effects of unnecessary alarms. While some of the effects and their causal relations are self-evident or common sense in

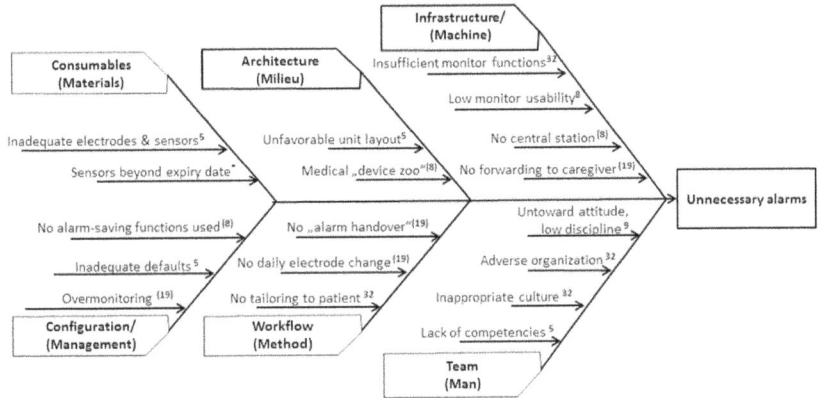

Figure 1: Two levels of the root cause model of unnecessary alarms; references in parentheses denote "inferred" causes, one cause marked with "*" was only mentioned during focus group sessions

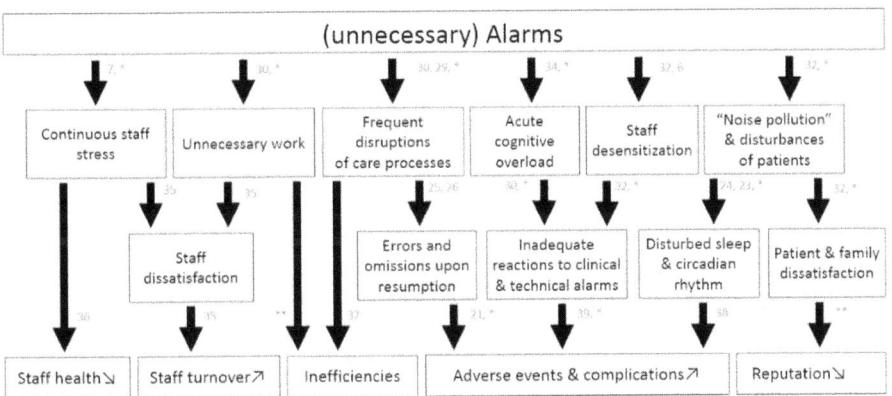

Figure 2: Potential impacts of unnecessary alarms. Not all causal relations are shown. Impacts mentioned during focus groups sessions are marked with "*", self-evident impact is marked with "**", only part of the supporting evidence from literature is referenced due to space limitations.

the literature, others may be less obvious. For instance, the relationship between disruptions of care processes and increased error rates has been demonstrated for some tasks in Healthcare settings (e.g. [20]), but only a few of them included ICU nurses [21].

Please note that, for a better readability, not all identified causal relationships are explicit shown in the figure. The impact of interruptions on stress, perceived workload and job satisfaction, for instance, is well established, but not depicted in the figure.

4. Discussion and Conclusion

Comprehensive models of both the contributing causes to unnecessary alarms and effects of these alarms are needed to guide the development of systematic approaches to address alarm fatigue. In the literature, we found only root cause models for particular units and events [22], but none that would aspire to cover the entire breadth of causal factors. Two general models, one for causes and one for effects of unnecessary alarms were developed, based on a scoping review and expert interviews. The cause model shows that the root causes are located in very diverse areas: While some causes are related to technology and technical infrastructure, others stem more from the workflow/process domain. Another, often overlooked source of problems is associated with the ICU as a sociotechnical system and people working in a team: Their attitude and discipline, technical and clinical competencies as well as collaboration and communication within the team. The two models allow to causally link root causes to undesirable consequences, avoiding the need to establish a consented and measurable model of Alarm fatigue as a condition of individual healthcare workers. The obvious fact that any of the diverse root causes may be present or absent in a unit also explains the fact that Alarm fatigue so far defeated many attempts of a unified solution: Only if the concrete unit at hand is understood regarding all of the possible root causes, one can try to improve the situation with reasonable hope of success. It must be noted that while the literature provides many recommendations to reduce unnecessary alarms, there seems to be a "blind spot" regarding actionable advice to influence behavioral factors of caregivers and teams.

Further work is needed to map the impacts of unnecessary alarms to indicators which are routinely measurable on an ICU and which cover all (or most of) the dimensions of the effect model. Work on a first set of such indicators has already started in the AlarmRedux project. These indicators will also allow transitioning from generic and unconditional advice dominating the literature (e.g. in *[19]*) to specific interventions addressing identified root causes.

Conflict of Interest

Dirk Hüske-Kraus is working at Philips Healthcare. Wolfgang Schlauch is working at Bitsea GmbH. The other authors state that they have no conflict of interests. All authors are part of the AlarmRedux-Project (www.alarmredux.de) founded by the Federal Ministry of Education and Research (BMBF). (Code: 16SV7501)

References

[1]　K.E. Raymer, J. Bergström, J.M. Nyce, Anaesthesia monitor alarms: a theory-driven approach, Ergonomics 55 (2012), 1487-1501.
[2]　F. Schmid, M.S. Goepfert, D. Kuhnt, et al., The wolf is crying in the operating room: patient monitor and anesthesia workstation alarming patterns during cardiac surgery, Anesthesia & Analgesia 112 (2011), 78-83.
[3]　ECRI INSTITUTE, Top 10 health technology hazards for 2013, Health Devices 41 (2012), 342-365.
[4]　M. Gorges, B.A. Markewitz, D.R. Westenskow, Improving alarm performance in the medical intensive care unit using delays and clinical context, Anesth Analg 108 (2009), 1546-1552.
[5]　AAMI FOUNDATION HTSI, Using Data to Drive Alarm System Improvement Efforts - The Johns Hopkins Hospital Experience 2012, http://www.premiersafetyinstitute.org/wp-content/uploads/Johns-Hopkins-White-Paper.pdf, Last Accessed: 23.3.17.
[6]　M. Imhoff and S. Kuhls, Alarm algorithms in critical care monitoring, Anesth Analg. 102 (2006), 1525-1537.
[7]　S. Siebig, S. Kuhls, M. Imhoff, et al., Intensive care unit alarms--how many do we need?, Crit Care Med 38 (2010), 451-456.
[8]　Association for the Advancement of Medical Instrumentation, A siren call for action, Summit Publications: Clinical Alarms, Arlington, VA, 2011, http://www.aami.org/publications/summits/2011_Alarms_Summit_publication.pdf, Last Accessed: 23.3.17.
[9]　K.C. Graham and M. Cvach, Monitor alarm fatigue: standardizing use of physiological monitors and decreasing nuisance alarms, Am J Crit Care 19 (2010), 28-34; quiz 35.

[10] C.W. Paine, V.V. Goel, et al., Systematic Review of Physiologic Monitor Alarm Characteristics and Pragmatic Interventions to Reduce Alarm Frequency, J Hosp Med 11 (2016), 136-144.

[11] K.J. Ruskin and D. Hueske-Kraus, Alarm fatigue: impacts on patient safety, Curr Opin Anaesthesiol 28 (2015), 685-690.

[12] ECRI INSTITUTE, Top 10 technology hazards for 2012. The risks that should be at the top of your prevention list, Health Devices 40 (2011), 358-373.

[13] S.T. Lawless, Crying wolf: false alarms in a pediatric intensive care unit, Critical care medicine 22 (1994), 981-985.

[14] L.L. Terry Fairbanks, et al., Citing reports of alarm-related deaths, the Joint Commission issues a sentinel event alert for hospitals to improve medical device alarm safety, ED Manag 26 (2013).

[15] M. Vockley, Plan, Do, Check, Act: Using Action Research to Manage Alarm Systems, Signals, and Responses, 2012, http://www.aami.org/htsi/SI_Series/Beth_Israel_2013.pdf, Last Accessed: 23.3.17.

[16] H. Arksey and L. O'Malley, Scoping studies: towards a methodological framework, International journal of social research methodology 8 (2005), 19-32.

[17] K.C. Wong, Using an Ishikawa diagram as a tool to assist memory and retrieval of relevant medical cases from the medical literature, Journal of medical case reports 5 (2011), 120.

[18] G. Montibeller and V. Belton, Causal maps and the evaluation of decision options—a review, Journal of the Operational Research Society 57 (2006), 779-791.

[19] AAMI Foundation, Clinical Alarm Management Compendium, 2015, http://www.aami.org/alarm_compendium.pdf, Last Accessed: 23.3.17.

[20] J.I. Westbrook, E. Coiera, W.T. Dunsmuir, et al., The impact of interruptions on clinical task completion, Qual Saf Health Care 19 (2010), 284-289.

[21] F.A. Drews, The frequency and impact of task interruptions in the ICU, Proceedings of the Human Factors and Ergonomics Society Annual Meeting, SAGE Publications, 2007, pp. 683-686.

[22] D. Del Dotto, Improving Telemetry Alarm Management at UMass Memorial Healthcare Center, Worcester Polytechnic Institute, 2013.

[23] J.G. Hofhuis, P.E. Spronk, H.F. van Stel, et al., Experiences of critically ill patients in the ICU, Intensive Crit Care Nurs 24 (2008), 300-313.

[24] R. Elliott, S. McKinley, P. Cistulli, M. Fien, Characterisation of sleep in intensive care using 24-hour polysomnography: an observational study, Crit Care 17 (2013), R46.

[25] J. Scott-Cawiezell, G.A. Pepper, R.W. Madsen, et al., Nursing home error and level of staff credentials, Clin Nurs Res 16 (2007), 72-78.

[26] J.I. Westbrook, A. Woods, M.I. Rob, et al., Association of interruptions with an increased risk and severity of medication administration errors, Arch Intern Med 170 (2010), 683-690.

[27] T.N. Wenham and D. Graham, Venous gas embolism: An unusual complication of laparoscopic cholecystectomy, J Minim Access Surg 5 (2009), 35-36.

[28] B. Van Rompaey, M.M. Elseviers, M.J. Schuurmans, et al., Risk factors for delirium in intensive care patients: a prospective cohort study, Crit Care 13 (2009), R77.

[29] E.M. Petersen and C.L. Costanzo, Assessment of Clinical Alarms Influencing Nurses' Perceptions of Alarm Fatigue, Dimens Crit Care Nurs 36 (2017), 36-44.

[30] J.S. Allen, K. Hileman, Simple Solutions for Improving Patient Safety In Cardiac Monitoring(2013).

[31] L. Varpio, C. Kuziemsky, C. MacDonald, W.J. King, The helpful or hindering effects of in-hospital patient monitor alarms on nurses: a qualitative analysis, Comput Inform Nurs 30 (2012), 210-217.

[32] L. Honan, M. Funk, M. Maynard, D. Fahs, J.T. Clark, Y. David, Nurses' Perspectives on Clinical Alarms, Am J Crit Care 24 (2015), 387-395.

[33] A. Rensen, M.M. van Mol, I. Menheere, et al., Quality of care in the intensive care unit from the perspective of patient's relatives: development and psychometric evaluation of the consumer quality index 'R-ICU', BMC Health Serv Res 17 (2017), 77.

[34] Drew BJ; Harris P; Zègre-Hemsey JK; et al.: Insights into the Problem of Alarm Fatigue with Physiologic Monitor Devices: A Comprehensive Observational Study of Consecutive Intensive Care Unit Patients. PLoS ONE 2014, 9(10), pp.

[35] Lu, Hong, Alison E. While, K. Louise Barriball. "Job satisfaction among nurses: a literature review." International journal of nursing studies 42.2 (2005): 211-227.

[36] B. Pikó Work-related stress among nurses: a challenge for health care institutions, Perspectives in Public Health, Vol 119, Issue 3, pp. 156 – 162.

[37] B.P. Bailey, J.A. Konstan: On the need for attention-aware systems: Measuring effects of interruption on task performance, error rate, and affective state. Comput Hum Behav (2006), 22(4), 685-708.

[38] Wenham T; Pittard A: Intensive care unit environment. 2009, 9(6), 178-183.

[39] Lacker C: Physiologic Alarm Management. Pa Patient Saf Advis 2011, 8(3), pp 105—8, http://patientsafetyauthority.org/ADVISORIES/AdvisoryLibrary/2011/sep8(3)/Pages/105.aspx

German Medical Data Sciences: Visions and Bridges
R. Röhrig et al. (Eds.)
© 2017 German Association for Medical Informatics, Biometry and Epidemiology (gmds) e.V. and IOS Press.
This article is published online with Open Access by IOS Press and distributed under the terms
of the Creative Commons Attribution Non-Commercial License 4.0 (CC BY-NC 4.0).
doi:10.3233/978-1-61499-808-2-112

IT Decision Making in German Hospitals – Do CEOs Open the Black Box?

Johannes THYE[a,1], Ursula HÜBNER[a], Jens HÜSERS[a] and Birgit BABITSCH[b]
[a] *Health Informatics Research Group, Hochschule Osnabrück, Germany*
[b] *Human Sciences, New Public Health, University Osnabrück, Germany*

Abstract. Health IT and communication systems are indispensable in German hospitals for clinical as well as administrative process support. However, IT is often regarded as a "black box" for hospital CEOs. Thus, the question arises how can CEOs decide if they do not know what is in the box? In order to answer this question, half-structured interviews with 14 German hospital CEOs were conducted. They revealed three principle decision processes: the supported decision, the joint decision and the corporate level decision. In all cases, the hospital CEO and the CIO interacted to reach the final decision, most strongly in the joint decision mode and least strongly in the corporate decision mode. Only the joint decision mode definitely forced the CEO to open the "black box" of IT. In the era of digitalisation, however, CEOs must develop better competencies to decide over complex matters.

Keywords. Chief executive officers, hospital, decision making, medical informatics

1. Introduction

Clinical processes in hospitals cannot be performed appropriately without the support of health IT [1-2]. Therefore, health IT is a matter of the boss, i.e. the chief executive officer (CEO) or top management team (TMT), which cannot be simply delegated. Ideally, CEOs or TMT work at eye level with the IT department, represented by the chief information officer (CIO)[2], to make decisions about IT investments. Nevertheless, IT is often regarded as "black box" by the CEO or TMT [2]. This could hold true for several reasons: Studies suggest that a considerable number of hospitals do not have enough IT staff. This underrepresentation of IT may lead the CEO or TMT to neglect IT issues. If IT is represented by a CIO and if, however, the CIO is not a member of the board of directors, IT topics are less discussed at board meetings and do not receive the same attention as other topics [3-6]. Furthermore, there is evidence that CEOs and CIOs may not share the same understanding of IT [3,7], that the TMT or CEO may underestimate the importance and the potential of IT or that misalignment between the hospital strategy and the IT strategy exists [3,8-9]. These circumstances can be interpreted as a symptom of CEOs and TMT members to treat IT as a "black box". Against this background, the question arises: How can decisions about hospital IT be made if the one who decides does not have the necessary insight? IT governance models offer behavioural archetypes: e.g. business monarchy, which required full understanding of IT matters, or IT monarchy,

---

[1] Corresponding Author, Johannes Thye, M.A., research fellow, Hochschule Osnabrück, Caprivistraße 30A, 49076 Osnabrück, Germany; E-mail: johannes.thye@hs-osnabrueck.de.

[2] We use the term CIO for all persons in a leading IT role irrespectively of their position as board member.

which goes along with full decision power of the CIO [8]. Also the model of a strategic CIO - CEO partnership [3] emphasises aspects like trust, position of the CIO in the TMT, shared IT vision as factors that could impact the process of decision making. The IT decision process in hospitals leads to a multiple-criteria and a multi-stakeholder approach, which requires the stakeholders to possess fundamental IT knowledge. In any case, the "black box" of hospital IT has to be opened in order to come to founded decisions, whoever makes these decisions in the end. In this study, the interaction or missing interaction of CEOs and CIOs should be analysed. The questions thus were:

- How can the IT decision making process be described and what kind of interactions exist between CEOs and CIOs in this process?
- What are factors associated with the decision making process?

This part of the study tries to answer these questions from the perspective of hospital CEOs, a perspective that has been often neglected. Therefore, a qualitative, hypothesis generating approach was chosen.

2. Methods

In order to answer these questions, half-structured interviews with German hospital CEOs were conducted to analyse the IT decision process in depth. A literature research on decision making and CEO - CIO communication was performed in common databases (ACM, SpringerLink, IEEE Xplore, PSYCINFO) to design the interview guideline. Keywords such as CEO, CIO, relationship, decision making, health IT and synonyms were combined to find relevant studies. The following topics were identified as major areas of interest: reporting structure and responsibility for deciding on major IT issues including the role of the CIO [5-7,9], IT governance and strategy [7-8,10] as well as the relationship with the CIO [3-4,7]. IT decision making in healthcare was found to be covered only poorly by the literature. As it can be assumed that hospitals as expert organisations, with their particular structures and groups of influential persons, form a particular environment of its own, results from studies outside healthcare cannot be transferred to hospitals one-on-one. To close potential knowledge gaps, qualitative interviews were chosen to explore the topic, thus to be able to address and discussed individual issues during the interview. According to the guideline developed, the interviews should start with demographic information (hospital: size, ownership, group, type, teaching status; interview partner: age, gender, education, graduation, position). Before touching the major part about the decision making process, the guideline planned a question about how important IT was for the interviewee. This opening question was meant to set the stage for the following questions on decision making, in particular: "Who decides about major IT events?", "How is this process initiated?" and "Is there any collaboration with the CIO?" and if yes "How do you collaborate with your CIO?". Further questions addressed groups who contributed ideas to the decision making process. Moreover, there were questions on factors affecting the decision making process. Finally, we provided room to add new important topics, which we had not covered before. All eight questions (without demographics) were open and included the option to add new aspects.

We balanced the persons invited to the interview, who originated from a convenience sample, according to hospital size, affiliation to a hospital group (system affiliation), ownership and teaching status. Additionally, we tried to include interview partners with different degrees and gender to maximise the variety in the sample. The guideline was sent to all participants prior to the interview. The recruiting process was stopped when all types of interviewees could be included and when the findings from the interviews saturated. The interviews were recorded and transcribed with MAXQDA 12. Data were analysed deductively based on main and subcategories derived from the literature and expert discussions. Furthermore, categories were inductively added during coding.

3. Results

A total of 14 interviews was conducted from 30th May to 11th October 2016, of which twelve were face-to-face interviews and two telephone interviews. The interviews lasted between 30 and 75 minutes.

Table 1: Hospital demographics

Ownership	Hospital size	System affiliation	Teaching status
Public [n=3]	Up to 299 beds [n=3]	Yes [n=7]	University hospital [n=1]
Private [n=3]	300 to 599 beds [n=7]	No [n=7]	Other teaching status [n=10]
Not-for-profit [n=8]	More than 600 beds [n=4]		No teaching hospital [n=3]

Participants were located in Lower Saxony [n=6], North Rhine Westphalia [n=5], Eastern [n=2] and Southern Germany [n=1]. The age of the participants was between 32 years and 56 years (mean 46 years, SD 7.26). Female [n=2] as well as male [n=12] interview partners were represented. All participants had an economic background, of which four had an additional degree in nursing and one in medicine.

According to all interviews, the decision making process was initiated by an idea that was stimulated in many cases by a new law or by the IT department and also by the clinicians or TMT, however, to a lesser degree. Three principle decision making processes were reported in the interviews (Figure 1a). In the first type of processes, the final decision was made by the hospital CEO who received advice and preparatory help from the CIO. Often an external consultancy firm was additionally involved. The process was accompanied by jour fixe meetings and dedicated project meetings. The second type embraced a joint decision process that resulted in collaborative decisions of the inter-professional team involved. The collaboration consisted of the CEO, the CIO and additionally end users, typically clinicians or their representatives. The final decision was collaborative and preceded by jour fixe meetings and if applicable by workshops. The third type of decision processes was characterised by the influence of the holding or any other parent corporation that made the final decision. As the interviewees reported, the CEOs, CIOs or regional CIOs from the group could occasionally impact these decisions depending on the individual CEOs or CIOs power and the group size or structure. In most of the cases, decisions made at corporate level had to be implemented: "We have a group strategy and as individual hospital we cannot deviate from it ..." [interview 9]. In 79% [n=11]) of the cases, either type one or type three held true, whereas a joint decision was made only in 21% [n=3] of the cases. As seen in decision types one and two, there was an interaction between CEO and CIO on a regular basis. Most of the organisations (86% [n=12]) had fixed weekly or biweekly meetings. A majority of the CIOs was integrated into the TMT meetings: 50% [n=7] of the CIOs on a permanent basis, 14% [n=2] at least on call. The other CIOs [n=5] meet the CEO only on a jour fixe, at project or informal meetings.

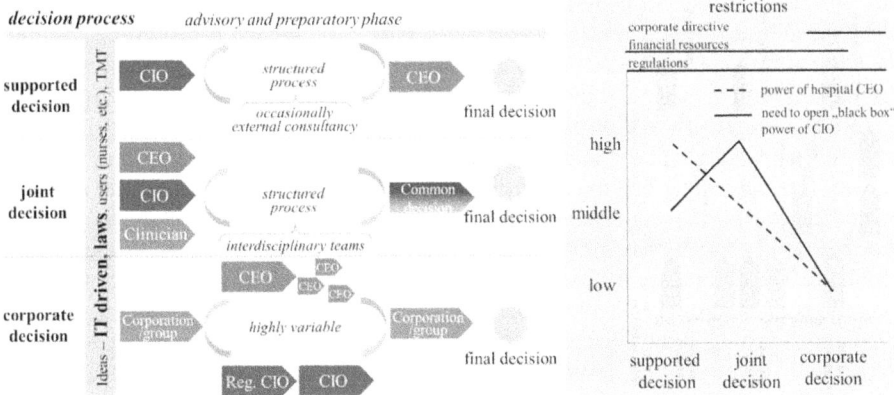

Figure 1a: IT decision making processes   **Figure 1b:** Hypotheses generated by this study

As the interview showed, the importance of IT was recognised by most CEOs. Statements like "without IT nothing works in our hospital" [interview 2] or "when IT collapses it is a disaster" [interview 14] underlined this notion. The interviewees reported that there existed an IT strategy, which was derived from the hospital or group strategy in most cases. Nevertheless, some hospitals reacted ad hoc when changes and resulting problems occurred. CEOs in this study mentioned "clinical process support", "user satisfaction" and "legal regulations" as most frequent reasons for implementing new IT systems or improving existing ones. According to the interviews, CEOs regarded financial resources [n=10], corporate guidelines [n=7] and laws [n=6] as most important circumstances restricting their freedom of decision. Two interviewees emphasised "trust between CEO and CIO" to be crucial because the information given by the CIO could not be verified by the CEO due to missing IT knowledge.

4. Discussion

We conducted qualitative interviews to investigate the decision making process in German hospitals in order to identify core mechanisms and attitudes. Qualitative interviews offer the advantage to add evolving questions and extend the guideline in an individual way if necessary. Previous studies, which had focused on business IT and the relationship between CEO and CIO, could only partly mark out the field. The interviews, which were conducted in a sample representing many different kinds of hospitals, revealed three types of processes how decisions about IT investments are made: the supported decision, the joint decision and the corporate level decision. The first type represents a case with the greatest power of the CEO who seeks help from the CIO but in the end decides herself/himself. The second type reflects a shared decision approach which allows other stakeholders, i.e. the CIO and the clinicians, to contribute at eye level. In this case, the hospital CEO still possesses power to shape the final decision. The last type, finally, is characterised by the weakest position of the CEO, who has to bow to the corporate directive. It is also the last type, where the hospital CEO does not have any need to open the "black box" of IT. The first type of decision making is ambiguous with regard to the "black box" as the CEO receives help from the CIO. In this case, the CEO either fully trusts the CIO, as the interviewees remarked, and does not open the "black box" or the CEO tries to understand what the CIO proposed and has to obtain at least some insight into what happens in the "black box". The second decision type requires the CEO to fully understand at a high level how IT works in order to be prepared for the discussions with the CIO and the clinicians. These considerations lead to the hypotheses as shown in Figure 1b. All decision types are obviously independent of the importance of IT for the CEO as all the interview partners unanimously emphasised how essential IT was. It is interesting that many participants in this study mentioned better IT support of clinical workflows and increased user satisfaction as ignition for the IT decision process. However, only the joint decision type seemed to be appropriate for solving these problems. The dominance of financial arguments over matters of the "black box", i.e. IT matters, is most strongly visible in the first decision type and we can assume that it is even more existing in the third type, when the decision is made at corporate level. CEOs in our study expressed the desire for more business thinking of the CIO, which reveals the wish for smoother discussions about financial issues. This qualitative study is mainly limited by its perspective that only covers the CEO's one. However, as CEOs are the main decision makers, as this study supported, their views are of paramount importance.

5. Conclusion

This study revealed three types of IT decision making. Only one of them definitely forces the CEO to open the "black box" of IT. In the era of digitalisation, however, CEOs must develop better competencies to decide over complex matters, such as IT.

6. Conflict of Interest

There are no competing interests.

References

[1] Kuperman G. Reflections on AMIA-looking to the future. J Am Med Inform Assoc **20** (2013), e367. http://dx.doi.org/10.1136/amiajnl-2013-002435

[2] Simon A. Die betriebswirtschaftliche Bewertung der IT-Performance im Krankenhaus am Beispiel eines Benchmarking-Projektes. In: Schlegel H, editor. Steuerung der IT im Klinikmanagement. Vieweg + Teubner Verlag, Wiesbaden, 2010. 73-90.

[3] Hütter A, Arnitz T, Riedl R. Die CIO/CEO-Partnerschaft als Schlüssel zum IT-Erfolg. HMD – Praxis der Wissenschaftsinformatik **50** (2013), 103-111. http://dx.doi.org/10.1007/BF03340858

[4] Feeny DF, Edwards BR, Simpson KM. Understanding the CEO / CIO Relationship. MIS Quarterly **16** (1992), 435-448. http://dx.doi.org/10.2307/249730

[5] Banker RD, Hu N, Pavlou PA, Luftman J. CIO Reporting Structure, Strategic Positioning and Firm Performance. MIS Quarterly **35** (2011), 487-504. http://dx.doi.org/10.2139/ssrn.1557874

[6] Moghaddasi H, Sheikhtaheri A. CEO is a Vision of the Future Role and Position of CIO in Healthcare Organizations. J Med Syst **34** (2010), 1121-1128. http://dx.doi.org/10.1007/s10916-009-9331-4

[7] Krotov V. Bridging the CIO-CEO gap: It takes two to tango. Business Horizons **58** (2015), 275-283. http://dx.doi.org/10.1016/j.bushor.2015.01.001

[8] Weill P, Ross JW. IT Governance. Harvard Business School Press, Boston, 2004.

[9] Köbler F, Fähling J, Leimeister JM, Krcmar H. How German Hospitals Govern IT – An Empirical Exploration. Proceedings of the 17th European Conference on Information Systems (ECIS); Verona, Italy (2009), 317. http://aisel.aisnet.org/ecis2009/317

[10] Johnson AM, Lederer AL. IS Strategy and IS Contribution: CEO and CIO Perspectives. Information Systems Management **30** (2013), 306-318. http://dx.doi.org/10.1080/10580530.2013.832962

German Medical Data Sciences: Visions and Bridges
R. Röhrig et al. (Eds.)
© *2017 German Association for Medical Informatics, Biometry and Epidemiology (gmds) e.V. and IOS Press.*
This article is published online with Open Access by IOS Press and distributed under the terms
of the Creative Commons Attribution Non-Commercial License 4.0 (CC BY-NC 4.0).
doi:10.3233/978-1-61499-808-2-117

Cognitive Performance of Users Is Affected by Electronic Handovers Depending on Role, Task and Human Factors

Mareike PRZYSUCHA[a,1], Daniel FLEMMING[b], Georg SCHULTE[a],
Ursula HÜBNER[a]

[a] *Health Informatics Research Group, University AS Osnabrück, Germany*
[b] *Katholische Stiftungsfachhochschule Munich, Germany*

Abstract. Patient handovers are cognitively demanding, crucial for information continuity and patient safety, but error prone. This study investigated the effect of an electronic handover tool, i.e. the handoverEHR, on the memory and care planning performance of nurse students (n=32) in a randomised, controlled cross-over design with the factors handover task and handover role. On a descriptive level, handover recipients could improve their memory performance with electronic support, handover givers their performance of writing care plans. Statistically meaningful differences occurred, however, only when the participants were givers. Without handover experience and with low fluency to word problems, givers performed badly in the most demanding of the handover tasks. Final recommendations, however, can only be made after replicating this study in a clinical setting with mixed groups.

Keywords. handover, electronic health record, memory, care planning, cognition

1. Introduction

Handovers are cognitively demanding [1], crucial for information continuity [2] and patient safety [3] but also prone to information corruption [4]. Although they form a specific clinical scenario of its own, they also share many elements with other clinical scenarios such as ward rounds and case conferences [5]. All these scenarios are challenging for information givers with regard to summarising the clinical case and presenting the information in a succinct manner as well as for information recipients with regard to understanding the clinical case and being able to make use of this information for patient care [5]. Handovers at the change of shifts are well-studied showing that handover performance depends on the handover experience [6] and on cognitive abilities to make clinical judgements [7]. Recalling the relevant patient information is one of the major prerequisites for making the right decisions and planning adequate clinical interventions [8]. As attention and perception precede any memory performance, the presentation of handover information becomes a vital factor as could be demonstrated by Hertzum and Simon [9], who installed wide screen monitors for use in handover situations. Based on these deliberations, an electronic health care record system for

---

[1] Corresponding Author, Ursula Hübner, Hochschule Osnabrück, Health Informatics Research Group, D-49009 Osnabrück, Germany; E-mail: u.huebner@hs-osnabrueck.de.

handovers, the handoverEHR, was developed, tested regarding usability and improved accordingly [10]. This study aims at investigating the effect of the handoverEHR on the memory and care planning performance of nurses depending on whether the information about the clinical case was presented in text form (list) or in graphical form (map). Furthermore, we were interested to study potential differences between handover givers and recipients and the effect of human factors that might function as confounding variables.

2. Methods

Study design. In order to achieve these objectives, a randomised controlled cross-over study was conducted, in which the following three experimental conditions were realised: a) handovers without any support (WITHOUT) (control group), b) handovers, in which the information was presented in lists that were generated by the handoverEHR (LIST), and c) handovers, which were supported by cognitive maps produced with the help of the handoverEHR (MAP), see Fig. 1. All study participants had to take part in all conditions both in the role of handover givers and as handover recipients. The participants were randomly allocated to one of the three experimental groups to start with. Thus these groups differed with regard to the sequencing of the experimental conditions in order to avoid a systematic timing effect. There was a wash-out phase of at least three months in between. The handover sessions took place in groups of four participants, who either handed over a patient (GIVER) or received the handover (RECIPIENT). As there were four patients to be handed over per experimental session, each of the group participants was a giver in one case and a recipient in the other three cases. The cases to be handed over were realistic and similar regarding the amount and complexity of information. This design, thus, entailed two factors with repeated measures, with handover task (WITHOUT, LIST and MAP) as first factor and handover role (GIVER and RECIPIENT) as second one.

Sample. A total of 32 study participants was recruited from a convenience sample of nursing students of the University of Applied Sciences Osnabrück in their third study year, who finished all three experimental phases. There were 23 females and 9 males with an average age of 22.04 ± 2.69 years and 2.87 ± 0.53 years of nursing experience.

Study protocol. All study participants answered a questionnaire with potentially confounding variables, i.e. age; experience in nursing (years), in handovers and in using an electronic patient record system; self-confidence, capability in handing over patients and fluency of writing care plans according to the nursing process. Participants in the LIST and MAP groups (Fig. 1) were given a one-hour introduction and training phase that included using lists, developing maps and presenting them on a 50" monitor. After each of the four handovers per session, the givers and the recipients wrote down the information items that they recalled. Furthermore, both givers and recipients developed a care plan for the incoming shift based on all information provided. The study took place in a lab environment to control for external factors.

Data analysis. In case of givers, items recalled were classified as correct, incorrect or missing with regard to the initial case description, in case of recipients, they were classified in comparison to what the givers actually said. The care plans of givers and recipients were compared to a gold standard care plan, which had been developed by a nursing expert (DF). In addition, the analysis of the recipients' care plans considered potential information deficits of the recipients due to missing handover information.

Similar to the items recalled, the items in the care plans were classified as correct, incorrect or everyday knowledge of nurses.

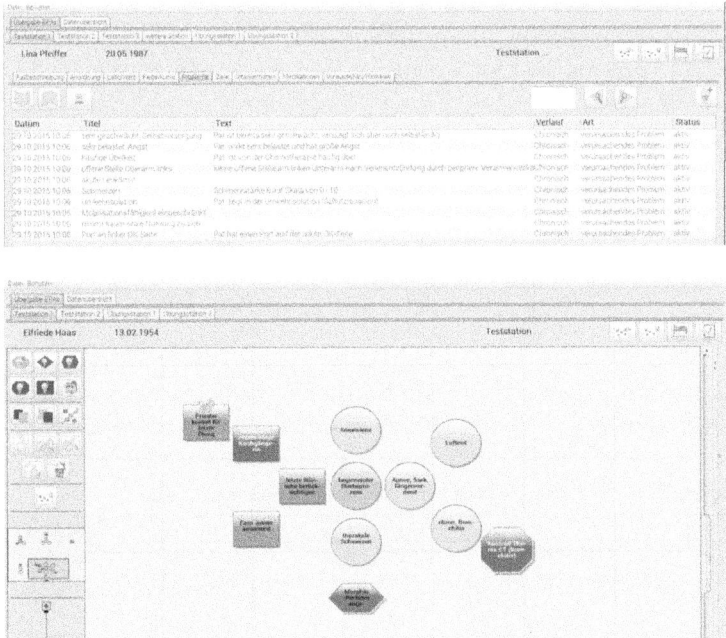

Figure 1: Screenshot LIST (above) and MAP (below). Circles denote problems and are associated with goals, interventions, medication and recommendations/advice [10]

As these classifications required expert knowledge, they were performed with the help of an independent nursing expert (GS). Data were analysed with the General Linear Model function integrated in SPSS Statistics Version 24. Alpha was set at 0.05.

3. Results

Memory. Table 1 shows the mean relative frequency of correctly recalled items for the two roles and the three experimental tasks. GIVERs received the overall best results when handing over information WITHOUT any help and the overall worst result when presenting the clinical cases as cognitive MAPs. In contrast, RECIPIENTs recalled items WITHOUT help much worse than GIVERs and increased their performance in the LIST and MAP condition compared to WITHOUT. This interaction between role and task was significant (F(2;62)=6.78, p=0.002), i.e. however, only GIVERs differed significantly (LIST vs. MAP and WITHOUT vs. MAP).

When differentiating between persons with handover experience (n=15) and no handover experience (n=17), the results revealed a significant interaction between handover type, role and experience (F(2;60)=3.31, p=0.043) as shown in Table 2. Again only GIVERs differed significantly, with experience between WITHOUT and LIST or MAP, without experience between LIST and MAP.

Table 1: Average percentage of correctly recalled items ± standard deviation ($n = 32$)

MEMORY		WITHOUT	LIST	MAP
Correct	GIVER	56% ± 18	50% ± 18	41% ± 18
items	RECIPIENT	46% ± 12	50% ± 11	49% ± 14

In most cases, persons without experience had lower values than those with experience (Tab. 2).

Table 2: Average percentage of correctly remembered items ± standard deviation ($n = 32$) for persons with handover experience, i.e. always or often (n=12) and no handover experience, i.e. seldom or never (n=17)

MEMORY	handover experience	WITHOUT	LIST	MAP
GIVER	yes	63% ± 20	44% ± 15	45% ± 16
	no	51% ± 17	54% ± 13	39% ± 20
RECIPIENT	yes	48% ± 9	52% ± 10	48% ± 14
	no	45% ± 15	48% ± 12	49% ± 15

Planning. There were no significant overall effects of the handover types, the handover role and their interaction on the relative number of correct planning items (Tab. 3).

Table 3: Average percentage of correctly planned items ± standard deviation ($n = 32$)

PLANNING		WITHOUT	LISTS	MAPS
Correct items	GIVER	89% ± 13	92% ± 11	89% ± 18
	RECIPIENT	88% ± 9	86% ± 17	85% ± 12

Breaking down these results for groups of persons who rated their own fluency to word potential problems as high (n=24) or low (n=8), showed a significant interaction between handover role and fluency ($F(1;30)=11.82$, $p=0.002$) and likewise a significant interaction between handover type, handover role and fluency ($F(2;60)=4.09$, $p=0.02$). A pairwise comparison revealed significantly higher values in the MAP condition for GIVERs with a high fluency than those with a low fluency.

Table 4: Average percentage of correctly planned items ± standard deviation ($n = 32$) for persons with high (n=24) and low fluency to word potential problems (n=8)

PLANNING	fluency	WITHOUT	LIST	MAP
GIVER	high	88% ± 14	92% ± 12	93% ± 12
	low	89% ± 11	93% ± 11	74% ± 27
RECIPIENT	high	88% ± 10	84% ± 12	84% ± 13
	low	92% ± 6	93% ± 6	89% ± 11

4. Discussion

This study investigated a) the influence of two types of electronic support on memory and care planning in handovers compared to no support and b) the influence of the handover role either as giver or recipient. The two types of electronic support differed with regard to the degree of novelty, complexity and visual support. The handover roles differed regarding the degree of using the handoverEHR actively.

The overall finding of this study was that the memory performance of GIVERs declined from the conditions WITHOUT, over LIST to MAP, while the performance of the RECIPIENTs nearly stayed the same. When planning, GIVERs benefited from the

MAP only when they were highly fluent wording potential problems. In the other case their performance deteriorated, which resulted in a significant difference in the MAP condition. This study included a homogeneous group of nurse students, which is both a strength (smaller variability) and a limitation (lower validity).

5. Conclusion

Analysed on a descriptive level, handover recipients can improve their memory performance with electronic support, handover givers their performance of writing care plans. Statistically meaningful differences occurred, however, only when the participants were GIVERs. Without handover experience and with low fluency to word problems, GIVERs performed badly in the MAP condition, the most demanding task. Final recommendations, however, can only be made after replicating this study in a clinical setting with age and experience mixed groups.

6. Conflict of Interest

The authors state that they have no conflict of interests.

Acknowledgment

This study was funded by the State of Lower Saxony Germany (grant: ZN 2819).

References

[1] M.D. Cohen, B. Hilligoss & A.C. Kajdacsy-Balla Amaral, A handoff is not a telegram: an understanding of the patient is co-constructed, *Critical Care (London, England)* **16**(1) (2012), 303.
[2] R. Randell, S. Wilson, P. Woodward, & J. Galliers, Beyond handover: supporting awareness for continuous coverage, *Cognition, Technology & Work* **12**(4) (2010), 271–283.
[3] L.J. Donaldson, S.S. Panesar & A. Darzi, Patient-Safety-Related Hospital Deaths in England: Thematic Analysis of Incidents Reported to a National Database, 2010–2012, *PLoS Medicine*, **11**(6) (2014).
[4] M.J.W. Thomas, T.J. Schultz, N. Hannaford & W.B. Runciman, Failures in Transition: Learning from Incidents Relating to Clinical Handover in Acute Care, *Journal for Healthcare Quality*, **35**(3) (2013), 49–56.
[5] C.E. Kuziemsky & L. Varpio, A model of awareness to enhance our understanding of interprofessional collaborative care delivery and health information system design to support it, *International journal of medical informatics*, **80**(8) (2011), e150–160.
[6] M.F. Rayo, A.F. Mount-Campbell, J.M. O'Brien, S.E. White, A. Butz, K. Evans & E.S. Patterson, Interactive questioning in critical care during handovers: a transcript analysis of communication behaviours by physicians, nurses and nurse practitioners, *BMJ Quality & Safety*, **23**(6) (2014), 483–489.
[7] B.W. Pickering, K. Hurley & B. Marsh, Identification of patient information corruption in the intensive care unit: using a scoring tool to direct quality improvements in handover, *Crit Care Med.* **37**(11) 2009, 2905-12.
[8] S.P. Marshall, Schemas in Problem Solving, *Cambridge University Press* (1995).
[9] M. Hertzum & J. Simonsen, Positive effects of electronic patient records on three clinical activities, *International Journal of Medical Informatics*, **77**(12) (2008), 809–817.
[10] D. Flemming, M. Przysucha, U. Hübner, Cognitive Maps to Visualise Clinical Cases in Handovers. Design, Implementation, Usability, and Attractiveness Testing, *Methods Inf Med*, **54**(5) (2015), 412–423.

German Medical Data Sciences: Visions and Bridges
R. Röhrig et al. (Eds.)
© *2017 German Association for Medical Informatics, Biometry and Epidemiology (gmds) e.V. and IOS Press.*
doi:10.3233/978-1-61499-808-2-122

Technical Environment for Developing the SNIK Ontology of Information Management in Hospitals

Konrad HÖFFNER[a,1], Franziska JAHN[a], Christian KÜCHERER[b], Barbara PAECH[b],
Birgit SCHNEIDER[a], Martin SCHÖBEL[a], Sebastian STÄUBERT[a] and Alfred
WINTER[a]

[a] *IMISE, University of Leipzig, Härtelstraße 16-18, 04107 Leipzig, Germany*
[b] *Software Engineering Group, Heidelberg University, Institute for Computer Science,*
Im Neuenheimer Feld 205, 69120 Heidelberg, Germany

Abstract. The SNIK project converts textbooks about information management in hospitals to a domain ontology that provides a shared vocabulary for institutions to model and integrate processes, data and infrastructure. To accommodate user groups with different requirements and technical backgrounds, and to support incremental and cooperative development, we create a system architecture to publish, visualize, browse and query the ontology, as well as to evaluate and improve the data quality.

Keywords. Health Information Management, Ontology, Hospital Information System

1. Introduction

1.1. Introduction

Knowledge about hospital information systems and their management (HIM) is mainly available through textbooks, articles, frameworks, standards and experts working in this field. In order to structure and formalize the HIM knowledge, we developed *SNIK* (German: *Semantisches Netz des Informationsmanagements im Krankenhaus*), an ontology that integrates terms, definitions and relations of strategic, tactical and operational information management, Information Technology (IT) service management and IT governance with a special focus on healthcare [1]. SNIK is manually extracted from HIM textbooks and is modelled as a *Resource Description Framework (RDF)* graph, which represents machine processable knowledge about arbitrary concepts in the form of *triples,* which specify binary relations between resources. An *RDF resource* is uniquely represented by a *Uniform Resource Identifier (URI)* and can be an individual, a property (relation) or a class (set of individuals). Each triple has the form "(subject, property, object)". For example, we encode the sentence "Activity diagrams are part of UML." as the triple (ActivityDiagram, subClassOf, UmlDiagram). As the SNIK ontology relates to abstract textbook knowledge and not to any concrete hospital, SNIK does not contain individuals. SNIK consists of 1936 classes, 63 properties and 63916

---

[1]Corresponding Author, E-mail: konrad.hoeffner@imise.uni-leipzig.de.

triples in version 0.3.3. We used SNIK in teaching to help health informatics students acquire and practice the terminology of HIM [2]. SNIK also can be used for requirements engineering and software development [15]. In the following, we present the requirements, concept and implementation of the SNIK system architecture to provide quality assurance, visualizations and services for querying and browsing the ontology.

1.2. Requirements

Different technical challenges have to be considered when providing a complex ontology for user groups with different backgrounds, but also during its incremental and cooperative development: (1) Convert manually created extraction tables to an RDF ontology. (2) Integrate a new subontology into SNIK. (3) Enable users to interact with the ontology without installing specialized tools. (4) Assure the quality of the ontology.

2. State of the art

The system architecture of SNIK is inspired by successful Semantic Web projects: DBpedia [3] is the RDF conversion of Wikipedia. Due to its size and generality, there is a large amount of interlinks to DBpedia, making it a central part of the Semantic Web. Besides millions of instances, DBpedia also contains a handcrafted ontology. The data is available over a SPARQL[2] endpoint, an RDF browser and as RDF dumps. Healthcare science also has a prominent [14] status in the Semantic Web with transformations of databases such as PubMed [4], Drugbank [5] and SIDER [6].

3. Concept

We fulfill the requirements listed in section 1.2 by introducing a system architecture that consists of established libraries, Semantic Web tools, and development platforms. We thus also provide a blueprint for developers and maintainers of other large ontologies. In particular, (1) to enable RDF conversion, we configure a CSV to RDF conversion tool and (2) we use a link discovery framework to integrate new subontologies into SNIK. (3) A *graph-based visualization* gives an overview and emphasizes relations, while an *RDF browser* provides details about particular resources. A *SPARQL endpoint* answers formal queries and enables the usage and development of other tools and services. (4) To ensure a high data quality, quality management determines objective quality criteria that are used both to compute quality scores and to find offending triples.

---

[2] Recursive Acronym for *SPARQL Protocol and RDF Query Language*

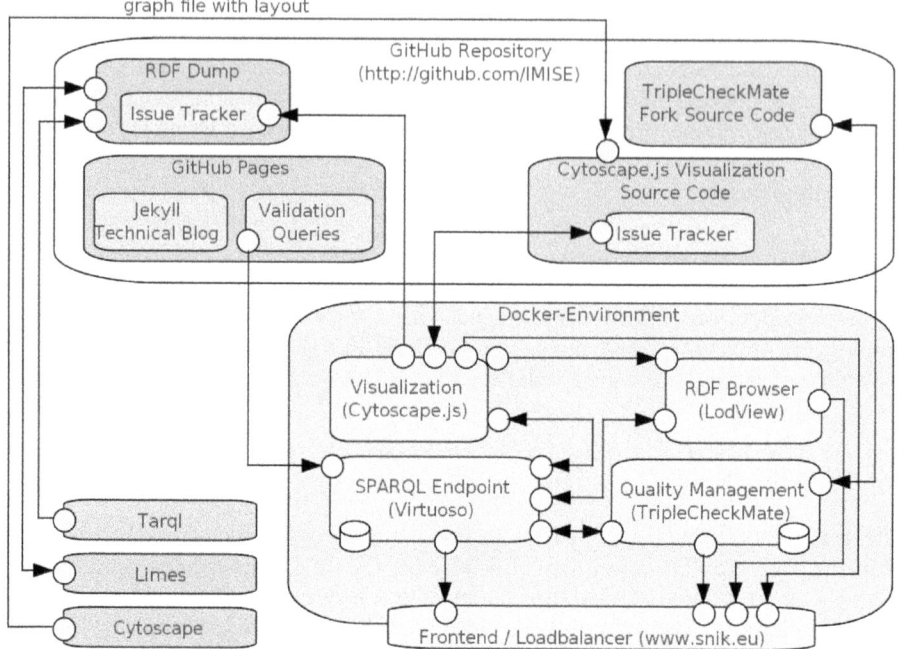

Figure 1. SNIK system architecture 3LGM² model [12]. Rounded rectangles depict application components, arrows pointing from circle to circle illustrate communication over interfaces. For initial setup, all application components are involved, but violet components have to run once. The green components are running at normal operation. To perform an update, the blue components are active and also the green components are affected.

4. Implementation

The components of the SNIK system architecture and their relations are shown in Figure 1. The applications are provided as Docker containers if possible to ease setup, deployment and portability. First, the knowledge extracted from information management textbooks to tabular data by domain experts needs to be converted to RDF. To set up a new subontology, we convert the tables using *Tarql*[3] with a mapping configuration file[4]. On update, we upload the serialized RDF to our public *Git repository* and *SPARQL endpoint*[5]. We serialize the ontology from the endpoint to a table, which we import and layout in Cytoscape, and then move to the visualization repository. We publish subsequent releases both periodically, after the initial release accompanying the quality assurance efforts, and also when significant user feedback is accumulated through the issue tracker and implemented. After quality control according to quality criteria defined in [7], we also create link candidates between the subontologies using *LIMES*, the *Link Discovery Framework for Metric Spaces* [8] with the *RDF dump* and a mapping configuration. A high confidence mapping consists of all class pairs that have a label in common. A lower confidence mapping consists of all class pairs having a label pair with

---

[3] http://tarql.github.io
[4] https://github.com/IMISE/snik-csv2rdf
[5] OpenLink Virtuoso 7.20.3217, supports SPARQL 1.1

trigram similarity of 0.8 or higher. Both mappings are manually verified where unrelated pairs are discarded. The remaining ones are categorized using relations from the Simple Knowledge Organization System (SKOS) [9]. Non-ontologists interact with the ontology over the RDF browser and the visualization. The browser queries the SPARQL endpoint to resolve the URI of a resource[6] to a HTML page with properties of the resource and links to others. A machine-processable RDF description of a single resource is available as well. It is implemented as a fork of LodView[7] with minor modifications.

The visualization is based on the Cytoscape.js library, a JavaScript version of Cytoscape [10]. The library shows the ontology as a graph and calculates the shortest paths between classes. For teaching, we created the "spiderworm", which combines the shortest path between two classes with all connected nodes of the target class [2]. Additional custom functionality includes a search using exact string matching with the class labels from the SPARQL endpoint, a collection of filters to simplify the graph, and access to the RDF browser description of a class. Modelling errors can be reported to the RDF dump issue tracker by sending the user to a pre-filled issue template. Users can also report visualization problems itself through the issue tracker of the visualization.

While the issue tracker mostly handles issues that are incidentally noticed, we also offer a TripleCheckMate [11] instance for dedicated quality control of specific or randomly chosen classes queried from the SPARQL endpoint. TripleCheckMate was originally developed to evaluate the data quality of DBpedia instances, but it is configurable enough that we could adapt a fork with small changes to our ontology and to evaluate classes instead of instances. Evaluation results are saved in a SQL database. Domain and range statements as well as Web Ontology Language (OWL) restrictions are also automatically verified using SPARQL queries.

5. Lessons learned

Developing a JavaScript visualization based on Cytoscape.js instead of using the Cytoscape desktop application allowed us to have custom functionality with little development time, easy deployment and updates, and no installation requirement. Using Tarql with custom mapping configuration files saved us considerable costs for software development, adaption and maintenance compared to a self-developed solution. Trough hosting our code bases and ontologies on GitHub, we take advantage of public access, history, simultaneous editing, releases, issue trackers, and outside code patch suggestions. Collecting data quality issues automatically through SPARQL queries, from dedicated manual fact checking over TripleCheckMate, and from incidental observations over the issue tracker connection in the visualization, maximizes data quality improvements.

6. Conclusion

With the help of Semantic Web technologies and Docker, we developed a modular and flexible architectural environment to deal with a growing ontology. Users benefit from easy access over a multi-view web interface and different possibilities to interact with the ontology and to jointly improve its quality. Nevertheless, for using the provided

---

[6]such as http://www.snik.eu/ontology/meta/Top
[7] http://lodview.it/

features and maintaining the ontology, active users are needed. Therefore, we have to promote the SNIK ontology on data portals and social media for it to be actively used by medical informatics students, lecturers and software developers.

7. Conflict of Interest

The authors state that they have no conflict of interests.

8. References

[1]   Schaaf M, Jahn F, Tahar K, Kücherer C, Winter A, Paech B. Entwicklung und Einsatz einer Domänenontologie des Informationsmanagements im Krankenhaus. In: INFORMATIK 2015 Lecture Notes in Informatics (LNI). Bonn: Gesellschaft für Informatik e.V. (GI); 2015. p. 753–65.

[2]   Jahn F, Schaaf M, Kahmann C, Tahar K, Kücherer C, Paech B et al. An Ontology-Based Scenario for Teaching the Management of Health Information Systems. In: Exploring Complexity in Health: An Interdisciplinary Systems Approach: Proceedings of MIE2016 at HEC2016. Amsterdam: IOS Press; 2016. p. 359–63 (Stud Health Technol Inform; vol. 228).

[3]   Bizer C, Lehmann J, Kobilarov G, Auer S, Becker C, Cyganiak R and Hellmann S. DBpedia - A crystallization point for the Web of Data. *Web Semantics: Science, Services and Agents on the World Wide Web. Amsterdam: Elsevier Science Publishers B. V.* 7 154–65; 2009

[4]   Roberts R J. PubMed Central: The GenBank of the published literature. In: *Proceedings of the National Academy of Sciences of the United States of America* 98 381–2; 2001

[5]   Law V, Craig K, Djoumbou Y, Jewison T, Guo A C *et al.* DrugBank 4.0: Shedding New Light on Drug Metabolism. *Nucleic acids research* 42 D1091-7; 2014

[6]   Kuhn M, Letunic I, Jensen L J and Bork P. The SIDER database of drugs and side effects. *Nucleic acids research* 44 D1075-9; 10.1093/nar/gkv1075; 2016

[7]   Zaveri A, Rula A, et al. Quality assessment for Linked Data: A Survey. *Semantic Web* 1 1–5; 2012

[8]   Ngomo A-C N and Auer S 2011 LIMES - A Time-Efficient Approach for Large-Scale Link Discovery on the Web of Data *IJCAI-11: In: Proceedings of the twenty-second international joint conference on artificial intelligence.* Menlo Park: AAAI Press; *2011.* pp 2312–7

[9]   Miles A. SKOS: Requirements for Standardization. In: *Proceedings of the 2006 International Conference on Dublin Core and Metadata Applications*; 2006. pp 55–64

[10]   Schaaf M, Jahn F, Tahar K, Kücherer C, Winter A, Paech B. Visualization of Large Ontologies in University Education from a Tool Point of View. In: Exploring Complexity in Health: An Interdisciplinary Systems Approach: Proceedings of MIE2016 at HEC2016. Amsterdam: IOS Press; 2016. p. 349–53 (Stud Health Technol Inform; vol. 228).

[11]   Kontokostas D et al. TripleCheckMate: A Tool for Crowdsourcing the Quality Assessment of Linked Data. *Knowledge Engineering and the Semantic Web.* Berlin Heidelberg: Springer; 2013.

[12]   Winter A, Brigl B, Wendt T. Modeling Hospital Information Systems (Part 1): The Revised Three-Layer Graph-Based Meta Model 3LGM^2. Methods Inf Med 2003; 42(5):544–51.

[13]   Merkel D. Docker: Lightweight Linux Containers for Consistent Development and Deployment. Linux Journal. Houston: Belltown Media; 2014 (vol. 239), 2.

[14]   Cheung K, Prud'hommeaux E, Wang Y, Stephens S. Semantic Web for Health Care and Life Sciences: A Review of the State of the Art. : 111-113. Brief Bioinform; 2009. 10 (2): pp 111–113.

[15]   Kücherer, C. Use of Domain Ontologies to Improve Requirements Quality. In: Requirements Engineering: Foundation for Software Quality. Berlin Heidelberg: Springer; 2017.

German Medical Data Sciences: Visions and Bridges
R. Röhrig et al. (Eds.)

doi:10.3233/978-1-61499-808-2-127

Factors Influencing the Implementation and Distribution of Clinical Decision Support Systems (CDSS)

Benjamin R. KUX [a,1], Raphael W. MAJEED [a,b],
Janko AHLBRANDT [a,c] and Rainer RÖHRIG [a,b]

[a] *Justus-Liebig-University Giessen, Germany*
[b] *Carl von Ossietzky University Oldenburg, Germany*
[c] *Ruprecht-Karls University Heidelberg, Germany*

Abstract. Clinical Decision Support Systems (CDSS) can have positive effects on quality of care measures, yet have not gained widespread traction in healthcare. This study sought to determine and evaluate barriers and facilitators to CDSS implementation and distribution. Based on 768 systems identified in a literature review we conducted semi-structured telephone interviews with 54 system developers in 16 countries. Qualitative analysis led to the identification of 66 key factors influencing implementation. Central issues evolved around CDSS properties, quality and integration, as well as usability, user related factors, internal marketing, resource issues and collaborations with emphasis partly on topics differing from existing research. Additionally, evidence pointed to regional differences regarding implementation hurdles. Recent regulatory requirements were deemed less of a barrier to system adoption than expected, even though lacking expertise in this area was surprisingly common among interview partners.

Keywords. Clinical Decision Support Systems, Health Information Systems, Barrier, Medical Devices, Medical Device Legislations

1. Introduction

The growing complexity of medical care contributes to a high number of preventable adverse events in patient care worldwide [1]. Great efforts have been made in recent years, with varying success, to improve patient safety and promote evidence based medicine [2]. Computer systems that assist with clinical decision making (CDSS) have repeatedly proven their ability to have a positive impact on quality of care measures [3]. Governments and legislators in various countries strive to advance the use of CDSS. Yet as of today these systems have failed to gain widespread traction in healthcare [4].

A large body of literature exists that cites hurdles and facilitators for the implementation of Health Information Technology (HIT) and specifically CDSS. These include various models for the adoption of new technologies [5], systematic reviews of case reports [6], Delphi studies [7] and other surveys of experts [8], as well as field work [9] and user surveys [10]. Limitations of current research include a strong focus on Anglo-American studies [11] in a domain that is very much influenced by cultural

---

[1] Corresponding Author: Benjamin.R.Kux@med.uni-giessen.de.

factors, methodical inadequacies of many systematic reviews [11] and a general pronounced fragmentation in this field of research [12]. Additionally, the impact of potential implementation barriers like recent regulatory requirements regarding the classification of software as a medical device, have not been studied systematically. This study therefore sought to identify and evaluate obstacles and facilitators to the implementation and distribution of CDSS in a comprehensive multinational study.

2. Methods

We conducted semi-structured telephone interviews with CDSS developers, who have published papers on their systems between 2002 and 2012. Potential interview partners were identified using a Medline search based on proven search strategies. 768 CDSS were identified after reviewing more than 70,000 titles. Owing to language barriers, we focused on developers situated in Europe and North America. 150 potential interview partners were contacted via E-Mail. Acknowledging the aforementioned dominance of Anglo-American studies on CDSS implementation hurdles, 120 (80%) of the contacted developers were based in Europe. Researchers in both regions were selected randomly.

Interviewees were queried on their CDSS implementation experiences and factors aiding or hindering that process using open questions (Table 1). Additionally, we collected data on three often-cited barriers, namely requirements imposed by legislators, issues regarding knowledge management, as well as challenges concerning lacking standards for sharing CDSS content. Developers were also questioned on the current implementation status of their projects, resources consumed by the development, their role in the development process and their professional background. Interviews were conducted in either German or English. All interviews were fully transcribed. For evaluation, we resorted to qualitative methods developed by Mayring [13], which combine both deductive techniques and practices rooted in grounded theory.

3. Results

3.1. Response Rate and Descriptive Statistics

136 out of 150 (90%) E-Mails reached their recipients. 63 (46%) developers replied to our invitation for an interview. In total 54 interviews were conducted between August and December 2014. The average interview time amounted to 16 minutes. Nine experts replied late (3), deemed themselves non-specialists (2) or were not able to find time for an interview (4). Interviews were conducted with experts from 16 different countries, with the majority based in Germany (13), the Netherlands (7), the US (7), Italy (6) and Canada (6). 42 (78%) of the interview partners were male. Most experts possess either a medical degree (28) or work as computer scientists (16). On average, the developers looked back on 22 years of working experience and 17 years of experience with HIT. A vast majority of the developed CDSS were knowledge-based systems (48 or 89%). The sample included CDSS that provided guidance in therapeutic decisions (24 or 44%), drug prescription (13 or 24%), diagnosis (13 or 24%) and prevention (3 or 6%) in a variety of different medical specialties. The majority of CDSS was developed or deployed in teaching hospitals (36 or 67%). 21 (39%) of all systems were integrated with existing HIT. 54% of the selected systems (29) required data input by medical personal.

7 (13%) of the CDSS generated actionable output. 19 (35%) of the systems had undergone evaluation. The implementation rate amounted to 50% at the time of the respective CDSS publications (27) and had dropped to 41% at the time of the interviews (22) with eight new installations and 13 out of 27 systems that had ceased operation. 19 (35%) of the developers had plans to implement their system again in the future.

3.2. Qualitative Analysis

Table 1 aggregates the main factors influencing CDSS implementation and distribution according to the interviewed developers. The cited barriers and facilitators to implementation were pooled, as a majority perceived these to be two sides of a coin.

Table 1. Factors with an influence on successful CDSS implementation

Category	Influencing Factor
System (83*)	Quality (16), properties (15), workflow integration (12), usability (12), EMR integration (8), transparency (7), maintenance (3), availability (3), updates (2), security (2), scalability (2), performance (1)
User (46)	Time (9), project involvement (9), motivation (5) , relevance (5), loss of influence & control (4), output acceptance (3), IT know-how (2), job security (2), information overload (2), resistance to change (1), incentives (1), expectations (1), utility (1), general acceptance (1)
Management/ decision makers (26)	Internal marketing (16), organization (3), external marketing (3), HR planning (1), economic benefit (1), hierarchies (1), implementation (1)
External partners (13)	Collaboration (10), external funds (1), investors (1), marketing (1)
Resources (13)	Funding (10), data (1), know how (1), human resources (1)
Politics/Legal framework (13)	Regulation (8), funding (3), liability (1), patents (1)
Existing IT (12)	Performance (3), data availability (3), interfaces (2), standards (2), standards regarding data structures (1), general conditions (1)
Scientific community (11)	Evaluation (5), grants (3), publications (2), guideline development (1)
Project team (10)	Interdisciplinarity (5), training (3), preferences (2)
Public (4)	NGOs (2), patients (2)
Competition (1)	Collaborations (1)

* Number of supporting statements

Looking at regional differences in adoption barriers, management related factors are quoted more often by developers in the US than in Western Europe. Here, system related aspects like quality and CDSS properties are deemed relatively more important. Furthermore, regulatory aspects are mentioned solely by interviewees from Northern and Western Europe. A specific inquiry into this topical issue reveals that only 33% of the developers see regulation as a barrier for the implementation of their system with a larger number acknowledging a challenge for CDSS adoption in general. 30% of the queried experts could not comment on the issue, as they were not familiar with current regulatory practice. Reasons for not being personally affected by regulation included CDSS developments before the passing of current legislation (6), systems that allegedly do not meet the definition of a medical device (6), CDSS that are still in a development stage (5) and missing relevant national laws (1). In the EU, software has to be certified as an active medical device, if the developer intends its use for the diagnosis, therapy, prevention or monitoring of diseases. Nonetheless, only 5% of the sampled systems have received certification. 85% of the interviewees have no plans to this end. Another often-mentioned barrier to long-term implementation is the maintenance of the CDSS knowledge base. However, 69% of the developers do not perceive this as a problem. They cite CDSS in small and static domains, along with maintenance work as part of the general internal guideline development process in hospitals as reasons.

4. Discussion

As part of this survey a wide range of factors influencing successful CDSS implementation were identified. Low adoption rates among interviewees show the need for detailed knowledge regarding CDSS adoption challenges. System quality is seen as one of the key elements for effective implementation. On that score, it became apparent that frequently the depiction of complex medical decision processes still presents a major challenge for developers. Common over-alerting and the realization that CDSS can potentially also do harm, add to the picture of a domain that still has to overcome substantial challenges. System properties are deemed almost equally important for successful adoption. In this regard, conflicting goals exist between small and simple CDSS in clearly defined domains that are easy to develop and maintain and the user demand for complex integrated solutions. The inadequate focus on the respective target groups by developers stands in close connection to calls for early user involvement in the CDSS development process. In this context, the interview partners see usability, transparency and time investment by the client as the key factors for user acceptance of the system. Many developers described barriers within the organization and the considerable resources needed to convince decision makers of a CDSS project. This is aggravated by the fact that these are often not one time investments by the developers, but rather part of a constant effort, where the raison d'être of a system has to be constantly explained and demonstrated in a dynamic organization. The majority of the interviewees develop CDSS in a university setting. In this context, collaboration with industry partners is often vital for implementation and distribution due to monetary constraints and limited legal and marketing expertise. Especially European scientists point out that system distribution and migration regularly exceeds both the resources and the goals of university research groups. This problem is somewhat less pronounced in the US, where CDSS development often occurs within health maintenance organization that migrate systems into their own clinics. Higher implementation rates in the US fit into this picture. Regulatory issues are among the most frequently cited implementation factors, though they are actively mentioned only by European developers, which can in part be attributed to currently unclear regulation intents by the FDA in the US. Overall, low concern about regulatory issues comes as a surprise given the potential consequences of a classification of software as a medical device, but can partly be explained by low overall adoption rates and plans for implementation.

Strengths of this study include its wide scope with interview partners from more than a dozen countries with often significant differences with regard to cultural and socioeconomic factors and the design of their healthcare systems. The sample was drawn from a comprehensive literature review. Despite a satisfactory response rate of 40%, a non-response-bias is likely. The qualitative methods used for data classification are highly formalized and allow for a standardized treatment of the data. At the same time the transfer of complex information into a rigid system of categories may have led to a loss in both meaning and context. Similarly, when conversing with non-native speakers, language barriers could have produced suboptimal data. Compared to existing literature, this study in part emphasizes different aspects with regard to CDSS implementation hurdles, for the first time adding the unique perspective of system developers in an international survey. Spreckelsen et al. report similar barriers, albeit with emphasis on user related and technical issues. [13] Paré et al. focus more on usability and project-based aspects compared to this study. [14] Partly differing barriers were also identified by Ash et al. [9], Moxey et al. [6] and Brenders et al. [7] The cited differences may in part be explained by input from experts with different backgrounds, a change in implementation barriers over time, regional differences with regard to adoption factors, a focus on different HIT, as well as differing qualitative methods.

5. Conclusion

Successful CDSS implementation depends on a wide variety of complex factors with potentially relevant regional differences. Surprisingly, regulatory aspects as a potential key barrier to the uptake of CDSS are currently not given much consideration by many developers. In light of the forthcoming profound changes in the EU with the planned passing of the Medical Device Regulation in 2017, European CDSS projects are likely going to face additional implementation challenges in the future.

6. Conflict of Interest

The authors state that they have no conflict of interests. The data is part of the doctoral thesis of BRK.

References

[1] James, JT, A New, Evidence-based Estimate of Patient Harms Associated with Hospital Care, *Journal of patient safety* 9 (2013), 122–128.
[2] Clancy, CM, Ten years after To Err is Human, *Am J Med Qual* 24 (2009), 525–528.
[3] Jaspers, MWM; Smeulers, M et al., Effects of clinical decision-support systems on practitioner performance and patient outcomes, *JAMIA* 18 (2011), 327–334.
[4] Wu, HW; Davis, PK et al., Advancing clinical decision support using lessons from outside of healthcare: an interdisciplinary systematic review, *BMC Med Inform Decis Mak* 12(2012), 90-99.
[5] Ammenwerth, E; Iller, C et al., IT-adoption and the interaction of task, technology and individuals: a fit framework and a case study, *BMC Med Inform Decis Mak* 6 (2006), 3-15.
[6] Moxey, A; Robertson, J et al., Computerized clinical decision support for prescribing: provision does not guarantee uptake, *JAMIA* 17(2010), 25–33.
[7] Brender, J.; Ammenwerth, E et al., Factors influencing success and failure of health informatics systems--a pilot Delphi study, *Methods Inf. Med* 45 (2006), 125–136.
[8] Jenders, RA; Osheroff, JA et al., Recommendations for clinical decision support deployment: synthesis of a roundtable of medical directors of information systems, *MIA Annu Symp Proc* (2007), 359–363.
[9] Ash, JS; Sittig, DF et al., Multiple perspectives on clinical decision support: a qualitative study of fifteen clinical and vendor organizations. *BMC Med Inform Decis Mak* 1 (2015): 35-46.
[10] Patterson, ES; Doebbeling, BN et al.,Identifying barriers to the effective use of clinical reminders: bootstrapping multiple methods, *J Biomed Inform* 38 (2005), 189–199.
[11] Mair, FS; May, C et al., Factors that promote or inhibit the implementation of e-health systems: an explanatory systematic review, *Bull World Health Organ* 90 (2012), 357–364.
[12] Bagozzi, RP, The Legacy of the Technology Acceptance Model and a Proposal for a Paradigm Shift, *J. Assoc. Inf. Syst.* 8 (2007), 244–254.
[13] Spreckelsen, C; Spitzer, K et al., Present situation and prospect of medical knowledge based systems in German-speaking countries: results of an online survey, *Methods Inf. Med.* 51 (2012), 281–294.
[14] Pare, G; Sicotte, C et al., Prioritizing the risk factors influencing the success of clinical information system projects. A Delphi study in Canada, *Methods Inf. Med.* 47 (2008), 251–259.

German Medical Data Sciences: Visions and Bridges
R. Röhrig et al. (Eds.)

doi:10.3233/978-1-61499-808-2-132

Disseminating a Standard for Medical Records in Emergency Departments Among Different Software Vendors Using HL7 CDA

Dominik BRAMMEN[a,b,1]; Heike DEWENTER[c], Volker THIEMANN[d],
Raphael W MAJEED[d], Tingyan XU[d], Kai U HEITMANN[e], Felix WALCHER[a], Sylvia
THUN[c], Rainer RÖHRIG[d]

[a] *Department of Trauma Surgery, Otto-von-Guericke-University Magdeburg, Germany*
[b] *Department of Anesthesiology, Otto-von-Guericke-University Magdeburg, Germany*
[c] *Hochschule Niederrhein, University of Applied Sciences, Krefeld, Germany*
[d] *Department of Medical Informatics, Carl von Ossietzky University Oldenburg,
Germany*
[e] *Heitmann Consulting and Services e.K., Hürth*

Abstract. A standardized medical record for the emergency department (GEDMR) was released in Germany, but only sparsely and randomly implemented by emergency department (ED) electronic health record (EHR) vendors. A reason for this may be a lacking common language between the medical and the Health Information Technology (HIT) domain. HL7 clinical document architecture (CDA) may leverage this communication gap. This paper reports on the effects of a professional medical association record standard on EHR vendors and the German ED-EHR market. Standard records and data standards are developed and published by different institutions either on governmental, healthcare agency or medical association level. There are some standard records, especially by US cardiology associations, transformed into HL7 C-CDA. GEDMR was modeled as HL7 CDA with the use of interoperable terminologies like LOINC and SNOMED CT. Being part of an emergency department data registry development project, local deployment at 15 project hospitals receiving sufficient funding was performed. Two major ED-EHR vendors adapted GEDMR within their product including CDA export. 106,868 CDAs were produced in six hospitals until now. Four local implementations with four different ED-EHRs were developed, producing 42,256 CDAs. Five additional vendors are adapting or developing an ED-EHR. The GEDMR-CDA implementation guide with funding for implementation in project hospitals had a significant impact on the German ED-EHR market. Within two years after release, a broadening and increasingly self-enforcing support by German ED-EHR vendors is notable.

Keywords. Medical Records; Health Level Seven/Standards; Electronic Health Records; Emergency Medicine, Emergency Department

---

[1] Corresponding author, Otto-von-Guericke-University Magdeburg, Department of Anesthesiology, Leipziger Str. 44, 39120 Magdeburg, Germany; E-mail: dominik.brammen@med.ovgu.de

1. Introduction

1.1. Introduction

Special data sets and pro formas for different medical specialties including emergency medicine are published by professional associations [1] or governmental authorities [2]. Even if emergency department (ED) data standards are defined by standardization organizations like Health Level 7 (HL7) [3], the implementation by electronic health record (EHR) vendors is fragmentary. This is especially true for Germany. Although the professional association for Emergency Medicine in Germany, the "German Interdisciplinary Association of Critical Care and Emergency Medicine" (DIVI), did release a standard record in 2010 called German Emergency Department Medical Record (GEDMR) [4] defining data standards and structure in six modules, only parts of the standard were implemented randomly by EHR vendors or individual implementations were established in single hospitals. A reason for this may be a lacking common language between the medical and the Health Information Technology (HIT) domain. HL7 Clinical Document Architecture (CDA) has the ability to represent professional association recommendations [5] leveraging this communication gap.

With the public funded research project "Improvement of Health Care Research in Emergency Medicine in Germany through Development of a National Emergency Department Registry" a HL7 CDA of the GEDMR was considered as the central interface between different ED-EHRs in multiple project hospitals and the data registry allowing timely data access with minimal barriers [6]. In a first project step, a CDA specification for the basic module of the GEDMR applicable to all ED patients was developed. Structured data was modelled in a machine-processable way (CDA Level 3) allowing for automatic secondary use of recorded data.

1.2. Requirements

After balloting, the guide should be adopted by different ED-EHR vendors thus developing a GEDMR compatible software version with CDA export capabilities. We report on the impact of a HL7 CDA version of a professional medical association record standard on ED-EHR vendors and the ED-EHR market in Germany.

2. State of the art

There are many ways, how standard records and data standards for EDs can be developed. Either, they are derived from national professional associations [7] or interdisciplinary and interprofessional institutions on a governmental or healthcare agency level [8], sometimes even by standards development organizations like HL7 [9]. Often, data sets for special emergency medicine related diseases are published by involved professional associations [10].

In Germany, the requirement for an ED standard record and data standard was first assumed by a working committee to the medical professional association DIVI in 2010 [4,11]. Finally, the GEDMR as a standard record and data standard was published with support by other professional associations for EDs. No institution established by national healthcare agencies or government compiles ED standards in Germany.

To our knowledge, no data standard published by a professional medical association for emergency medicine in Europe is represented by a HL7 CDA specification at the moment. For the US realm, there is a specification for a prehospital emergency service patient care report developed with support from the National EMS Information System (NEMSIS) [12]. Besides this, there is a comprehensive health policy statement by multiple US cardiological associations defining data standards, workflow integration, structured reporting and standard representation with HL7 C-CDA and IHE [13]. The importance of standard information and standard documentation for EHRs is therefore widely recognized [14].

Before our project, no actual implementation of the GEDMR standard record was available on the German EHR market. There were some individual implementations of the GEDMR with local EHRs, performed within two widely used hospital information systems by local enhancement developments without support or acknowledgement of the vendor.

3. Concept

The German ministry for research and education (BMBF) approved in 2011 a grant for the development of a national ED data registry using interoperability terminologies and technologies like HL7 CDA, LOINC or SNOMED CT. The project schedule included the modelling of medical domain standard pro forma GEDMR published by DIVI with CDA, the development of a data warehouse and the implementation of the GEDMR-CDA as an interface between the ED-EHR and a local registry data warehouse [15]. It was planned to recruit 15 project hospitals collecting routine ED-data in their already implemented ED-EHR for the transfer into the registry. Selection of project hospitals was based on willingness and capability. Either in-house development, local project management skills to support and push vendor or preexisting disposition of ED-EHR-vendor to support the project were decisive factors and funded by a reasonable amount of funding. Besides development of a German ED data registry, the introduction of standardized interoperability technologies into the German ED-EHR market was a primary project objective.

In Germany, only a limited number of HL7 CDA implementation guidelines exists while HL7 V2 is the main communication standard for hospital information exchange. The most significant CDA specification was started in 2005 by different German software vendors resulting in the German "Physician Note" (Arztbrief) with concurrent updates. This specification was in part adopted by the Association of Statutory Health Insurance Physicians providing only header information for transfer between primary care physicians with no support for any other content than a PDF/A. With the adoption, the physician note CDA gained support by an authority of the German health system. Other CDA implementations with structured content in Germany cover special scenarios being used primarily within research projects. In the US, the HL7 initiative for a Consolidated Templated implementation guide in cooperation with Integrating Healthcare Enterprise (IHE) and Health Information Technology Standards Panel (HITSP) led to a family of consolidated CDAs. The contained CDAs are acknowledged by the "Meaningful Use" program actually in stage 3 incentivizing the use of C-CDAs with EHR vendors. The BMBF fund represents a much smaller scale public funded incentive for implementing CDA in daily routine in emergency care in Germany.

4. Implementation

The first version of the implementation guideline was published on 18th of November 2015 on http://aktin.art-decor.org. Notification of the participating ED-EHR vendors followed immediately. Within one year, one Hospital Information System (HIS) vendor with a significant market share, (AGFA Healthcare GmbH, Germany) and one best-of-breed vendor (e.care BVBA, Belgium) customized their ED-EHR-System for GEDMR data standard and implemented a CDA-Export. As six EDs within the project use these systems, six hospitals are collecting the data elements of the standard GEDMR. Until March 2017, 1,850 CDAs from two AGFA Orbis installations and 106,868 CDAs from four e.care installations were exported in total. The exported numbers differ due to different implementation dates and different functionalities in retrospective data export. Four additional hospitals with different EHRs (Cerner medico, Telekom i.s.h.med, COPRA COPRA, IMESO ICUData) implemented an in-house development exporting 42,256 CDAs until now. Finally, three more vendors are adapting their ED-EHR. Two additional vendors are actually developing their GEDMR compliant version in two project hospitals. Besides funded project hospitals and thus indirectly funded vendors, two further vendors are developing a GEDMR compliant version with CDA export functionality to meet the emerging demand of the market. Based on the supporting vendors and their distribution on the German hospital market, approximately 80 % of the estimated 1,000 German EDs have the opportunity to implement a GEDMR compliant ED-EHR. An ad-hoc survey revealed roughly 10 % installed GEDMR compliant ED-EHR from different vendors at the moment.

5. Lessons learned

The GEDMR-CDA implementation guide, together with funding for implementation in project hospitals, had a significant impact on the German ED-EHR market. Within two years after release, a broadening and increasingly self-enforcing support by German ED-EHR vendors is notable. The combination of demand by EDs and an available data standard implemented in the language of the HIT business met the apparently existing needs. Besides enforcement by governmental authorities or large scale incentive programs like the US "Meaningful Use" program, the chosen approach was very effective in disseminating a professional medical association data standard and medical record among ED-EHR vendors. In terms of the research project, collecting data from participating EDs was the primary goal allowing for individual implementations of the GEDMR-CDA within existing ED-EHRs.

The chosen approach has its drawbacks. At least two vendors representing at least a 10 % market share are intentionally not supporting the GEDMR-CDA. Despite existing funding, one vendor has already implemented a GEDMR compliant ED-EHR but is not willing to implement a CDA-based interface justifying his decision with insufficient funding and insufficient return of investment. After acquisition and uncertain product future, the other vendor is neither able to develop an own solution nor willing to adopt an already available individual solution from one project hospital. It remains unclear if the vendor support for CDA will continue after project and funding completion. Until now, the implemented solutions are not evaluated for patient and data completeness. This evaluation will be the next project step for building a registry based on routine data export using HIE interoperability standards.

6. Conclusion

With a HL7 CDA implementation guide as leverage and implementation funding as stimulus, a medical professional associations' data standard can be established with EHR vendors in Germany. The HL7 CDA implementation guide operates as a shared language between HIT domain and medical domain facilitating misconceptions.

7. Conflict of Interest

The authors received funding from the German Ministry for Research (BMBF) (01KX1319A), (01KX1319B), (01KX1319C). DB is Co-Chair of Emergency Care Working Group, HL7 International. KH is CEO and ST is chair of HL7 Germany. FW is Chair of DIVI GEDMR Working Group.

References

[1] J.L. Hall, J.J. Ryan, B.E. Bray, et al., Merging electronic health record data and genomics for cardiovascular research, Circ. Cardiovasc. Genet. 9 (2016) 193–202.

[2] C. Polling, A. Tulloch, S. Banerjee, et al., Using routine clinical and administrative data to produce a dataset of attendances at Emergency Departments following self-harm, BMC Emerg. Med. 15 (2015) 15.

[3] J.C. McClay, P.J. Park, M.G. Janczewski, et al., Standard for improving emergency information interoperability: the HL7 data elements for emergency department systems., J. Am. Med. Inform. Assoc. (2015) 1–7.

[4] M. Kulla, M. Baacke, T. Schöpke, et al., Kerndatensatz „Notaufnahme" der DIVI, Notfall + Rettungsmedizin. 17 (2014) 671–681.

[5] R.H. Dolin, and L. Alschuler, Approaching semantic interoperability in Health Level Seven, J. Am. Med. Informatics Assoc. 18 (2011) 99–103.

[6] J.M. Hirshon, M. Warner, C.B. Irvin, et al., Research Using Emergency Department-related Data Sets: Current Status and Future Directions, Acad. Emerg. Med. 16 (2009) 1103–1109.

[7] G. Innes, M. Murray, and E. Grafstein, A consensus-based process to define standard national data elements for a canadian emergency department information system, CJEM. 3 (2001) 277–283.

[8] S.E. Gray, and C.F. Finch, Assessing the completeness of coded and narrative data from the Victorian Emergency Minimum Dataset using injuries sustained during fitness activities as a case study, BMC Emerg. Med. 16 (2016) 24.

[9] J. McClay, L.H. Langford, P. Park, et al., HL7 Version 3 Specification: Data Elements for Emergency Department Systems (DEEDS), Release 1 - US Realm, http://www.hl7.org/implement/standards/product_brief.cfm?product_id=326. (2013) 1–112. (accessed March 8, 2017).

[10] C.P. Cannon, A. Battler, R.G. Brindis, et al., American College of Cardiology key data elements and definitions for measuring the clinical management and outcomes of patients with acute coronary syndromes. (Acute Coro, J. Am. Coll. Cardiol. 38 (2001) 2114–30.

[11] F. Walcher, M. Kulla, S. Klinger, et al., [Standardized documentation in emergency departments with the core dataset of the DIVI]., Unfallchirurg. 115 (2012) 457–63.

[12] A. Walden, J.L. Ockham, S.R. Ockham, et al., HL7 Implementation Guide for CDA ® Release 2 – Level 3: Emergency Medical Services; Patient Care Report , Release 1 – US Realm, (2014) 1–181.

[13] T.A. Sanborn, J.E. Tcheng, H.V. Anderson, et al., ACC/AHA/SCAI 2014 health policy statement on structured reporting for the cardiac catheterization laboratory: A report of the american college of cardiology clinical quality committee, 2014.

[14] L.G. Jensen, and C. Bossen, Factors affecting physicians' use of a dedicated overview interface in an electronic health record: The importance of standard information and standard documentation, Int. J. Med. Inform. 87 (2016) 44–53.

[15] J. Ahlbrandt, D. Brammen, R.W. Majeed, et al., Balancing the need for big data and patient data privacy - an IT infrastructure for a decentralized emergency care research database., Stud. Health Technol. Inform. 205 (2014) 750–4.

German Medical Data Sciences: Visions and Bridges
R. Röhrig et al. (Eds.)

doi:10.3233/978-1-61499-808-2-137

Requirements Analysis for a Clinical Decision Support System Aiming at Improving the Artificial Nutrition of Critically Ill Patients

Christina SCHÜTTLER[a,1], Marc HINDERER[a], Stefan KRAUS[a], Anne-Katharina
LANG[b], Hans-Ulrich PROKOSCH[a] and Ixchel CASTELLANOS[b]

[a] *Medical Informatics, Friedrich-Alexander-Universität Erlangen-Nürnberg*
[b] *Department of Anaesthesiology, University Hospital Erlangen*

Abstract. *Background:* Nutrition support is an important aspect regarding the care
of critically ill patients. Malnutrition affects the recovery process negatively.
However, the impact on the clinical outcome is often underestimated in complex
clinical settings due to several factors hindering optimization of nutrition. *Objective:* To identify the requirements for a clinical decision support system that enables the medical staff to improve its patients' nutritional status. *Methods:* A literature review and interviews with two senior physicians were conducted to refine the
requirements for the support system as well as to determine the inclusion criteria
for a subsequent intervention study. *Results:* The analysis resulted in: (i) the identification of 4 measurement parameters for the assessment of the nutrition status; (ii)
the graphical layout in adherence to the standards-based implementation approach
for the creation of multi-patient dashboards; (iii) the definition of the study group.
The nutrition dashboard will be implemented and integrated based on the set requirements, followed by an intervention study evaluating the dashboard's efficacy.

Keywords. Nutritional status, intensive care unit, clinical decision support

1. Introduction

Nutrition support is an important factor in the care of critically ill patients. In particular,
patients in intensive care units (ICU) may suffer from malnutrition and its related complications. Barr et al. reported a prolonged duration of mechanical ventilation by an
average of 9.5 days in the study group before the implementation of a nutritional management protocol [1]. Further possible consequences may include a prolonged ICU stay
as well as an increased morbidity and mortality rate [1, 2].

Since healthcare providers have become increasingly aware of the benefits of an
adequate nutritional balance, several approaches are pursued to avoid energy deficiency
and malnutrition [3, 4]. For this purpose, clinical decision support (CDS) systems have
been designed and integrated in clinical environments in order to provide close monitoring and additional information supporting medical staff [4, 5]. The University Hos-

---

[1] Corresponding Author: Christina Schüttler, Wetterkreuz 13, 91058 Erlangen, Germany. E-mail: christina.schuettler@fau.de

pital Erlangen is a tertiary care hospital with approximately 1.400 beds and 12 ICUs that utilize a commercial patient data management system (PDMS, Integrated Care Manager, ICM©, Dräger Medical, Lübeck, Germany) which was introduced in 2006 [9]. Our local PDMS installation, besides allowing for electronic clinical documentation, provides support for several CDS functions based on Arden Syntax Medical Logic Modules (MLMs) which are in use in clinical daily routine [6, 10]. However, to the present day there are no MLMs that address nutrition. Local intensivists at our largest surgical ICU with 35 beds expressed a clinical demand for such an integrated nutritional monitoring. Thus, we set out to implement a CDS function in form of a multi-patient nutrition dashboard.

The purpose of this paper is to describe the requirements analysis for developing a nutrition dashboard that is tailored to the needs of the local ICU setting. The findings of this research provide the basis for upcoming refinements and adjustments to the users' needs. Furthermore, this work is intended to lay the groundwork for an intervention study evaluating the dashboard's efficacy on practitioner performance and clinical outcomes.

2. Methods

Our investigation comprised the requirements analysis of both the graphical layout of the outer dashboard structure and the CDS functions to be provided by the specific contents.

We analyzed the guidelines of the German Society for Nutritional Medicine and the European Society for Clinical Nutrition and Metabolism in order to identify relevant clinical parameters for the artificial feeding of intensive care patients, such as nutritional requirements, parameters for measuring a patient's nourishment, and outcome parameters. Two senior physicians from the local ICU who have experience in artificial nutrition of intensive care patients reviewed and revised the identified parameters. They added additional parameters, such as medical conditions requiring a reduced or elevated nutrient intake.

Subsequently, we conducted semi-structured interviews with these two physicians as representatives of the primary user group focusing on two issues. The first one referred to the requirements of an electronic nutrition dashboard in the specific ICU with respect to technical and clinical features and the preferred design of the user interface. Based on a literature research, wireframes of possible variations of the dashboard layout were prepared in order to discuss different content presentations. The second issue concerned the inclusion criteria for the planned subsequent clinical trial aiming at evaluating the efficacy of the nutrition dashboard.

3. Results

The performed analyses and interviews defined the specifications for the content requirements and the graphical layout for the dashboard as well as the inclusion criteria for the intervention study.

The display elements required by our local physicians include the nutritional target values regarding calorie requirements, proteins, carbohydrates, and fats. Calculations of the total energy demand are based on the recommendations extracted from the relevant literature and the conducted expert interviews. The basal metabolic rate will be calculated by the Harris-Benedict (HB) equation. The caloric requirements can additionally be adjusted by stress factors related to specific medical conditions (Table 1). The requirements of proteins, carbohydrates and fats originate from the university hospital's current standard operating procedure (SOP) and are presented in Table 2.

Table 1. Relevant stress factors that reduce or elevate the nutrition intake.

Medical condition	Factor	Affected nutrients
Sepsis	1,3	Calorie
Peritonitis	1,4	Calorie
Polytrauma	1,3 – 1,5	Calorie
Acute liver failure, liver cirrhosis	1,2 – 1,3	Calorie
Tertiary burns	1,7 – 2,0	Calorie
Short bowel syndrome	0,85 – 1,5	Calorie
Fever	+ 0,1/°C	Calorie
Renal failure	1,2 – 1,5	Proteins

Table 2. Requirements of proteins, carbohydrates and fats in accordance to the SOP of the local ICU.

Parameters	Formula	% of total energy
Proteins	0,8 – 1,5 g/kg/d	10 – 15
Carbohydrates	3 – 3,5 g/kg/d	50 – 60
Fats	0,7 – 1,3 g/kg/d	20 – 35

A ward overview focusing on the nutritional status of all patients currently on ICU should be integrated within a full screen, providing structured information on the present nutrition status of all patients and highlighting critical situations in order to allow medical staff to easily notice issues and optimize nutrition. The basic design will conform to a straightforward standards-based implementation approach for the creation of multi-patient dashboards with a tabular structure containing one row per patient [6]. This row will include patient name, bed position, and the most relevant data arranged in cells. The design of the nutrition dashboard (Figure 1) is intended to include three levels:

(1) *Matrix illustration*: indicates if a patient fulfills the defined nutritional requirements or if he is outside of this range. For this purpose, the dashboard displays (a) the actual nutritional intake of the day; (b) the percentage of the calculated total nutritional target for the day; (c) the applied stress factor; and (d) a color highlighting to signal if the daily status is within the recommended range (green) or not (red).

(2) *Tooltip*: is displayed when the cursor hovers over a specific button (mouseover). It shows a short summary of the patient data and the underlying calculations for the nutritional target value.

(3) *Detailed info box*: provides the most detailed documentation of the nutritional status (e.g. graphics, progress monitoring, etc.) by clicking on the patient's indicator panel.

The main criterion for inclusion in the intended study is the sole reception of artificial nutrition support. Thus, we will enroll patients whose length of ICU stay exceeds seven days while simultaneously receiving parenteral nutrition.

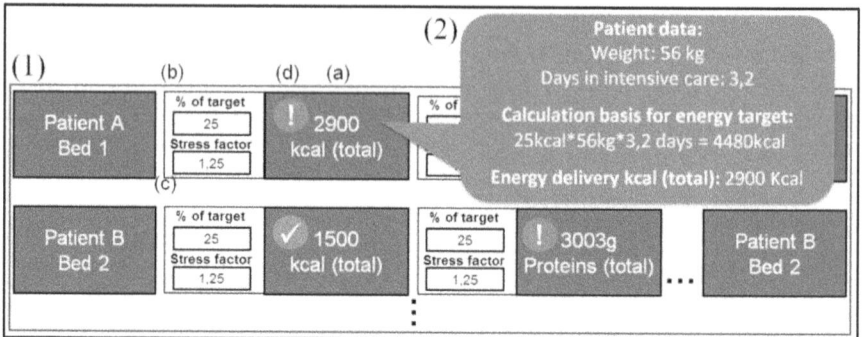

Figure 1. First exemplary draft of the layout of the dashboard: matrix illustration (1) and tooltip (2).

4. Discussion

Nutritional care is an important part of inpatient care and a crucial issue in ICUs. Overlooking this aspect might deteriorate the clinical outcome, such as mortality, morbidity, infectious disease complications, and length of ventilation or hospitalization [1, 2].

The occurrence of an unbalanced nutritional status in the hospital and particularly in the ICU is frequently due to the fact that various factors affect the metabolic process in a way that might be underestimated by medical staff. This includes stress factors related to certain medical conditions (Table 1) as well as thermal factors that need to be considered [4, 7]. Moreover, interruptions of artificial feeding caused by diagnostic or therapeutic tasks can have a negative impact by simply interrupting nutrition intake. Furthermore, the HB formula has its limitations (e.g. regarding weight history and ethnicity) and therefore may need to be adjusted [11].

In order to avoid malnutrition due to lack of awareness of nutrition standards or insufficient monitoring, different approaches have been described. Some organizational and educational efforts have aimed to implement and improve nutritional strategies in routine intensive care. These efforts include the work of expert groups consisting of nurses and physicians who developed nutritional management protocols, charts, guidelines and forms in the clinical information system (CIS). In this context, computer-aided support systems prove to be superior to paper-based forms due to the required calculations for a balanced nutrition [4, 8]. Berger et al. described a computerized information system that operates without additional manual input of the relevant parameters; instead, it extracts them from the local CIS. This results in a time-reduced and error-reduced nutritional monitoring [5].

We plan to embed the dashboard into the graphical user interface of the local PDMS, with user-driven activation. While the first of the three levels described above will provide a concise and automated generated overview, the third one is intended to offer more extensive background information; the second level presents an intermediate stage. Thus, the three tiers enable the user to obtain the necessary information and simultaneously avoid information overload. This seems advantageous in comparison to information systems that display all information on a single sheet [5].

Our prototype is limited to monitor artificial nutrition by calculating and visualizing the nutritional status and highlighting patients that do not comply with previously defined thresholds. It is not intended as an active alerting system with automatic pop-ups or acoustic warnings, since these features were undesired by the interviewed physicians. Reactions to such warnings are not extremely time-critical and an alert might be considered a nuisance. Moreover, the dashboard is not intended as order-entry system or for computed prescription in contrast to some other systems [4, 5, 8].

The underlying architecture of the nutrition dashboard will be implemented in Arden Syntax, resembling a proof of concept that has already been successfully implemented in the local PDMS [6].

After specifying both the medical requirements for calculating the nutritional need and the graphical interface to operate the nutrition dashboard, the next steps will be the implementation and further refinements (e.g. interviews with other user groups such as the nursing staff and nutritionists) of the nutrition dashboard, followed by the integration into the PDMS of the local ICU and a subsequent intervention study to evaluate the effect of the CDS functions on the quality of nutritional supply.

5. Conflict of Interest

The authors state that they have no conflict of interests.

Acknowledgement

The present work was performed in fulfillment of the requirements for obtaining the degree "Dr. rer. biol. hum." from the Friedrich-Alexander-Universität Erlangen-Nürnberg (FAU) (CS).

References

[1]   J. Barr, M. Hecht, K.E. Flavin et al., Outcomes in Critically Ill Patients Before and After the Implementation of an Evidence-Based Nutritional Management Protocol, *Chest* 125 (2004), 1446-57.
[2]   C.M. Martin, G.S. Doig, D.K. Heyland et al., Multicentre, cluster-randomized clinical trial of algorithms for critical-care enteral and parenteral therapy (ACCEPT), *CMAJ* 2 (2004), 197-204.
[3]   P. Singer, G.S. Doig, C. Pichard, The tight calorie control study (TICACOS): a prospective, randomized, controlled pilot study of nutritional support in critically ill patients, *Intensive Care Med* 37 (2011), 601-609.
[4]   R.J.M. Strack van Schijndel, S.D.W. de Groot, R.H. Driessen et al., Computer-aided support improves early and adequate delivery of nutrients in the ICU, *Neth J Med* 67 (2009), 388-393.
[5]   M.M. Berger, J.-P. Revelly, J.-B.Wasserfallen et al., Impact of a computerized information system on quality of nutritional support in the ICU, *Nutrition* 22 (2006), 221-229.
[6]   S. Kraus, C. Drescher, M. Sedlmayr et al., Using Arden Syntax for the creation of a multi-patient surveillance dashboard, *Artif Intell Med* (2015), http://dx.doi.org/10.1016/j.artmed.2015.09.009.
[7]   J.J. Lunn., M.J. Murray, Nutritional Support in Critical Illness, *Yale J Biol Med* 71 (1998), 449-456.
[8]   P. Porcelli, A Survey of Neonatal Parenteral Nutrition Design Practices in North Carolina, *J Perinatol* 24 (2004), 137-142.
[9]   I. Castellanos, T. Bürkle, H.-U. Prokosch et al., Concept for the hospital-wide implementation of a patient data management system at a large clinical center-an interdisciplinary challenge, *Anästh Intensivmed* 50 (2009), 618-29.
[10]   I. Castellanos, S. Kraus, D. Toddenroth et al., Using Arden Syntax Medical Logic Modules to reduce overutilization of laboratory tests for detection of bacterial infections - Success or failure?, *Artif Intell Med* 25 (2015), S0933-3657. http://dx.doi.org/10.1016/j.artmed.2015.09.005.
[11]   C.C. Douglas, J.C. Lawrence, N.C. Bush et al., Ability of the Harris Benedict formula to predict energy requirements differs with weight history and ethnicity, *Nutr Res* 27 (2007), 194-199.

German Medical Data Sciences: Visions and Bridges
R. Röhrig et al. (Eds.)
© 2017 German Association for Medical Informatics, Biometry and Epidemiology (gmds) e.V. and IOS Press.
This article is published online with Open Access by IOS Press and distributed under the terms
of the Creative Commons Attribution Non-Commercial License 4.0 (CC BY-NC 4.0).
doi:10.3233/978-1-61499-808-2-142

Antecedents of CIOs' Innovation Capability in Hospitals: Results of an Empirical Study

Jan-David LIEBE[a,1], Moritz ESDAR[a], Johannes THYE[a], Ursula HÜBNER[a]

[a] *Health Informatics Research Group, Osnabrück University AS, Germany*

Abstract. CIOs' innovation capability is regarded as a precondition of successful HIT adoption in hospitals. Based on the data of 142 CIOs, this study aimed at identifying antecedents of perceived innovation capability. Eight features describing the status quo of the hospital IT management (e.g. use of IT governance frameworks), four features of the hospital structure (e.g. functional diversification) and four CIO characteristics (e.g. duration of employment) were tested as potential antecedents in an exploratory stepwise regression approach. Perceived innovation capability in its entirety and its three sub-dimensions served as criterion. The results show that CIOs' perceived innovation capability could be explained significantly ($R^2=0.34$) and exclusively by facts that described the degree of formalism and structure of IT management in a hospital, e.g. intensive and formalised strategic communication, the existence of an IT strategy and the use of IT governance frameworks. Breaking down innovation capability into its constituents revealed that "innovative organisational culture" contributed to a large extent ($R^2=0.26$) to the overall result sharing several predictors. In contrast, "intrapreneurial personality" ($R^2=0.11$) and "openness towards users" ($R^2=0.18$) could be predicted less well. These results hint at the relationship between working in a well-structured, formalised and strategy oriented environment and the overall feeling of being capable to promote IT innovation.

Keywords. CIO, innovation capability, intrapreneurship, strategic cooperation

1. Introduction

Health information technology (HIT) innovations are considered to be an intrinsic component of hospital success [1]. This said, HIT innovations are less about specific IT applications, but about building "digital options" through complex integrated and multifunctional systems [1, 2]. In expert organisations like hospitals, this goal can only be achieved by making the right IT investments and by considering the complex network of social, organisational and technical aspects that surround successful HIT implementation [3]. Chief information officers (CIOs) stand at the heart of corresponding management activities [4]. Their perceived ability to initialise, implement and institutionalise new and suitable HIT solutions can be defined as *innovation capability* [5], a construct composed of latent personal and organisational characteristics. These are in detail: an *innovative organisational culture* and the CIOs'

---

[1] Corresponding Author, Jan-David Liebe, Osnabrück University of AS, Health Informatics Research Group, PO Box 1940, 49009 Osnabrück, Germany; E-mail: j.liebe@hs-osnabrueck.de.

intrapreneurial personality and *openness towards users* [6]. Innovative organisational culture describes a working environment that nurtures unorthodox thinking, which is based on shared values, basic underlying assumptions and observable artifacts [7, 8]. With regard to HIT, innovative organisational culture can be characterised by shared visions about the future role of HIT, by a supportive hospital board (HB) and by a certain degree of flexibility in organisational structures, processes and work routines [3, 6]. Intrapreneurial personalities were originally characterised as "(..) dreamers who do. Those who take hands-on responsibility for creating innovation of any kind, within a business" [9]. Intrapreneurial hospital CIOs' can be characterised as being risk-affine and pro-active in regard to new HIT solutions [6, 10]. They are inclined to compensate a lack of decision-making power with entrepreneurial thinking and actions [6, 10]. Openness towards users can be defined by a strong orientation to clinicians' needs, the willingness to cooperate with users in IT project and by the awareness of social standing and professional autonomy [3, 5, 6].

In a previous study, we reported about developing an *innovation capability* score for hospital CIOs [6]. Based on this, it seems to be promising for researchers and practitioners (i.e. hospital managers) to explore antecedents of CIOs' innovation capability. In HIT adoption research, several approaches to explain the origin of innovations theoretically and empirically can be found [11,12]. Various studies focus on the status quo of IT management, which surrounds HIT implementation, e.g. the sophistication of strategic cooperation between CIO and HB, the use of IT governance frameworks or the existence of an IT strategy [10]. While other studies investigate the influence of structural hospital characteristics like size, functional differentiation, teaching status or ownership on HIT implementation [11]. Finally, there is a large body of research on individual characteristics to explain innovativeness (e.g. qualification in terms of working experience or degree) [12]. Considering these diverse research streams, this study intends to explore antecedents of the CIOs' innovation capability in hospitals.

2. Methods

The study was based on data captured in a nationwide survey among 1284 CIOs in German hospitals between February and April 2016 [13]. It furthermore builds on a composite score to measure the perceived *innovation capability* of CIOs [6]. This score, which consists of the three sub-scores *innovative organisational culture*, *intrapreneurial personality* and *openness towards users,* was found to be reliable and valid [6]. In order to explore the antecedents of the CIOs' innovation capability in this study, we performed four stepwise regression analyses. The composite score and its three sub-dimensions served as criterion. Sixteen attributes that described the status quo of IT management, the structure of the hospital and individual characteristics of the CIO were entered as predictors. The status quo of IT management was operationalised by eight items: (1) number of frequently communicated strategic information between CIO and HB as a measure of communication intensity, (2) communication environment of CIO and HB (e.g. coffee breaks vs. official meetings) as a measure of formalisation, (3) use of a management cockpit to visualise strategic information, (4) use of IT governance frameworks, (5) existence of an IT strategy, (6) membership of a nurse and/or (7) a physician in the HB to measure participation and (8) status as reference hospital as a measure for a formalised cooperation with IT vendors. Structural hospital demographics were measured by four items: (1) number of in-patient beds as a measure of size, (2) number of clinical units as a measure of functional diversification, (3) teaching status and (4) ownership (private vs public). Individual characteristics of the CIO were measured also by four items: (1) work experience (in years), (2) duration of employment (in years), (3) clinical background of the CIO (e.g. nursing) and (4) academic degree. We tested for normal distribution and homoscedasticity of the residuals as well as for multicollinearity (by calculating the variance inflation factor (VIF)). Data were analysed with SPSS 24®.

3. Results

Data from 142 CIOs (response rate 11.1%) were included in the analysis after the original data set (n=176 [13]) was adjusted for missing data. CIOs in the final sample were responsible for 17.6% of all German hospitals (n=344) [14]. Table 1 and Table 2 show descriptive statistics of all items that were included in the regression models.

Table 1. Descriptive statistics of binary items (n=142)

Item	Yes	No
Formalisation (CIO and HB rather communicate in formal meetings)	57.0%	43.0%
CIO uses a management cockpit to visualise strategic information	14.8%	85,2%
IT governance frameworks (e.g. COBIT, ITIL) are used	35.2%	64.8%
An IT strategy exits	76.8%	23.2%
Formalised cooperation with IT vendors (status of a reference hospital)	42.3%	57.7%
A nurse is member of the HB	59.9%	40.1%
A physician is member of the HB	71.8%	28.2%
Hospital is a teaching hospital	56.3%	43.7%
Hospital is privately owned	12.7%	87.3%

Table 2. Descriptive statistics of metric items (n=142, [1]value range 1 to 100)

Item	Mean	SD	Min.	Max.
Communication intensity (freq. communicated information)	2.6	0.5	1.0	3.9
Functional diversification (number of clinical units)	9.2	8.0	1.0	45.0
Size (number of beds)	414.0	321.0	45.0	1563.0
CIOs' work experience (years)	14.0	8.3	0.0	35.0
CIOs' duration of employment (years)	11.7	7.8	0.0	32,0
Composite score: innovation capability[1]	56.0	12.4	28.2	87.9
Sub-score: innovative organisational culture[1]	43.8	21.1	0.0	100.0
Sub-score: intrapreneurial personality[1]	42.3	15.0	36.2	100.0
Sub-score: openness towards users[1]	74.7	14.1	0.0	86.7

The stepwise inclusion of the 16 predictors resulted in four significant regression models. Five predictors, assigned to status quo of IT management, significantly explained 34 % variance of *innovation capability*. Four of these predictors also significantly explained 26 % of *innovative organisational culture*. *Openness towards users* was significantly explained (18 %) by three predictors (number of clinical units, physician HB member, academic degree) and *intrapreneurial personality* (11 %) by the two IT management related variables "formalisation" and "IT governance" (Table 3). Residuals were normally distributed and showed no signs of heteroscedasticity, neither did the calculated VIF indicate multicollinearity.

4. Discussion

The main finding of this study is that CIOs innovation capability can be significantly explained by a formalised, intense, professional and strategic cooperation between the CIO and the hospital board. In hospitals, as in other organisations, technological innovations require the redirection of resources that would otherwise be allocated to non-IT related strategic objectives [5].

Table 3. Stepwise regression models (n=142)

	Innovation capability		Innovative org. culture		Intrapreneurial personality		Openness towards users	
	Cor. R^2= .34		Cor. R^2=.26		Cor. R^2=.11		Cor. R^2=.18	
	Beta	VIF	Beta	VIF	Beta	VIF	Beta	VIF
Status quo of IT management								
Communication intensity	0.23	1.23	0.27	1.22	-	-	-	-
Formalisation	0.31	1.13	0.24	1.10	0.26	1.03	-	-
Use of mgmt. cockpit	0.15	1.11	0.15	1.08	-	-	-	-
Use of IT governance	0.19	1.08	-	-	0.20	1.03	-	-
Existence of IT strategy	-	-	0.15	1.08	-	-	-	-
Reference hospital	-	-	-	-	-	-	-	-
Physician is HB member	0.12	1.03	-	-	-	-	0.15	1.01
Nurse is HB member	-	-	-	-	-	-	-	-
Structural hospital demographics								
No. of beds	-	-	-	-	-	-	-	-
No. of clinical units	-	-	-	-	-	-	0.19	1.15
Teaching hospital	-	-	-	-	-	-	-	-
Private ownership	-	-	-	-	-	-	-	-
Individual characteristics of the CIO								
Professional activity	-	-	-	-	-	-	-	-
Duration of employment	-	-	-	-	-	-	-	-
Academic degree	-	-	-	-	-	-	0.19	1.06
Clinical background	-	-	-	-	-	-	-	-

It can be assumed that an intense and formal exchange of strategic information in association with the use of IT based management cockpits, supports the lobbying in favour of HIT initiatives. A sophisticated strategic cooperation might furthermore lead to optimal trade-offs between clinical and technical requirements [3, 10]. This assumption is supported by the fact that CIOs perceive their innovation capability to be higher if a physician is part of the hospital board. Working together on establishing strategic IT initiatives might provide opportunities to educate each other about technical and clinical requirements [10]. In addition, clinicians in top management teams might act as "boundary spanners" to champion IT initiatives on the frontline level [3]. The certainty to be backed by clinical champions may furthermore facilitate the perceived capability to implement and institutionalise new HIT in clinical practice [5]. The ability to refer to hospital wide accepted IT strategy and to IT governance frameworks could have similar effects on certainty in actions [4]. Structural hospital characteristics, which were found to determine HIT adoption rates [11], could not explain innovation capability. Thus, CIOs' perceived innovation capability seems to be rather a function of proper management conditions than of size, teaching status or ownership. This study is limited with regard to the response rate of 11.1% that might have caused a non-response bias in our sample. The results therefore require further validation. Future research approaches could peruse additional predictors for *intrapreneurial personality* and *openness towards users* (e.g. the "big five" personality traits [12]) to better explain the perceived *innovation capability* as a whole.

5. Conclusion

This study is the first step towards a deeper understanding of CIOs' perceived innovation capability in hospitals and its antecedents. These insights help paving the way for establishing an innovation culture in healthcare organisations.

6. Conflict of Interest

The authors state that they have no conflict of interests.

7. Acknowledgement

We would like to thank Franziska Jahn and Alfred Winter (University Leipzig) as well as Christian Kücherer and Babara Peach (University Heidelberg) for their cooperation in the data collection phase. This study was funded by BMBF (grant: 16OH21026.).

References

[1] Chaudhry B, Wang J, Wu S *et al.* Systematic review: impact of health information technology on quality, efficiency, and costs of medical care. Annals of internal medicine 2006; 144:742-752.
[2] Hübner U. What Are Complex eHealth Innovations and How Do You Measure Them? Methods of information in medicine 2015; 54:319-327.
[3] Cresswell K, Sheikh A. Organizational issues in the implementation and adoption of health information technology innovations: an interpretative review. Int journal of medical informatics 2013; 82:e73-e86.
[4] Haux R, Winter A, Ammenwerth E, Brigl B. How to Strategically Manage Hospital Information Systems. In: Strategic Information Management in Hospitals. Springer; 2004. pp. 177-220.
[5] Avgar AC, Litwin AS, Pronovost PJ. Drivers and barriers in health IT adoption: a proposed framework. Applied clinical informatics 2012; 3:488-500.
[6] Esdar M, Liebe JD, Weiß JP, Hübner U. Exploring Innovation Capabilities of Hospital CIOs: An Empirical Assessment. Stud Health Technol Inform. 2017;235:383-387.
[7] Schein E, H. Organizational culture. American Psychologist 1990; 45:109–119.
[8] Khazanchi S, Lewis MW, Boyer KK. Innovation-supportive culture: The impact of organizational values on process innovation. Journal of Operations Management 2007; 25:871-884.
[9] Pinchot G. Building the intrapreneurial environment. In Pinchot G. (Hrsg): Intrapreneuring: Why you don't have to leave the corporation to become an entrepreneur. Harper&Row, New York, 1985:4-74.
[10] Bradley RV, Byrd TA, Pridmore JL *et al.* An empirical examination of antecedents and consequences of IT governance in US hospitals. Journal of Information Technology 2012; 27:156-177.
[11] Greenhalgh T, Robert G, Macfarlane F *et al.* Diffusion of innovations in service organizations: systematic review and recommendations. Milbank Quarterly 2004; 82:581-629.
[12] Patterson F, Kerrin M, Gatto-Roissard G. Characteristics and behaviours of innovative people in organisations. Literature Review prepared for the NESTA Policy & Research Unit 2009:1-63.
[13] Kücherer C, Liebe JD, Schaaf M, Thye J, Paech B, Winter A, Jahn F. The Status Quo of Information Management in Hospitals-Results of an Online Survey. In: Mayr HC, Pinzger M (Hrsg.): Informatik 2016. Lecture Notes in Informatics (LNI), 2016; 259:1-15.
[14] Bundesamt S. Gesundheit. Grunddaten der Krankenhäuser Fachserie 12 Reihe 6.1.1. 2015.

German Medical Data Sciences: Visions and Bridges
R. Röhrig et al. (Eds.)
© *2017 German Association for Medical Informatics, Biometry and Epidemiology (gmds) e.V. and IOS Press.*
doi:10.3233/978-1-61499-808-2-147

Identification of Measures and Indicators for the IT Security of Networked Medical Devices: A Delphi Study

Stefan LEBER [a,1] and Elske AMMENWERTH [a]

[a] *Institute of Medical Informatics, UMIT – University for Health Sciences, Medical Informatics and Technology, Hall in Tirol, Austria*

Abstract. The networking of medical devices or systems in a hospital network is the foundation for modern medical diagnostics and therapy. This, however, makes possible numerous hazards that could lead to risks for patients, clinical processes or data and information. The aim of the work was to develop a catalogue of measures and indicators for the effective support of the IT risk management process in a health facility. Through a qualitative and quantitative Delphi study among 21 experts, it was possible to identify an initial 51 practice-relevant measures of IT risk management that a hospital should implement. Additionally, 27 indicators were defined which can be used to measure the impact of these measures. Of the 51 measures, 35 were seen as especially important, particularly organizational measures. Of the 27 indicators, six were seen as especially important, particularly indicators to measure networking effectiveness. The study also investigated the impact of the measures on the indicators. A case study is planned to investigate the practicability of the identified measures and indicators.

Keywords. Risk management, networked medical devices, computer security, data security, computer communication network, Delphi study

1. Introduction

Vulnerabilities in infusion pumps that are deliberately exploited by computer hackers. A patient monitor alarm that is not transmitted to the physician due to a network configuration error. A sudden failure of the IT-network that prevents retrieval of urgently needed X-ray images from the archives. The networking of medical devices and systems in a hospital network is of increasing importance, as more and more medical devices are designed to be able to exchange data and information with other medical devices and with clinical information systems [1]. However, technical faults, human error, deliberate actions or organizational failures can influence the data flow in such a way so as to jeopardize the security of data and information and of clinical processes or the safety of patients. To counteract these hazards, hospitals must implement a systematic IT risk management process for networked medical devices and systems (medical IT risk management) [2, 3].

---

[1] Corresponding author: Stefan Leber, Institute of Medical Informatics, UMIT – University for Health Sciences, Medical Informatics and Technology, Eduard Wallnöfer Zentrum 1, 6060 Hall in Tirol, Austria, stefan.leber@edu.umit.at.

There are several existing standards (e.g. ISO/IEC 27000-series, ISO 15408, ISO 18045, ISO 31000, etc.) that provide method, process or practice recommendations on information security management and for the realization of IT risk management. EN 80001-1 is the standard for application of risk management for IT-networks incorporating medical devices. The implementation of the standard in practice, however, is rather complex [2, 4]. The reasons for this are the lack of concrete and practice-relevant measures [4] or indicators giving information whether and to what degree the intended results were achieved.

The aim of the present work was to develop a *catalogue of measures* which, on the basis of empirical knowledge of experts, can provide concrete, practice-relevant measures for the implementation of IT risk management for networked medical devices and systems, as well as a *catalogue of indicators* which can be used to measure the impact of the measures. Another aim was to determine the influence of the individual measures on the individual indicators. It was not an aim to compare the empirical knowledge of the experts with current standards.

2. Methods

A Delphi study was conducted among 21 experts whose work involves the IT risk management for networked medical devices (e.g. hospital IT managers, IT risk managers, biomedical engineers, etc.) and whose specific practical or empirical knowledge makes them suited to apply their understanding and their interpretations to define and assess the wanted measures and indicators [5].

2.1. First survey round - Qualitative expert surveys to identify practice-relevant measures and indicators

A written and fully anonymised survey was conducted over a period of 75 days. In ten open-ended questions, respondents were asked about their personal views and experiences regarding the risks of networked medical devices in a hospital network. At first, the participants were requested to provide their opinion on current news reports (e.g. the hacking of respirators or infusion pumps). The respondents were then asked to add those hazards they considered to be important from their own experience. This was followed by a discussion of possible measures and indicators for IT risk management. The final discussion centred on the question if and how much this jeopardizes patient safety or the security of data and information or clinical processes.

The 21 answers of this qualitative written survey were analysed using a qualitative content analysis. The procedure corresponded to the process model of summarizing inductive category formation as described by Mayring [6]. In the process, a list of relevant measures of IT risk management and a list of possible indicators, among other things, were extracted.

2.2. Second survey round - Quantitative expert surveys to confirm the results of the first survey round and to identify the correlations between measures and indicators

The anonymised survey was conducted over a period of one month. The survey comprised a total of 20 closed-ended questions. Using a four-point scale ranging from "*No importance*" to "*Very high importance*" (cf. Figure 1), the experts were now asked to assess those measures and indicators which in the preceding qualitative survey round had been cited as necessary in the implementation of medical IT risk management. The experts were also asked whether they saw a correlation between measures and indicators and how strong they suspected this correlation to be.

During the processing of the data, a simple descriptive frequency analysis (mean, standard deviation and frequency distribution) was conducted for each measure, indicator and correlation estimate. The results of the first survey round were deemed confirmed if the measure or indicator was assessed to be important by a simple majority of >50% of the experts (mean > 2.5). A further distinction in measures and indicators with very high and with moderate importance was made thereafter. Here the cut-off also was 50% (cf. Figure 1).

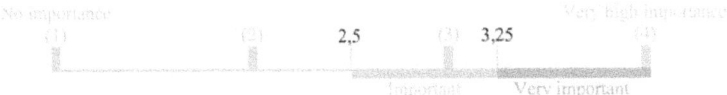

Figure 1. Scale for the assessment of the indicators and measures.

3. Results

In the first survey round, 27 indicators for measuring the IT risk management for networked medical devices or systems in a hospital network as well as 51 measures to implement the IT risk management were identified. Measures and indicators were each assigned to six categories (cf. Figures 2 and 3).

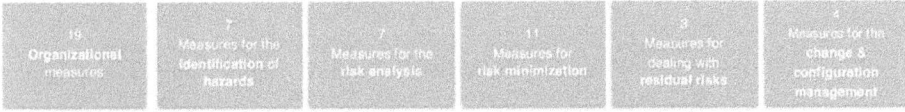

Figure 2. The six measure categories (incl. number of incorporated measures).

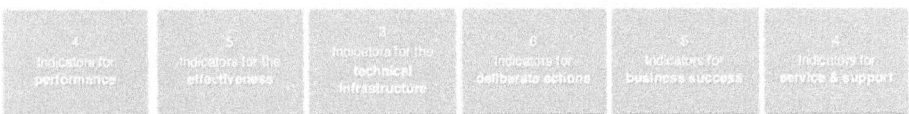

Figure 3. The six indicator categories (incl. number of incorporated indicators).

In the second survey round, all of the indicators and measures except for one indicator and one measure were confirmed as important by the experts. 35 measures and 6 indicators were seen as "very important" (cf. Table 1 and 2).

Table 1. The important measures (a selection).

Category	Measure
Organisation	- Interface between biomedical engineering and IT department must be ensured
	- Areas of impact and validity must be defined
	- All networked medical devices/systems must be registered
	- Roles and tasks of the risk manager must be clearly defined
	- Risk management processes must be developed and implemented
	- A company-wide coordinated procurement process must be established
	- External laws and regulations must be taken into consideration
	- A manager with responsibility must be appointed and employed
	- A risk management file must be created
	- Roles and tasks of the manufacturer must be unambiguously resolved

Category	Measure
Identification of hazards	- Complete network description and documentation must be made - Risk management activities must be regularly reflected - Ask manufacturer about possible risks in IT networking - Ask users which risks could arise - Identify networking purpose and use to identify hazardous situations - Create or adapt hazard catalogue (e.g. BSI baseline protection)
Risk analysis	- Document risk analyses and evaluations - Define degrees of severity for patient safety - Define degrees of severity for data and information security - Define risk matrix, i.e. different risk levels - Define degrees of severity for process effectiveness
Risk minimization	- Technical infrastructure must be kept state of the art - Interface and communication standards must be used at all times - Fundamental general IT security must be ensured - Risk-minimizing measures must be examined and documented - System communication as often as possible in a virtually separate network
Residual risks	- Residual risks must be documented and traceable - Residual risks must be systematically estimated and justified
Change and configuration management	- Systematic change and configuration processes must be developed - Frequent changes should be defined as standard processes (routine) - Large changes or new additions should be organized as project - All changes and configurations must be approved

Table 2. The important indicators (a selection).

Category	Indicator
Networking effectiveness	- Number of emergency power events triggered by the failure of networked medical devices/systems - Number of errors to patient data through ineffective networking (e.g. no HL7 or DICOM) of a medical device/system - Number of incidents in which patient and examination data were not available
Deliberate actions	- Number of unauthorized data changes and unauthorized access events - Number of covert or unrecognized connections - Number of hacker attacks

In six correlation estimates, >90% of the experts agreed that a correlation exists between measure and indicator categories (cf. Figure 4). The majority of the experts stated that the measures defined as very important have the strongest influence on an indicator category. About 30% of the experts were of the opinion that all measures are equally important and approx. 10% of the experts believe that all measures must be implemented before an impact on the indicator can be registered.

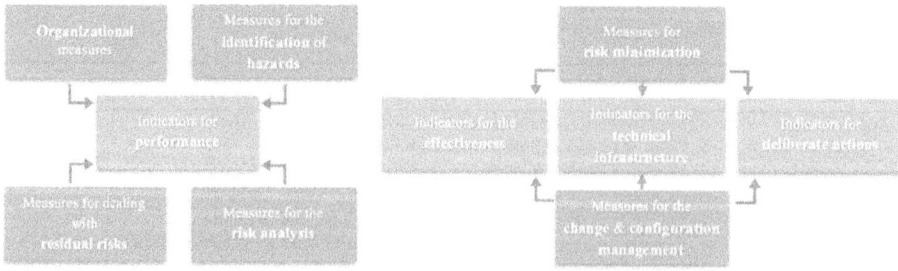

Figure 4. Correlations of measure and indicator categories.

4. Discussion

The mix of qualitative and quantitative expert surveys in a Delphi study is a suitable method for ascertaining the desired practice-relevant measures and indicators. The oral survey that had originally been planned in the first survey round could not be conducted due to numerous spontaneous cancellations. This may be due to the reactivity effects [7], namely the fear of the respondents of embarrassment or of being judged by the interviewer. We thus changed the method to a non-reactive written survey. This decision proved its worth: the participant rate was high with 21 experts.

The experts were agreed after already two survey rounds which measures and indicators are important. A third survey round, as would have been possible in a Delphi study, was therefore no longer necessary. Overall, especially the measures to ensure data and information security were found important. The efficiency and the reliability with which the network services are available as well as the number of deliberate actions which can occur were found to be the most important indicators. The difficulties in the practical implementation of IT risk management for networked medical devices or systems described in many publications [2, 3] and practice reports [2, 4] should be greatly reduced using the identified measures and indicators.

5. Conclusion

The study yielded measures and associated indicators for IT risk management that were unanimously considered by experts to be very important. The practicability of the identified measures and indicators must still be verified in case studies. An essential prerequisite for this is the creation of a catalogue of measures and indicators offering concrete and detailed implementation recommendations. In this context, the current standards for information security management an IT risk management should also be considered. The case study must investigate whether the measures are implementable and the indicators are measurable, as well as which financial, organizational and technological costs are required.

Conflict of interest

The authors state that they have no conflict of interests.

References

[1] Deutsche Krankenhausgesellschaft e.V, *Anwendung des Risikomanagements für IT-Netzwerke, die Medizinprodukte beinhalten*, Dt. Krankenhaus Verlagsgesellschaft mbH, Düsseldorf, 2011.
[2] J. Ahlbrandt, R. Röhrig, Safety first! managing risks for a daisy chain of medical devices connected to the IT-network - first experiences applying IEC 80001-1, *Stud Health Technol Inform,* 2013, 192:982.
[3] P. Williams, A. Woodward, Cybersecurity vulnerabilities in medical devices: a complex environment and multifaceted problem, Med Devices (Auckl). 2015; 8: 305–316.
[4] A. Gärtner, *Verteilte Alarmsysteme*, TÜV Media GmbH, Köln, 2016.
[5] A. Bogner, B. Littig, W. Menz, Interviews mit Experten, VS Verlag, Wiesbaden, 2014.
[6] P. Mayring, *Qualitative Inhaltsanalyse*, Beltz Verlag, Weinheim und Basel, 2015.
[7] W. Hussy, M. Schreier and G. Echterhoff, *Forschungsmethoden für Psychologie und Sozialwissenschaften*, Springer Verlag, Berlin Heidelberg, 2015.

German Medical Data Sciences: Visions and Bridges
R. Röhrig et al. (Eds.)
© 2017 German Association for Medical Informatics, Biometry and Epidemiology (gmds) e.V. and IOS Press.
This article is published online with Open Access by IOS Press and distributed under the terms
of the Creative Commons Attribution Non-Commercial License 4.0 (CC BY-NC 4.0).
doi:10.3233/978-1-61499-808-2-152

Extending the Query Language of a Data Warehouse for Patient Recruitment

Georg DIETRICH[a,1] Maximilian ERTL[c], Georg FETTE[a,b], Mathias KASPAR[b],
Jonathan KREBS[a], Daniel MACKENRODT[d], Stefan STÖRK[b] and Frank PUPPE[a]

[a] *Chair of Computer Science VI, Würzburg University, Germany*
[b] *Comprehensive Heart Failure Center, University Hospital Würzburg, Germany*
[c] *Service Center Medical Informatics, University Hospital Würzburg, Germany*
[d] *Institute for Clinical Epidemiology, Würzburg University, Germany*

Abstract. Patient recruitment for clinical trials is a laborious task, as many texts have to be screened. Usually, this work is done manually and takes a lot of time. We have developed a system that automates the screening process. Besides standard keyword queries, the query language supports extraction of numbers, time-spans and negations. In a feasibility study for patient recruitment from a stroke unit with 40 patients, we achieved encouraging extraction rates above 95% for numbers and negations and ca. 86% for time spans.

Keywords. Information Extraction, Data Warehouse, clinical trials, text queries.

1. Introduction

A comparison of electronic health record (EHR) systems showed that patient recruitment is not a standard feature and that clinical research has not been in the focus of the EHR vendors [1]. Clinical Data Warehouses (CDW) like I2B2 [2] or PaDaWaN [3] are very suitable for patient recruitment for clinical trials with inclusion and exclusion criteria. Steps towards an automatic identification of patients for clinical trials by parsing the natural language description of the criteria has been designed [4] and attempted [5]. Both approaches queried existing structured data only.

But a data warehouse also consists of unstructured data like textual reports and discharge letters, that - with the exception of search engine technologies [6] - is hardly usable for this task without preprocessing. There are many attempts to extract structured information from unstructured documents with various approaches (e.g. [7], [8], [9] for German texts). However, such information extraction approaches must be done when the data is loaded into the data warehouse and require a lot of engineering work for preprocessing. Therefore, a query option where rules for search criteria can be stated ad hoc even on unstructured data would be an attractive feature for a data warehouse.

However, this topic has not been studied well for CDWs. The text query features of I2B2 are not published officially, but the documentation shows, that text data can be queried with the "like" operator of SQL[2]. That is similar expressive as wildcard queries.

---

[1] Corresponding Author, Georg Dietrich, Chair of Computer Science VI, Würzburg University, Am Hubland, 97074 Würzburg, Germany; E-mail: georg.dietrich@uni-wuerzburg.de.
[2] http://community.i2b2.org/wiki/display/DevForum/Text+search+in+i2b2

This search is a filter, it does not extract data. In addition, it is much faster to query an indexed document than to use the SQL like operator processing the entire text.

This paper describes a query extension for the CDW PaDaWaN of the University Hospital Würzburg and a feasibility study in which patient recruitment will be done with complex ad-hoc queries for patients from a stroke unit. The input is a query containing the inclusion and exclusion criteria and the output is a list of suitable patients. It is intended, that an alert is generated, when a new potential participant has been found for the clinical trial. Challenging criteria for the recruitment include a rule condition on the duration from onset of the stroke till admission at the hospital and some exclusion criteria like atrial fibrillation.

2. Methods

The automatic patient recruitment system is a pipeline consisting of a query tool for the CDW that produces a spreadsheet with all relevant information which is then logically processed by an interpretation layer. The outcome are patients which are a candidates for recruitment (Figure 1).

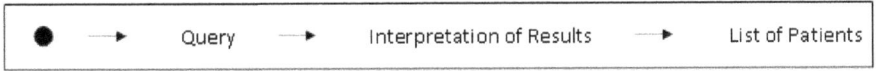

Figure 1. Pipeline of the recruitment system.

PaDaWaN uses as storage engine the index library Lucene[3] containing both structured and unstructured data. That's a big advantage for dealing with textual queries. During the index process, every piece of information runs through a data type specific pipeline for preprocessing before it is added to the index. The pipeline for text data contains basic NLP operations like stemming, stop word removal and ignoring case sensitivity.

The most important development took place in three different stations in the query progress. First we added a useful **preprocessing** function, second we added several powerful **query features** and third we modified the **result presentation** to make these improvements usable for further processing.

The additional preprocessing function is used to identify all negations and pseudo negations in a text by using a modified version of the negex algorithm [10]. The text is segmented in noun phrases which are classified whether they contain a negation or not.

Furthermore, discharge letters get segmented into sections like history, physical examination, lab data, etc. that are queryable separately afterwards.

The additional query features include basic, but strong functions like boolean retrieval, wildcards and phrase query. Boolean retrieval returns texts that contain some given words and can be combined using the logical operators *and, or, not*. Wildcards can be used at any position of a token to represent any characters. A phrase query matches a sequence of words like e.g. "Vorhofflimmern" (atrial fibrillation):
vhf OR vorhofflimm* OR vfli OR vofli OR fvhli

---

[3] https://lucene.apache.org/core/

A more advanced feature is a context specific query providing control over the order and proximity of the given terms. The input are two or more words that must be in a context to each other in the queried text, like e.g.:
[Flimmern Vorhof]

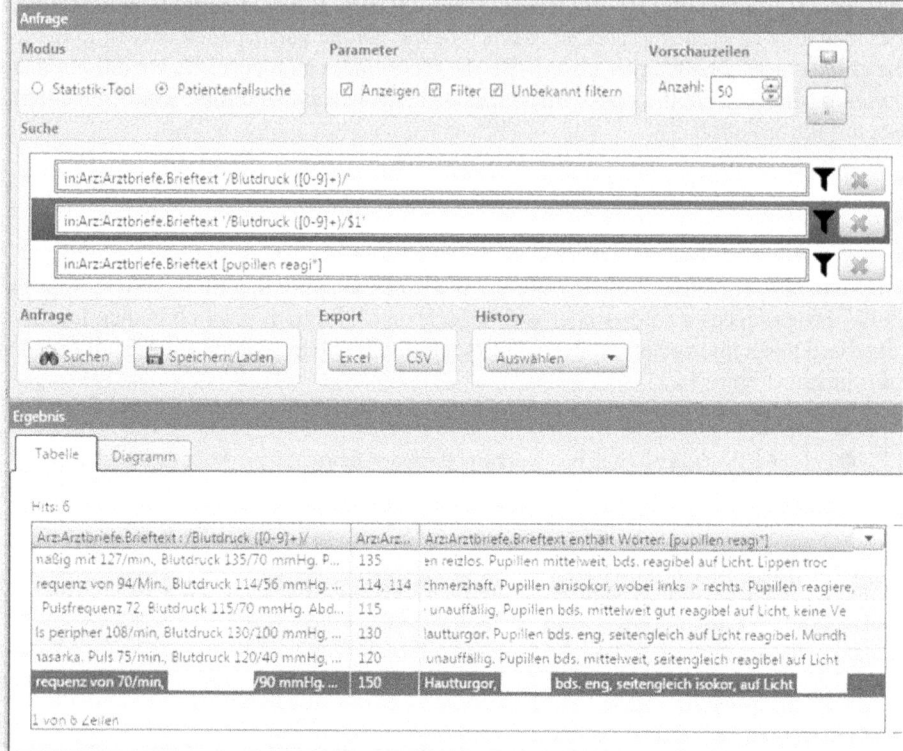

Figure 2. Example query in the PaDaWaN web app: First column shows a regex query which is displayed with context in the result snippet, second shows the extracted value of the regex query. The last column shows a context sensitive query with a wildcard.

Another powerful feature is the query with regular expressions (regex). The user can define a regex using the standard syntax including predefined character classes, quantifiers, alternatives and grouping. For subsequent processing the format of the output can be defined, too: the whole expression with context, just the expression or even a single group, e.g. a number, e.g.:
/parameter ([0-9]+)/$1

The expression is defined between the slashes. In this example, it must start with the string "parameter". The brackets define a group, here *[0-9]+* which represents a number. *$1* refers to the first group in the regex, the number. So the output of this regex is just the number that can be further processed by rules (see interpretation of results in Figure 1).

For dealing with the extraction of dates, many such expressions are necessary. To increase the usability a subquery mechanism allows splitting big queries into smaller groups. They can be stored separately and then referenced from other queries. That allows an incremental creation of complex queries.

The result presentation visualizes the results for the diverse query features. The hits of the given query terms are highlighted in matching documents from which small snippets are generated similar to Google. Optionally, the underlying entire text (i.e. the report) can be opened and the hit is highlighted in that as well. Each column of the result can also be exported in a CSV or Excel format (see Figure 2).

The query language is kept simple so that the physicians can use the tool on their own. They work together with technical experts for complex queries.

The interpretation layer in Figure 1 is a simple rule framework which transforms words like *noon* to *12 pm* or computes time differences between two timestamp.

3. Results

We evaluated the performance on 40 patient cases in the context of a stroke study recruitment task with emphasis on four different query features: standard keyword search, search with negations (atrial fibrillation negated), extraction of a numerical value (used by rules in the interpretation layer) and extraction of two timestamps of a day (used by the interpretation layer to compute a time span and compare it with a threshold). For this study we used no structured data, all information was extracted from text documents. Not all desired data was given within each patient case document, therefore we give the number of relevant documents in addition in Figure 3.

	Documents	Correct extractions	%
Standard keyword search	40	40	100
Keyword search with negations	40	39	97,5
Extraction of numerical values	39	38	97,4
Extraction of the time of a day	30	26	86,6

Figure 3. Evaluation results for four different query types within the feasibility study for patient recruitment

4. Discussion

Our solution to deal with negations in texts was to restrict the scope of the query to just two sections instead of the entire discharge letter. Otherwise, more errors would have been made than 1 in 40 documents. However, we used knowledge about the particular use case. Another way facing this problem is to improve the negation identification in general at preprocessing time, but this is still very challenging [11, 12, 13, 14].

The biggest challenge in the feasibility study was the computation of the duration of symptoms. To achieve that two dates have to be parsed and subtracted. Errors were made by mapping words like *"morning"* or *"since awake"* to the specific date and time, because some words were not covered by the rules and the resolution of other dates was incorrect. For this use case, working with time intervals would be simpler and sufficient, because only the classification of the duration of two dates matters. For instance, the duration between since *"awake"* and *"noon"* could be categorised into "less than 10 hours".

5. Conclusion

This paper presents a lightweight but powerful instant information extraction method approach for recruiting patients for a clinical study. It allows to gain information from unstructured texts. The engineering process takes minutes instead of weeks or month, when the data is preprocessed by an information extraction approach.

Further development will be done to add features and to expand the expressive power. One specific goal of future work is the integration of the interpretation layer into the query tool, which is currently a post-processing step. Then the system would e.g. be able to perform interval arithmetic or complex calculations like BMI = weight / height^2.

6. Conflict of Interest

The authors have no conflict of interests.

References

[1] Schreiweis B, Trinczek B, Köpcke F, Leusch T, Majeed R, Wenk J, Bergh B, Ohmann C, Röhrig R, Dugas M, Prokosch H. Comparison of Electronic Health Record SystemFunctionalities to support the patient recruitmentprocess in clinical trials. International Journal of Medical Informatics, 83(11), 860-868, 2014
[2] Murphy S, Weber G, Mendis M, Gainer V, Chueh HC, Churchill S, Kohane I. Serving the Enterprise and beyond with Informatics for Integrating Biology and the Bedside (i2b2), J Am Med Inform Assoc. 17(2) (2010) 124-130.
[3] Dietrich, G., Fell, F., Fette, G., Krebs, J., Ertl, M., Kaspar, M., Störk, S. Puppe, F.: Web-PaDaWaN: Eine Web-basierte Benutzeroberfläche für ein klinisches Data Warehouse (2016). HEC 2016, Joint Conference of GMDS, DGEpi, IEA-EEF, EFMI, DocAbstr. 421, 2016.
[4] Majeed R, Röhrig R.Identifying patients for clinical trials using fuzzy ternary logic expressions on HL7 messages. Stud Health Technol Inform, 169, 170-174, 2011
[5] Lonsdale DW, Tustison C, Parker CG, Embley DW. Assessing clinical trial eligibility with logic expression queries. Data & Knowledge Engineering; 66(1): 3–17, 2008
[6] Dietrich, G.; Fette, G.; Puppe, F.: A Comparison of Search Engine Technologies for a Clinical Data Warehouse. in CEUR Workshop Proceedings, T. Seidl, Hassani, M., Beecks, C. (eds.) (2014). (Vol. 1226) 235-242.
[7] Starlinger J, Kittner M, Blankenstein O, Leser U. How to Improve Information Extraction from German Medical Notes, it - Information Technology 58 (10/2016).
[8] Krieger H.-U., Spurk C., Uszkoreit H., Xu F., Zhang Y., Mueller F., and Tolxdorff T. Information extraction from german patient records via hybrid parsing and relation extraction strategies. In LREC, pages 2043-2048, 2014.
[9] Toepfer M., Corovic H., Fette G., Kluegl P., Stoerk S., and Puppe F. Fine-grained information extraction from german transthoracic echocardiography reports. BMC medical informatics and decision making, 15(1):1, 2015.
[10] Chapman W, Bridewell W, Hanbury P, Cooper GF and Buchanan BG, A simple algorithm for identifying negated findings and diseases in discharge summaries. Journal of Biomedical Informatics. Volume 34, Issue 5, October 2001, Pages 301-310
[11] Wu S, Miller T, Masanz J, Coarr M, Halgrim S, Carrell D, Clark C. Negation's Not Solved: Generalizability Versus Optimizability in Clinical Natural Language Processing. 2014. PLOS ONE 9(11)
[12] Mutalik P, Deshpande A, Nadkarni PM. Use of general-purpose negation detection to augment concept indexing of medical documents: a quantitative study using the UMLS. J Am Med Inform Assoc. 2001 Nov-Dec;8(6):598-609.
[13] Huang Y, Lowe HJ. A novel hybrid approach to automated negation detection in clinical radiology reports. J Am Med Inform Assoc. 2007 May-Jun;14(3):304-11. Epub 2007 Feb 28.
[14] Sohn S, Wu S, Chute CG.; Dependency Parser-based Negation Detection in Clinical Narratives. AMIA Jt Summits Transl Sci Proc. 2012; 2012: 1–8.

German Medical Data Sciences: Visions and Bridges
R. Röhrig et al. (Eds.)

157

doi:10.3233/978-1-61499-808-2-157

Implementation of Task-Tracking Software for Clinical IT Management

Anne-Maria PUROHIT[a,1], Clemens BRUTSCHECK[a], Hans-Ulrich PROKOSCH[a], Thomas GANSLANDT[a] and Martin SCHNEIDER[a]

[a] *University Hospital Erlangen, IT Department*

Abstract. Often in clinical IT departments, many different methods and IT systems are used for task-tracking and project organization. Based on managers' personal preferences and knowledge about project management methods, tools differ from team to team and even from employee to employee. This causes communication problems, especially when tasks need to be done in cooperation with different teams. Monitoring tasks and resources becomes impossible: there are no defined deliverables, which prevents reliable deadlines. Because of these problems, we implemented task-tracking software which is now in use across all seven teams at the University Hospital Erlangen. Over a period of seven months, a working group defined types of tasks (project, routine task, etc.), workflows, and views to monitor the tasks of the 7 divisions, 20 teams and 340 different IT services. The software has been in use since December 2016.

Keywords. Health information management, information management, Project management

1. Introduction

1.1 Introduction

The IT Department of the University Hospital Erlangen, Germany, has 130 employees in seven divisions. The work is organized in functional teams (systems technology, hospital information systems, and desktop services, among others) as well as in cross-functional and interdisciplinary project teams. Several tools are in use for project and task planning and controlling - from paper-based Post-it notes, to Excel lists, MS outlook tasks, Microsoft (MS) SharePoint lists, MS Project plans, and so forth. Double documentation is unavoidable in keeping the to-do lists of individual employees and project plans (if they exist) updated. The status of routine tasks and projects is often only available to one team - unclear dependencies between projects and routine activities follow. Another issue is controlling tasks, which are often discussed and assigned in meetings and require the employee to transfer them to their own to-do lists. Our goal was therefore to implement task-tracking software to manage all IT projects and tasks across teams. A key goal is a comprehensive project list that shows all activities of the IT department at first glance.

---

[1] Corresponding Author: Anne-Maria Purohit, IT Department/Med. IK-Zentrum, University Hospital Erlangen, Glückstraße 11, 91052 Erlangen, Germany; E-mail: anne-maria.purohit@uk-erlangen.de

1.2 Requirements

- R1: The tool should be used for managing projects of different sizes as well as for managing routine operations (termed "functional tasks" in this paper). Tracking and controlling tasks from different sources (functional tasks, project tasks, task assigned in meetings, personal to-dos) in one database is required.

- R2: It should be possible to create different views of the task database for managers, individual users, project/functional teams, and for the whole IT department.

- R3: The tool should allow the user to communicate about tasks, to set a due date and workflow statuses, assign these to a team or a coworker, and document structured information like clients and stakeholders involved.

- R4: The documentation of project plans with different hierarchy levels (work breakdown structure) is required. The tool should allow building a schedule.

- R5: The user should be able to filter, search, and sort tasks by due date, assignee, IT service and status, and see all projects across departments and institutions.

- R6: Connection between tasks and documentation (project documentation, meeting notes, technical documentation, release notes, etc.) is required.

The documentation of tasks associated with changes to incidents and service requests (SR) was not planned (definition: see IT Infrastructure Library (ITIL) [1]). A help-desk system for first-level support is already in use, so we decided to set up the task-tracking systems for project tasks and as a next step include the documentation of incidents / SR in the new tool.

2. State of the art

There is a consensus among experts that problems in healthcare IT projects are more managerial than technical [2]. Most of health IT projects do not deliver what they should, are over budget or are late [3, 4]. Literature has proven that missing project management (PM) methods are one significant reason why IT implementations fail [5, 6, 7]. But the reality of many IT departments in healthcare is: too many simultaneous and dependent projects, insufficient PM skills of software engineers and a lack of professional PM tools [8, p. 32]. 45% of the IT-projects in German Hospitals are not reaching their set goals [8, p. 32]. And IT health care departments are most of the time organized as a combination of two or more types of organizational structures, such as the project-organization-structure and the functional organization structure [9]. So functions are moved from functional departments like "In-patient Clinical Applications" etc. to project teams. Allocation of resources is only possible if tasks on both sides are documented with the same quality. The implementation of a task-tracking software should solve these problems: one tool for all teams, which includes all health IT projects at the university hospital and specified standards for the documentation of tasks.

3. Concept

A working group of 15 key users and managers for selection and customization of a software tool for task-tracking and project management was founded in May 2016. Meetings were twice a month or weekly. The following specifications were created.

3.1 Task contexts

We identified four task contexts: projects, work in functional teams, committees and personal tasks. Because the organization has a matrix structure, we want to have both types of tasks in the system: functional objectives (reported to functional managers) and project tasks (reported to project managers). For the third source of tasks, "committees" were identified; for example, a management board, where members were assigned to tasks in every topic. Normally, the assignee needs to transfer the task by hand from a protocol to its own to-do list. The challenge for the new tool was to skip this step and create the task directly in the protocol and assign it to a personal to-do list. We only want to use one tool for organizing tasks, so the option to document sensitive tasks and personal reminders was required. The different tasks needed varying kinds of authorization, which are shown in Table 1.

Table 1. Task categories and the authorized employees.

Categories of tasks	Description	Authorized Employees
Project	Task from a project role (project member)	Project team
Routine	Tasks from a functional role, standard changes	Functional team
Personal	Personal tasks	The specific user only
Committees	Task assigned in specific meetings (not project meetings)	Member of the board meetings

The transfer of tasks from one space to another should be possible, as well as views and queries on multiple projects.

3.2 Types of issues and hierarchy

To plan and track projects, a hierarchy of tasks is needed. The working group agreed that three levels are necessary. The new system needs to link tasks and the related packages to accumulate the progress of a task package based on its subtasks. In the committee space it should be possible to document important decisions right next to tasks.

3.3 Views on the task pool

The main question was: what do different stakeholders want to know? Which views do we need in a tracking system? Here are some examples:

- A single **user** wants to see all of his or her project tasks and the tasks of the IT services he or she supports, as well as the tasks of colleagues in functional teams or project teams.
- The **project manager** wants to see all tasks in the project in a timeline and in a hierarchical structure, and to monitor progress and assign tasks.
- The **functional manager** wants an overview of all of his or her team's

projects, as well as all tasks belonging to the IT service this team is in charge of.

- The **CIO, portfolio manager** and **advisory boards** want to see an overview of all planned, ongoing and closed projects.
- The **customer** wants to see the progress of the project they are paying for.

To create views about tasks related to specific IT services, every routine task needs to refer to one of the 340 IT services that the IT department hosts. The system should be flexible enough that there may be views defined on the task pool, (for example, for a single team) as well as the ability to easily build queries on the task pool.

4. Implementation

We chose the commercial software product JIRA (Version 7.2.7, Atlassian, AUS, https://de.atlassian.com/) as the issue tracking tool to fulfill the requirements. We bought JIRA (for agile software development) and JIRA core (for project management). We chose JIRA because it satisfied our main requirements, and could also connect with our enterprise wiki Confluence (Version 5.9), since they are made by the same vendor, Atlassian.Atlassian. The benefit was the simplicity in linking together project documentation in Confluence and task tracking in JIRA.

4.1   Projects in JIRA

JIRA offers projects as containers for different kinds of tasks - every container has its own concept of authorization. To support cross-functional work and transfer tasks from team to team, a container named "Routine" was created. This container encompasses all functional tasks and standard changes of all seven teams. This container is only accessible for members of the IT department. Every long-term project with its own project team and documentation has its own container in JIRA. All project members as well as physicians and nurses are granted access. Committees have their own container with a separate permission scheme and issue security.

4.2   Issue types and workflows in JIRA

In JIRA, every kind of issue can be implemented: bugs, feature requests, risks etc. We implemented four issue types: epics as a large piece of work which encompasses many issues, tasks, subtasks, and decisions. Epics, tasks and subtasks have similar field screens: they have the same four-step workflow (New Tasks, Approved Tasks, in Progress, Done) and due dates are required to create chronological project plans. Defining and using compatible fields and workflows for tasks from different sources makes it possible to transfer them from one project to another. We developed an add-on together with Seibert Media to assign JIRA issues in Confluence without opening JIRA (ConJira, V1.1, Seibert Media).

4.3   Views and filters in JIRA

We implemented the aforementioned views. The IT service related to each task also contains the information of the department and the team, which is responsible for the service. Based on this information it is possible to create views for teams without explicit documentation of the team. We built a dashboard showing the individual tasks for each employee. The tasks of operational teams and project teams were organized in Kanban Boards. An add-on called "Structure" was implemented to maintain a big picture of all projects and to organize the hierarchy of issues in project plans.

5. Lessons learned

The usage of IT depends on ease of use, usefulness and attitude. First, the documentation of the task needs to be fast: for example, through using autocomplete to search for a specific service. Second, the utility for an employee needs to be clear: for example better information and communication with coworkers and customers. A system driven solely by management and accounting will fail. To improve users' morale, every team should be involved in the customization process and the tool should used routinely, both in and out of meetings. Pain points in this project were the missing integration with the help-desk system and missing Gantt chart functionalities. For both problems, we are considering purchasing suitable Atlassian Ad-ons.

6. Conclusion

The tool has been in use since December 2016. We now have around 200 small projects and six long-term projects in JIRA, with over 3000 documented tasks. Last month, we started configuring JIRA for non-technical teams. The tool is in use in team meetings and by management to monitor and prioritize tasks and projects.

7. Conflict of Interest

The authors state that they have no conflicts of interest.

References

[1]   Aguttter, C., ITIL foundation handbook, AXELOS, London, (2015).
[2]   Kaplan, B., Harris-Salamone, K., Health IT Success and Failure: Recommendations from Literature and an AMIA Workshop. J Am Med Inform Assoc 2009; **16** (2009): 291-299.
[3]   Heeks R . Health information systems: Failure, success and improvisation. Int J Med Inf, **75** (2006); 125–137.
[4]   Wears RL., Berg M., Computer technology and clinical work: Still Waiting for Godot. J Am Med Assoc; **293** (2005), 1261–1263.
[5]   Paré, G. ; Sicotte, C. ; Jaana, M. ; Girouard, D.: Prioritizing the Risk Factors Influencing the Success of Clinical Information System Projects. In: Methods of information in medicine, **47** (2008), 251-259
[6]   Fleuren, M.: Determinants of innovation within health care organizations: Literature review and Delphi study, 16 (2004), 107-123.
[7]   Asad Mir F., Pinnington, AH., Exploring the value of project management. **32** (2014), 202-217.
[8]   Böckmann B, Akce A., Effectiv-IT Wertschöpfung von IT, Fachhochschule Dortmund/University of Applied Sciences and Arts, (2011).
[9]   Usmani, F. What is a Matrix Organization Structure? https://pmstudycircle.com/2012/08/what-is-a-matrix-organization-structure/; last access: 2017-06-01, (2012).

6. Interoperability – Standards, Terminologies, Classification

German Medical Data Sciences: Visions and Bridges
R. Röhrig et al. (Eds.)

165

doi:10.3233/978-1-61499-808-2-165

Expert2OWL: A Methodology for Pattern-Based Ontology Development

Kais TAHAR[a,1], Jie XU[a], Heinrich HERRE[a]

[a] *Institute of Medical Informatics, Statistics and Epidemiology, Medical Faculty, Leipzig University*

Abstract. The formalization of expert knowledge enables a broad spectrum of applications employing ontologies as underlying technology. These include eLearning, Semantic Web and expert systems. However, the manual construction of such ontologies is time-consuming and thus expensive. Moreover, experts are often unfamiliar with the syntax and semantics of formal ontology languages such as OWL and usually have no experience in developing formal ontologies. To overcome these barriers, we developed a new method and tool, called *Expert2OWL* that provides efficient features to support the construction of OWL ontologies using GFO (General Formal Ontology) as a top-level ontology. This method allows a close and effective collaboration between ontologists and domain experts. Essentially, this tool integrates Excel spreadsheets as part of a pattern-based ontology development and refinement process. *Expert2OWL* enables us to expedite the development process and modularize the resulting ontologies. We applied this method in the field of Chinese Herbal Medicine (CHM) and used *Expert2OWL* to automatically generate an accurate Chinese Herbology ontology (CHO). The expressivity of CHO was tested and evaluated using ontology query languages SPARQL and DL. CHO shows promising results and can generate answers to important scientific questions such as which Chinese herbal formulas contain which substances, which substances treat which diseases, and which ones are the most frequently used in CHM.

Keywords. Ontology development, Biomedical Ontologies, Knowledge Representation, Herbal Medicine, TCM, Expert2OWL

1. Introduction and related works

The formalization of expert knowledge about a domain requires a formal specification of the terms and relations the knowledge is built upon. In this paper, we apply the term ontology for knowledge systems represented in a formal language, such as OWL [1]. The formalization of expert knowledge enables a broad spectrum of applications, among them eLearning and expert systems [2]. In this work, we analyze various textual information about Traditional Chinese Medicine (TCM) from public resources such as TCM textbooks and online encyclopedias [3-4] as a source of domain knowledge as well as TCM expert experiences. Our aim is to propose a method for supporting the structural acquisition of knowledge in these resources and its formalization within OWL 2 DL [1]. The formalization of domain knowledge by OWL ontologies has the potential to offer to experts significant benefits in their domain. However, most domain

---
[1] Kais Tahar, IMISE, University of Leipzig, Härtelstr. 16-18, 04107 Leipzig, Germany;
E-mail: kais.tahar@imise.uni-leipzig.de

experts lack skills in using formal languages such as OWL or DL and usually have no experience in developing formal ontologies [2,5]. Domain experts therefore risk spending too much time in constructing ontologies that are in many cases impractical. To overcome these problems, experts need a domain core ontology (DCO) that defines and inter-relates the basic entities to formalize their domain knowledge in a useful manner. For that reason, domain experts should collaborate with ontologists to develop well-founded ontologies by using top-level ontologies such as GFO [6]. In addition, domain experts need easy access to authoring and refinement processes so that a close and effective collaboration with ontologists can be established.

We analyzed several existing tools mentioned in [2,5] such as *Mapping Master*, *Populous*, and *Excel2OWL* for their potential to build the CHO from our spreadsheets, but we concluded that none of these tools could be applied to our project. Due to the fact that these tools do not support pattern design with arbitrary restriction quantifiers and do not cover complex expressions such as intersection sets and equivalent classes axioms, we developed a new method and tool, called *Expert2OWL*.

Throughout this paper, we use standard semantic web terminology that refers to formal descriptions of ontological entities [1,7]. The rest of the paper is organized as follows: Section 2 explains *Expert2OWL* as an ontology engineering method, Section 3 presents the results obtained by applying this method in the field of CHM and finally, Section 4 concludes with a discussion and an outlook on future work.

2. Methods

Expert2OWL provides efficient features to support the collaborative development of OWL ontologies using GFO. Essentially, this tool integrates the Excel spreadsheet as part of a pattern-driven ontology development and refinement process. *Expert2OWL* enables an automatic transformation of spreadsheet content into OWL axioms. Axioms for a domain are logical expressions, written in a formal language such as first-order logic or DL [1], which are valid in the considered domain. Relational propositions are expressions that specify certain relationships between entities of a given domain. Relational propositions can be either true or false, while axioms on the contrary are certainty propositions that have the highest logical value in a domain and therefore represent domain tautologies [8]. For this reason, we use domain core axioms (DCAs) in our method as a foundation for the formalization and analysis of domain knowledge. Essentially, *Expert2OWL* implements a method that separates the full axiomatization from the immediate compilation of graspable propositions that experts rated as significant and, hence, are assumed to be true in the considered domain (see Figure 1).

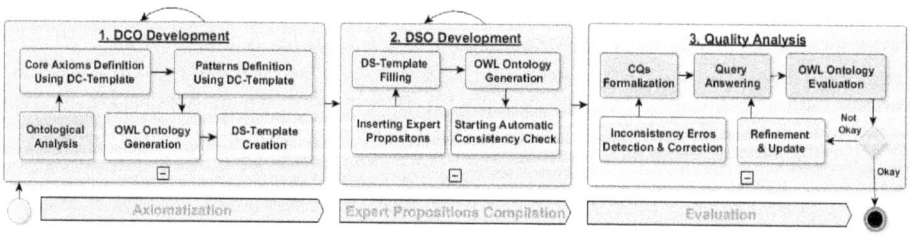

Figure 1. A pattern-based methodology for developing OWL ontologies using spreadsheets. The pale blue boxes show all tasks supported by the tool *Expert2OWL*.

These experts' propositions should be consistent with the defined DCAs. For example, in this work we collected propositions from TCM experts involved in the ontology development process. To automatically verify the consistency of these propositions, we implemented an inference engine that extends *Expert2OWL* with automated reasoning methods based on the previously declared DCAs. Our method is realized by a workflow that consists of three steps, called Axiomatization, Expert Propositions Compilation and Evaluation, which allow multiple iterations. This workflow is described using BPMN elements (see Figure 1). In the first step, ontologists develop a DCO based on interviews with domain experts by using a top-level ontology such as GFO. GFO provides a basic method for specifying the DCAs. The development of DCAs is the main and most creative task of the ontologist who collaborates with experts on this topic. We consulted TCM experts from the China Academy of Chinese Medical Sciences (CACMS) in Beijing, who provided answers to some important questions, such as the issues of compatibility of drugs and dose, the specification of meridians, and important information about clinical use cases including dosages of toxic herbal drugs. As a result, we developed an accurate and expressive DCO named GFO-CHO using *Expert2OWL*. GFO-CHO extends GFO with basic concepts, material objects, and symbolic structures illustrated in Table 1. The developed DCAs include axiom patterns, equivalent class axioms, disjoint class axioms, and embedding axioms. The Embedding axioms integrate the acquired knowledge in GFO (see Table 1).

Table 1. Embedding axioms for integrating the developed core ontology of Chinese Herbal Medicine in GFO.

GFO entities	GFO-CHO entities
gfo:concept	*gfo-cho:Chinese_herbal_fromula (CHF)* , *gfo-cho:TCM_therapeutic_use (TTU), gfo-cho:Health_problem (HP), gfo-cho:Disease, gfo-cho:Symptom, gfo cho:Drug_prescription (DP), gfo-cho:TCM_drug_prescription (TDP).*
gfo:Material_object	*gfo-cho:Budy_part (BP), gfo-cho:Meridian (M), gfo-cho:Plant (P), gfo-cho:Drug,, gfo-cho:Chinese_herbal_drug (CHD), gfo-cho:Substance (S).*
gfo: Symbol structures	*gfo-cho:Code (C), gfo-cho:ICD10_code (IC).*

We define axiom patterns as a specific type of DCA that is more complex and contain free variables. These complex patterns can be reused for assisting the implementation of experts' propositions such as semantic relationships between concepts or individuals (see Table 2). To support the development of these design patterns, *Expert2OWL* provides a domain core Template (DC-Template). This template offers a practical formalism for the specification of DCAs including pattern axioms with arbitrary restriction quantifiers. Using this template content, *Expert2OWL* generates an OWL ontology automatically. The resulting DCO contains OWL axiom patterns that restrict the basic types and relations within this domain. Based on these axiom patterns, *Expert2OWL* also creates a partly restricted domain specific template (DS-Template) automatically. This DS-Template is restricted with a drop down list (DDL) of binary relationships that point out the corresponding design patterns (see Table 2).

The second step – Expert Propositions Compilation – was also supported by *Expert2OWL*. During this step, experts compiled domain specific knowledge in the form of relational propositions that represent simple statements of the form SPO (subject predicate object). Hence, the structure of the DS-Template consists of three columns: one column for binary relations (predicate) and two columns for the relations' arguments. The domain expert selects the corresponding relationship from the DDL and adds a relational proposition regarding two domain entities (see Table 2). The variable Symbols *?X* and *?Y* are replaced with the first and second arguments of the domain expert's proposition. These arguments can be added arbitrarily because the consistency of each added propositions can be verified automatically using reasoning on axiom patterns of the developed DCO. The benefit of this modeling method is that it allows domain experts to describe the semantic network of CHM with relational propositions that are close to natural language sentences. This provides domain experts with an easy way to access the development process of formal ontologies without having to resort to learning a complex ontology language such as OWL. As a result, *Expert2OWL* generates a domain specific ontology (DSO) from the DS-Template.

Once the development process is finished, the next step is quality analysis, where the performance and quality of the developed ontology are evaluated and rapidly improved by using *Expert2OWL*. The earlier versions of CHO contained many inconsistency errors. *Expert2OWL* provides an inference engine that detects inconsistent expert's propositions and corrects them automatically. To evaluate the resulting ontology, we implemented several competency questions (CQs) [2] using SPARQL and DL[1].

Table 2. The first column shows exemplary relationships of the DDL. The second column illustrate the corresponding axiom patterns expressed in Manchester OWL Syntax with argument variables ?X and ?Y.

Relationships	OWL axiom patterns expressed in Manchester OWL Syntax
hasIngredient	*Class: ?X SubClassOf: CHF AND hasIngredient some ?Y*
	Class: ?Y SubClassOf: CHD
hasPlantSource	*Class: ?X SubClassOf: CHB AND hasIngredient only ?Y Class: ?Y SubClassOf: P*
hasMeridian	*Class: ?X SubClassOf: CHB AND hasMeridan only ?Y Class: ?Y SubClassOf: M*
relatedToCode	*Class: ?X SubClassOf: gfo:Entity AND relatedToCode some ?Y*
	Class:?Y AND SubClassOf: ID
instanceOf	*Individual: ?X Tpyes: ?Y Class: ?Y*
equivalentTo	*Class: ?X EquivalentTo: ?Y Class: ?Y*
hasProcedure	*Class: ?X SubClassOf: CHF AND Annotations:hasProcedure "?Y"*

3. Results

The proposed methodology was implemented as a tool named *Expert2OWL* and applied in the field of CHM. We consulted TCM experts and analyzed public textual resources [3-4] to discover important common basic entities and properties of Chinese herbal formulas and drugs such as prime ingredient, procedure, indication, dosage, disease, TCM therapeutic use, meridian, chemical compositions, and toxicity. As a result, *Expert2OWL* generates a formal CHO. It contains 2046 classes, 14 object properties, 1808 individuals and 16847 axioms that restrict CHO entities. A total of 4103 of these axioms were inferred automatically after inconsistency detection and correction with *Expert2OWL*. The resulting CHO is composed of two ontologies. The DCO contains 14 object properties and 131 DCAs, which are specified and implemented using *Expert2OWL* to integrate CHO entities in GFO. The DSO contains all essential individuals that instantiate 139 CHF, 193 CHD, 187 P, 576 S, 340 IC and 405 HP. All HPs including diseases and symptoms were coded in ICD-10 to promote the internationalization of CHM, and to harmonize it with Western medicine.

In addition, the expressivity of CHO was tested using multiple CQs implemented in SPARQL and DL. CHO yielded promising results and generated answers to important scientific questions. One example showed that Liquoric Root (甘草, Gan Cao) is the most frequently used herbal drug. It contains the substances glycyrrhetinic acid, glycyrrhizin, licochalcone, licorice extract and liquiritin. This drug was used in 65 CHFs and treats several health problems such as palpilations, dyspnoea and cough.

4. Discussion and outlook

A major benefit of our methodology compared with existing ones mentioned in [2,5] is that it provides features that support the collaborative development of new design patterns and enables the integration of the acquired knowledge in GFO. Furthermore, with *Expert2OWL* we can also separate the resulting DCO from the DSO. This enables us to expedite the development process of OWL ontologies and modularize the resulting ontologies. Another main advantage of our method is that it provides a general common formalism that is largely independent of the application case since the architecture of *Expert2OWL* stipulates the separation of the full axiomatization from the immediate compilation of domain specific knowledge in the form of relational propositions (see figure 1). Consequently, this method enables experts to subsequently change the DCAs including the restriction quantifiers consistently and easily in the DC-Template without redefining the Java source code. Furthermore, it provides automated detection and correction of inconsistency errors. Our approach thus offers to experts an easy and efficient way to build domain ontologies without resorting to complex ontology editing tools or even OWL syntax. Hence, *Expert2OWL* facilitates the domain experts' involvement in a collaborative ontology development process and reduces the required development time and costs. *Expert2OWL* can also be transformed into a web-based tool for real time collaborative ontology development so that multiple domain experts could share their filled templates and work simultaneously on the same content but from different PCs to generate consolidated domain ontologies. The resulting ontologies can be integrated into a knowledge base for analyzing Big Data using GFO. The benefit of using this top level ontology is the semantic interoperability that allows harmonizing related domain knowledge such as chemistry, pharmacy, medicine and biology. The embedded reasoner can infer implicit knowledge and detect inconsistency errors automatically.

In addition, the query answering method can be extended to build an ontology-based software that supports drug discovery from herbal medicine. The application of such a tool could effectively support and expedite drug research.

Acknowledgement.

We thank Dr. Yan Zhu from CACMS in Nanxiaojie 16, Dongzhimennei, Beijing for his support in clarifying various important notions in TCM.

References

[1] Hitzler P., Krötzsch M., Rudolph S., Sure Y., Semantic Web. Grundlagen. Springer, Berlin, 2008.
[2] Tahar K, Schaaf M, Jahn F, Kücherer C, Paech B, Herre H, Winter A. An approach to support collaborative ontology construction. *Studies in health technology and informatics* **228** (2016), 369-373.
[3] Zhu Zhenheng, Ming Chenchong, *Danxi's Mastery of Medicine*, China Bookstore press, Beijing, 1986.
[4] http://www.wiki8.com (accessed Mars, 3 2017)
[5] Jupp S et al., Populous: a tool for building OWL ontologies from templates, *BMC Bioinformatics* **13** (2012), S5
[6] Herre H: General Formal Ontology (GFO): A Foundational Ontology for Conceptual Modelling. In *Theory and Applications of Ontology: Computer Applications*, Springer, Netherlands; 2010, 297–345.
[7] Geroimenko V., *Dictionary of XML Technologies and the Semantic Web*, Springer, London, 2004
[8] Mendelson, E. *Introduction to Mathematical logic*, Van Nostrand, Princeton, 1964.

German Medical Data Sciences: Visions and Bridges
R. Röhrig et al. (Eds.)
© 2017 German Association for Medical Informatics, Biometry and Epidemiology (gmds) e.V. and IOS Press.
This article is published online with Open Access by IOS Press and distributed under the terms
of the Creative Commons Attribution Non-Commercial License 4.0 (CC BY-NC 4.0).
doi:10.3233/978-1-61499-808-2-170

Light-Weighted Automatic Import of Standardized Ontologies into the Content Management System Drupal

Christoph BEGER [a,b,1], Alexandr UCITELI [a] and Heinrich HERRE [a]

[a] *University of Leipzig, Institute for Medical Informatics, Statistics and Epidemiology*
[b] *University of Leipzig, University Hospital, Wachstumsnetzwerk CrescNet*

Abstract. The amount of ontologies, which are utilizable for widespread domains, is growing steadily. BioPortal alone, embraces over 500 published ontologies with nearly 8 million classes. In contrast, the vast informative content of these ontologies is only directly intelligible by experts. To overcome this deficiency it could be possible to represent ontologies as web portals, which does not require knowledge about ontologies and their semantics, but still carries as much information as possible to the end-user. Furthermore, the conception of a complex web portal is a sophisticated process. Many entities must be analyzed and linked to existing terminologies. Ontologies are a decent solution for gathering and storing this complex data and dependencies. Hence, automated imports of ontologies into web portals could support both mentioned scenarios. The Content Management System (CMS) Drupal 8 is one of many solutions to develop web presentations with less required knowledge about programming languages and it is suitable to represent ontological entities. We developed the Drupal Upper Ontology (DUO), which models concepts of Drupal's architecture, such as nodes, vocabularies and links. DUO can be imported into ontologies to map their entities to Drupal's concepts. Because of Drupal's lack of import capabilities, we implemented the Simple Ontology Loader in Drupal (SOLID), a Drupal 8 module, which allows Drupal administrators to import ontologies based on DUO. Our module generates content in Drupal from existing ontologies and makes it accessible by the general public. Moreover Drupal offers a tagging system which may be amplified with multiple standardized and established terminologies by importing them with SOLID. Our Drupal module shows that ontologies can be used to model content of a CMS and vice versa CMS are suitable to represent ontologies in a user-friendly way. Ontological entities are presented to the user as discrete pages with all appropriate properties, links and tags.

Keywords. Automatic data processing, biomedical ontology, information storage and retrieval, knowledge bases, metadata

1. Introduction

Drupal is an open source Content Management System (CMS). It was initially release in 2001 and ranks on the third place of all CMS ordered by market share with approximately 5%, according to Web Technology Surveys [1]. The benefit of using a CMS like Drupal is that users do not need any programming skills to create content on CMS based webpages. Drupal in its initial form, allows the user to create content as "node" with a

---

[1] Corresponding Author: **Christoph.Beger@imise.uni-leipzig.de**

comprehensive User Interface. Concrete nodes can be tagged by predefined vocabulary terms and the terms allow users to search for content with specific common features. Drupal profits from an active community, which develops many new functionalities via modules. Those modules can be installed in Drupal to enrich its features.

Leipzig Health Atlas (LHA) is an ongoing project at the University of Leipzig, funded by the German Ministry of Education and Research (reference number: 031L0026, program: i:DSem – Integrative Datensemantik in der Systemmedizin). The goal of LHA is to integrate information about finished projects, publications and corresponding data sets on a website to allow interested persons access of metadata and to possibly support upcoming scientific projects. In LHA we developed an ontology to describe mentioned entities, their properties and complex ties. After this step we uncovered the demand for a module which is capable of importing ontologies into Drupal.

At the time of writing this article there exists no reliable method to import ontologies into Drupal 8, which preserves hierarchies and properties of entities. Indeed, there is a Drupal module called Open Semantic Framework [2], but it is only available for version 7 and it does not incorporate ontological entities in Drupal's default database. Therefore if one wants to transfer data from an ontology into Drupal 8, it has to be done the manual way by creating content by hand. This deficiency is acceptable for small ontologies, but with growing size the required time increases to an unreasonable state.

The implementation of a Drupal module could simplify imports of ontologies significantly. Also, importing ontologies in Drupal could make them accessible to users without knowledge about ontologies, while motivating developers to model their content in ontologies, aware that those ontologies are easy to import in Drupal. Further, already existing and established ontologies/terminologies could be used to automatically create vocabularies in Drupal by extracting all required classes.

2. Methods

Based on the "Three ontology method" [3] we developed the Drupal Upper Ontology (DUO) as Task Ontology and integrated our LHA Ontology as Domain Ontology into it. DUO models concepts of Drupal's architecture, such as nodes, vocabularies and links.

2.1. The Drupal Upper Ontology

We developed an ontology which represents default components of Drupal (fields, nodes, files, vocabularies). The idea is to provide users predefined Drupal concepts which shall be specialized and instantiated in a domain ontology, so that the import module is able to map entities of the domain ontology into Drupal's database. Note that Drupal's fields (e.g. *title* or *content*) are represented in DUO as properties, node types (e.g. *Project* or *Publication*) and vocabulary tags (e.g. *Disease1*) as classes and concrete nodes (e.g. *Project1*) as individuals. Additional entities or files may be instantiated for reusability.

Figure 1 shows the structure of DUO and an exemplary Domain Ontology. The dashed connections between both ontologies symbolize instantiation, subclass and subproperty relations respectively. For integration and formal foundation of both, Task and Domain Ontology [3], we used the General Formal Ontology (GFO) [4] as Top-Level Ontology. In GFO sense we distinguish between symbolic structures (content of the pages, like text and images) and the entities (concepts or individuals, like concrete projects), that are represented by the symbolic structures. For the sake of simplicity we consider *duo:Entity, duo:Node* and *duo:File* as subclasses of *gfo:Individual* and *duo:Vocabulary* as a subclass of *gfo:Concept*. The precise ontological analysis of DUO entities is out of scope of this paper and will be covered in a separate publication.

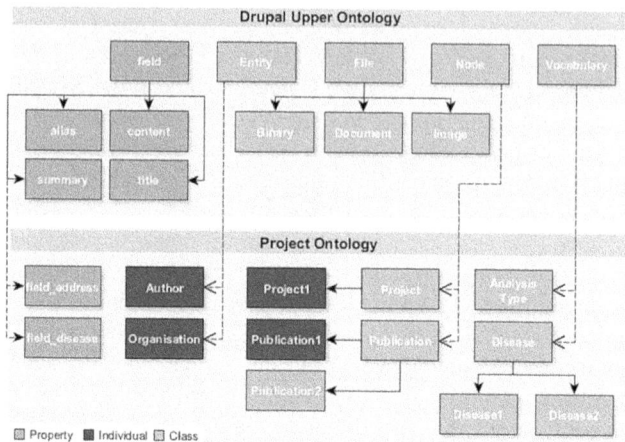

Figure 1. Structure of DUO as ER diagram with connections to a generic Domain Ontology.

2.2. Guideline for Ontology Conversion

In this section we explain how to modifying an existing or developing a new ontology to make it importable with our module. To avoid errors during the import process we defined some restrictions and requirements for an importable ontology. An ontology must import DUO, because only classes and properties which are defined by DUO and specialized or instantiated by the importing ontology itself are recognized. All remaining entities are ignored. Properties must match machine-readable field names in Drupal.

The next step concerns classifications of individuals (nodes) by concepts of vocabularies. To make the class hierarchies available as vocabularies you have to define a new subclass of *duo:Vocabulary* and assign all affected root classes to it. This allows the module to recognize vocabularies and their hierarchies.

Drupal is based on publishing pages with specific content. To denote individuals, which should be represented as page, assign them to a subclass of *duo:Node*. The subclass corresponds to Drupal's content type. It is also possible to import classes as Drupal pages. Additionally data respective annotation properties specify the values of node fields and object respective annotation properties denote links between node pages.

3. Results

We implemented a Drupal 8 compatible module[2], which is able to parse OWL or JSON files and imports extracted data by using Drupal's inbuilt API. Our module compensates Drupal's lack of an ontology import. Most ontologies can be easily transformed with small adjustments and resulting normalized ontologies are imported within a few steps.

---

[2] The module is available as download from the releases section of our GitHub repository: *https://github.com/Onto-Med/SOLID/releases*

The creation of the LHA metadata ontology was an ongoing process but very early iterations already consisted of approximately 100 classes, 200 individuals and 2000 axioms. Within a few minutes and with hardly any effort we imported mentioned metadata and implemented an automated pipeline, which periodically synchronized Drupal's database records and the ontology by using our module.

The Simple Ontology Loader in Drupal (SOLID) consists of components for file handling/parsing and data import. A file handler is used to parse uploaded files and transform the content into a PHP object. Depending on the file format, a factory serves the appropriate file handler. Additional file handlers can be added by inheriting *AbstractFileHandler*. At its current state the module implements two handlers, one for OWL (using the integrated EasyRdf library [5] of Drupal 8) and one for JSON. The JSON file is directly convertible to a PHP object and thus does not require conversions.

The file handler for OWL files extracts all classes beneath *duo:Vocabulary*. Direct children denote separate taxonomies and all children of these classes are hierarchical tags. In contrast to vocabularies, nodes can be individuals or classes, which instantiate direct subclasses of *duo:Node* or which are subclasses of them respectively. Their properties are stored as data, object or annotation properties. To extract the properties for an entity, the module iterates over all defined properties of the ontology. Imported properties are ignored, unless they are part of DUO. The module automatically resolves references to other individuals and extracts data depending on the instantiated class of the individual.

4. Discussion

Our module allows the import of any ontology (which imports DUO) without much effort. We expect that this novel way of presenting ontologies within Drupal will lower the barrier to access semantical structures, because ontological Entities and their relations are depicted with traditional websites and links. Furthermore the module enables ontology experts to model complex content of web portals as ontology and import them into Drupal.

Different approaches exist to combine semantics with CMS. For example Das et al. [6] introduced the Science Collaboration Framework (SCF), which supports web communities of the biomedical domain with semantical awareness. The authors describe a Drupal-based architecture, which can be enriched by gene ontologies. They mention proxies for referencing genes from multiple RDF-repositories, so that Drupal content is annotatable with those genes. Proxies are not generic, hence require implementations for each data source. The SCF enables annotation of existing Drupal content with ontology concepts, whereas SOLID allows to import semantically enriched content directly into Drupal so that its structures and properties are directly accessible by domain experts.

There are other domains where the amount of available data increases. For example according to [7] the recent "improvements in DNA sequencing have vastly increased the quantity and availability of genomic [...] data". Therefore, the authors of mentioned article developed the construction toolkit Tripal, which is a combination of Drupal and Chado, a database schema for storage of biological data. Where our import module transforms datasets into Drupal entities, Tripal brings a new database schema to store datasets and provides management, visualization and search capabilities. Both approaches are important in terms of data accessibility, but Tripal is more appropriate for domain experts for genomic data, where our module aims to present more general ontological data to non-domain experts.

Above mentioned articles are Drupal-based. Befa et al. [8] details an extension for the CMS Alfresco [9], which facilitates import and export of content as RDF/S ontology. The extension only supports data properties, whereas our module understands OWL syntax and allows the import of all property types. If a proper use case exists for Drupal content export as OWL, we may enhance our module with an export functionality.

In future, more and more sources of data will emerge and tools like SOLID will be necessary to improve the accessibility of highly domain specific data, which is also utilizable for other research areas.

5. Conclusion

Ontologies are available in a vast number to many domains, but they suffer from poor accessibility for non-ontologists. We developed a novel approach to overcome mentioned deficiency, by implementing a Drupal 8 module with import capabilities for ontologies. Our module enables an expert to present his ontologies to the general public, because ontological entities are transformed into Drupal nodes. Moreover, the module enhances the conception of a web portal, because complex entities and their relations can be easily modeled with an ontology. In consequence, the entities are importable with our module. All functionalities of DUO and SOLID were successfully validated with selected datasets of LHA. In time of writing this article, the design of the LHA Web Portal is not finished and thus is not available for public use.

6. Conflict of Interest

The authors state that they have no conflict of interests.

References

[1] W³ Techs, *Usage Statistics and Market Share of Content Management Systems for Websites, February 2017,* Q-Success, 2017. [Online]. Available: https://w3techs.com/technologies/overview/content_management/all. [Accessed 10 02 2017].
[2] Structured Dynamics LLC, *Open Semantic Framework*, Structured Dynamics LLC, 2017. [Online]. Available: http://opensemanticframework.org. [Accessed 10 02 2017].
[3] R. Hoehendorf, A.-C. N. Ngomo and H. Herre, *Developing Consistent and Modular Software Models with Ontologies*, Proceedings of the Eighth SoMeT_09, pp. 399-412, 2009.
[4] H. Herre, B. Heller, P. Burek, R. Hoehendorf, F. Loebe and H. Michalek, *General Formal Ontology (GFO) – A foundational ontology integrating objects and processes [Version 1.0.1]*, Leipzig, University of Leipzig, IMISE, 2007.
[5] N. Humfrey, *EasyRdf - RDF Library for PHP*, Available: http://www.easyrdf.org. [Accessed 10 02 2017].
[6] D. Sudeshna, L. Girard, T. Green, L. Weitzman, A. Lewis-Bowen and T. Clark, *Building biomedical web communities using a semantically aware content management system*, Brief Bioinform, pp. 129-138, December 2008.
[7] S. P. Ficklin, L.-A. Sanderson, C.-H. Cheng, M. E. Staton, T. Lee, I.-H. Cho, S. Jung, K. E. Bett and D. Main, *Tripal: a construction toolkit for online genome databases*, Database (Oxford), 29 Semptember 2011.
[8] M. Befa, E. Kontopoulos, N. Bassiliades, C. Berberidis and I. Vlahavas, *Deploying a Semantically-Enabled Content Management System in a State University*, Electronic Government and the Information Systems Perspective, EGOVIS 2010, Lecture Notes in Computer Science, no. 6267, 2010.
[9] Alfresco Software, Inc., *Activate Process and Content to Make Business Flow | Alfresco*, 2017. [Online]. Available: https://www.alfresco.com. [Accessed 8 May 2017].

German Medical Data Sciences: Visions and Bridges
R. Röhrig et al. (Eds.)

doi:10.3233/978-1-61499-808-2-175

Mapping Equivalence of German Emergency Department Medical Record Concepts with SNOMED CT After Implementation with HL7 CDA

Dominik BRAMMEN[a,b,1]; Heike DEWENTER[c,1], Kai U HEITMANN[d], Volker
THIEMANN[e], Raphael W MAJEED[e], Felix WALCHER[a], Rainer RÖHRIG[e], Sylvia
THUN[c]

[a] *Department of Trauma Surgery, Otto-von-Guericke-University Magdeburg, Germany*
[b] *Department of Anesthesiology, Otto-von-Guericke-University Magdeburg, Germany*
[c] *Hochschule Niederrhein, University of Applied Sciences, Krefeld, Germany*
[d] *Heitmann Consulting and Services e.K., Hürth*
[e] *Department of Medical Informatics, Carl von Ossietzky University Oldenburg,*
Germany

Abstract. Introduction: The German Emergency Department Medical Record
(GEDMR) was created by medical domain experts and healthcare providers
providing a dataset as well as a form. The trauma module of GEDMR was syntactically standardized using HL7 CDA and semantically standardized using different
terminologies including SNOMED CT, LOINC and proprietary coding systems.
This study depicts the mapping accuracy with aforementioned syntactical and semantical standards in general and especially the content coverage of SNOMED CT.
Methods: The specification of GEDMR (V2015.1) concepts with eHealth-
standards HL7-CDA, LOINC, SNOMED CT was analyzed. A content coverage
assessment was made using the ISO TR 12300 rating scheme, following descriptive analysis. Results: The trauma module of GEDMR contains 489 concepts, with
202 concepts expressed via HL7 CDA structure. It is possible to code 89 % of the
remaining concepts via SNOMED CT. 79 % provide an advanced level of semantic interoperability, as they represent the source information either lexically or as
an approved synonym. Discussion: The terminology binding problem is relevant
when combining different standards for syntactic and semantic interoperability
with best practice documents and reference specifications providing guidance. A
national license and extension for SNOMED CT in Germany as well as an ongoing
effort in contributing to the International Version of SNOMED CT would be necessary to gain full coverage for concepts in German Emergency Medicine and to
leverage the associated standardization process.

Keywords. health information exchange, SNOMED CT, Health Level Seven,
Logical Observation Identifiers Names and Codes, Emergency Medicine

---

[1] Corresponding authors: Dominik Brammen, Otto-von-Guericke-University Magdeburg, Department of
Anesthesiology, Leipziger Str. 44, 39120 Magdeburg, Germany; dominik.brammen@med.ovgu.de.
Heike Dewenter, Hochschule Niederrhein, FB Gesundheitswesen, Reinarzstrasse 49, 47805 Krefeld;
heike.dewenter@hs-niederrhein.de 2 shared first authors

1. Introduction

Syntactical and semantical interoperability is an essential prerequisite in the developing eHealth domain [1]. In this context, HL7 Clinical Documentation Architecture (HL7 CDA) is a leading document markup standard for creating syntactical and semantical standardized clinical documents [2]. Primarily, the standard provides the structure for syntactic interoperability, which is specified in the underlying HL7 Reference Information Model (RIM) [3]. Semantic interoperability can be achieved by reference terminologies like SNOMED CT used within CDA. Since the RIM specifies internal vocabularies for some structurally essential coded attributes, there are overlaps between CDA and SNOMED CT, which are resolved by guidance documents [4]. As there is no comprehensive adaption of SNOMED CT in Germany, national experiences with eHealth implementations combining HL7 CDA and the terminology are very limited [5].

The professional association the "German Interdisciplinary Association of Critical Care and Emergency Medicine" (DIVI), released a standard record for emergency departments in 2010 defining data standards. This German Emergency Department Medical Record (GEDMR) [6] was created by medical domain experts and healthcare providers defining a dataset and a form as technical artifact. As part of the governmental funded research project "Improvement of Health Services Research in Emergency Care in Germany by Establishment of a National Emergency Registry" two modules (basic and trauma) of the six-module GEDMR were syntactically standardized using HL7 CDA and semantically standardized using different terminologies including SNOMED CT, LOINC and proprietary code systems. The trauma module is to be investigated in this study.

Aim of this study is the actual realisation of the GEDMR-concepts with the differently named syntactical and semantical standards in general and especially the degree of equivalence of GEDMR concepts mapped with SNOMED CT.

2. Methods

The final implementation of the GEDMR (V2015.1) was analyzed. A HL7 CDA Release 2 specification of the trauma module was created, using the terminologies SNOMED CT and LOINC as well as HL7 Codes and proprietary codes when not coded otherwisely. The specification process was supported using the ART-DECOR® tool suite (http://www.art-decor.org) for collaboration between healthcare providers, terminologists and architects.

After extraction of all used concepts from the ART-DECOR database, their representation within the HL7 CDA was categorized. Used categories were "representation by HL7 CDA", "representation by LOINC" according to HL7 CDA recommendations, "representation by SNOMED CT" and "representation by proprietary codes" if no matching codes were found otherwise. For all concepts categorized "representation by SNOMED CT", a content coverage assessment was made using the ISO TR 12300 rating scheme "Degree of equivalence between source and target" [7]. As there is no valid German version of SNOMED CT available at present, concepts of the GEDMR had to be translated into English language for coding. No ethical vote was needed as neither humans nor personal data were included in this study.

3. Results

The trauma module of GEDMR contains 202 concepts with 287 sub-concepts in choice list items. Of these 489 concepts, 3 concepts were represented by pure CDA structure namely patient name, sex and date of birth. They are represented by XML-tags like <name> within the <patient> element of the record target. Further 199 concepts within the CDA were represented through Boolean expressions (yes/no), amounts of fluids/substances and timestamps. Of the remaining 287 concepts to be coded, Table 1 shows the chosen coding system according to best practice coding hierarchy HL7 CDA, LOINC, SNOMED CT.

Table 1. Analysis of terminology system used for concept coding within CDA (n=287)

Terminology System	Number of concepts	Percentage
Representation by HL7 CDA codes	8	3 %
Representation by LOINC	84	29 %
Representation by SNOMED CT	174	61 %
Representation by proprietary codes	21	7 %

While 92 concepts are represented by HL7 CDA or LOINC, 195 concepts are left for represention by SNOMED CT. Table 2 shows the contextual representation accuracy concerning these concepts, referring to the ISO TR 12300 rating. Concepts with no match in SNOMED CT were represented by proprietary codes (Table 1).

Table 2: Representation accuracy of SNOMED CT concepts suitable for the trauma module HL7 CDA (n=195)

Rating	Interpretation	Number of concepts	Percentage
1	Complete lexical match	129	66 %
2	Synonyme	25	13 %
3	Source broader than target	13	7 %
4	Target broader than source	7	3 %
5	No match	21	11 %

Assuming a direct comparison between source and target concept, there is a complete lexical match between 129 concepts, e. g. "Thoraxdrainage" (source), which means "chest drain" in English language, and |258643002|chest drain (physical object)| (target). Synonyms have been noted in 25 cases, e. g. "Analgosedierung", which means "analgosedation" in English, and |241712003|sedation with analgesic adjunct (procedure)|. The source concept has been found broader than the target concept in 13 cases, e. g. "Defibrillation", which means "defibrillation" in English, and |308842001|direct current defibrillation (procedure)|. The target concept has been noted broader than the source concept in 7 cases, e. g. "Kristalloide Infusionslösung", which means "crystalloid infusion solution" in English, and |51644004|electrolytic agent (substance)|.

Of chosen SNOMED CT concepts, 79 % percent provide either a complete lexical match or a synonyme respective the eligible GEDMR source concepts. 11 % of the chosen SNOMED CT concepts show broader expressions from both viewpoints, from source to target or from target to source. Thus, a successful coding rate of 89 % could be reached using SNOMED CT International for GEDMR concepts not coded with CDA or LOINC.

4. Discussion

Implementing data standards published by professional medical associations with HL7 CDA is one of the intended use cases [8]. For secondary reuse and machine processability of concepts, the underlying HL7 CDA structures and data types [2] as well as the usage of reference terminologies like LOINC and SNOMED CT are utilized in the CDA specifications. When implementing data standards in CDA, it is not directly obvious which coding system should be used for concept coding under certain circumstances. This terminology binding problem [9] is relevant when trying to achieve syntactic and semantic interoperability. HL7 provides guidance by best practice documents and reference specifications. For example, LOINC acts as an industry standard for encoding CDA Document Types for interoperability purposes according to the LOINC document ontology [10]. Further LOINC usage in CDA implementation guides refers to section heading codes (CDA Level 2). But also in the machine-readable clinical content (CDA entries), recommendations and reference specification practice are followed. Colloquially spoken, LOINC is the coding system used for asking questions ("which type of observation"), while SNOMED CT is used for coding clinical data being the answer to this question ("what coded result") [11].

As syntactic and semantic interoperability evolves world-wide, Germany has serious drawbacks without a national terminology for semantic interoperability being available to all participants of the health care system. SNOMED CT is the growing semantic interoperability standard in Europe and beyond. Many European countries are members of SNOMED International including 6 out of 9 direct neighbours to Germany.

Currently, of the concepts not coded by CDA or LOINC, 89 % can be coded successfully via SNOMED CT. 79 % provide an advanced level of semantic interoperability. Thus, a high coverage of GEDMR concepts with SNOMED CT lacking any national adaption is already possible. A German adaption including National Extensions to SNOMED CT is necessary for non-codeable concepts, with new questions arising. E. g., the *Severity score for illness or trauma* of the National Advisory Committee on Aeronautics (NACA) is used in the German Emergency Medical Service as well as in different European countries including member states of SNOMED International [12]. Adding the concept to a National Extension alone would not be sufficient as other countries may want to use this code as well. In other words, coordination is also desired on an European level.

As SNOMED CT human readable terms are primarily in English, sufficient competence regarding language and cultural differences is necessary to properly map German terms to English SNOMED CT concepts. For this work, a research license of SNOMED CT is available but the resulting CDA with SNOMED CT codes is intended to go in live-operation in at least 15 project hospitals. As Germany has no national license of SNOMED CT and thus a substantial license fee is involved for every participating hospital, we decided to replace all 174 sucessfully SNOMED CT-coded concepts with proprietary codes, until there is a national license available in Germany.

Therefore, for introduction of SNOMED CT in Germany, three prerequisites need to be fulfilled:

1. At least, a German license of SNOMED CT would be necessary on a national level to support the eHealth infrastructure.
2. A German extension of SNOMED CT including a translation would be necessary; this includes quality assurance methodologies and a national endorsement mechanism.

3. The remaining 11 % not matchable concepts have to be incorporated into SNOMED CT either as a German Language Reference Set, German National Extension or within the international core.

5. Conclusion

Coding of concepts within a HL7 CDA is subject to a hierarchical set of partly best practice rules. While some concepts are coded by CDA structure or coding system, section headings are usually coded using LOINC. The remaining clinical concepts were in 89 % successfully coded via SNOMED CT, with a high level of representation accuracy. A national license and extension for SNOMED CT in Germany as well as an ongoing effort in contributing to the International Version of SNOMED CT would be necessary to gain full coverage for concepts in German Emergency Medicine and sharing these concepts with other contributing countries.

Conflict of Interest

The authors received funding from the German Ministry for Research (BMBF) (01KX1319A), (01KX1319B), (01KX1319C). DB is Co-Chair of HL7 International Emergency Care Working Group. KH is CEO from HL7 Germany. FW is Chair of DIVI GEDMR Working Group, ST is chair of HL7 Germany.

References

[1] A. Aguilar, Semantic Interoperability in the context of eHealth, *Res. Semin. DERI Galway, December 15th.* (2005) 2–4.
[2] R.H. Dolin, L. Alschuler, S. Boyer, et al., HL7 Clinical Document Architecture, Release 2., *J. Am. Med. Inform. Assoc.* **13** (2005) 30–9. doi:10.1197/jamia.M1888.
[3] L. Vizenor, B. Smith, and W. Ceusters, Foundation for the Electronic Health Record: An Ontological Analysis of the HL7's Reference Information Model, **10** (2007) 5717.
[4] W.T. Klein, R. Hamm, D. Karlsson, et al., HL7 Version 3 Implementation Guide : TermInfo - Using SNOMED CT in CDA R2 Models, (2015) 1–157.
[5] H. Dewenter, and S. Thun, SNOMED CT und IHTSDO-Mitgliedschaft – Nutzen einer Referenzterminologie für Deutschland aus der Perspektive der Neuen Institutionenökonomik, in: E-Health Ökonomie, 2017: pp. 239–272.
[6] M. Kulla, M. Baacke, T. Schöpke, et al., Kerndatensatz „Notaufnahme" der DIVI, *Notfall + Rettungsmedizin.* **17** (2014) 671–681. doi:10.1007/s10049-014-1860-9.
[7] TECHNICAL REPORT ISO/TR 12300 - Health informatics - Principles of mapping between terminological systems, **2014** (2014).
[8] R.H. Dolin, and L. Alschuler, Approaching semantic interoperability in Health Level Seven, *J. Am. Med. Informatics Assoc.* **18** (2011) 99–103. doi:10.1136/jamia.2010.007864.
[9] A. Rector, R. Qamar, and T. Marley, Binding Ontologies & Coding systems to Electronic Health Records and Messages, in: O. Bodenreider (Ed.), Second Int. Work. Form. Biomed. Knowl. Represent., Baltimore: CEUR, 2006: pp. 11–19.
[10] Structured Documents Work Group, and Vocabulary Work Group, HL7 Implementation Guide: LOINC Document Ontology , Release 1, (2015) 1–88.
[11] A. Rico-Diez, S. Aso, D. Perez-Rey, et al., SNOMED CT Normal Form and HL7 RIM binding to normalize clinical data from cancer trials, in: 13th IEEE Int. Conf. Bioinforma. Bioeng., 2013.
[12] L. Raatiniemi, K. Mikkelsen, K. Fredriksen, et al., Do pre-hospital anaesthesiologists reliably predict mortality using the NACA severity score? A retrospective cohort study., *Acta Anaesthesiol. Scand.* **57** (2013) 1253–9. doi:10.1111/aas.12208.

German Medical Data Sciences: Visions and Bridges
R. Röhrig et al. (Eds.)
© *2017 German Association for Medical Informatics, Biometry and Epidemiology (gmds) e.V. and IOS Press.*
This article is published online with Open Access by IOS Press and distributed under the terms
of the Creative Commons Attribution Non-Commercial License 4.0 (CC BY-NC 4.0).
doi:10.3233/978-1-61499-808-2-180

From a Content Delivery Portal to a Knowledge Management System for Standardized Cancer Documentation

Danijela SCHLUE [a,1], Sebastian MATE [b], Jörg HAIER [c], Dennis KADIOGLU [d],
Hans-Ulrich PROKOSCH [b] and Bernhard BREIL [a]

[a] *Niederrhein University of Applied Sciences, Krefeld, Germany*
[b] *Medical Informatics, Univ. of Erlangen-Nürnberg, Erlangen, Germany*
[c] *The Nordakademie, Elmshorn, Germany*
[d] *University Medical Center Mainz, Germany*

Abstract. Heterogeneous tumor documentation and its challenges of interpretation of medical terms lead to problems in analyses of data from clinical and epidemiological cancer registries. The objective of this project was to design, implement and improve a national content delivery portal for oncological terms. Data elements of existing handbooks and documentation sources were analyzed, combined and summarized by medical experts of different comprehensive cancer centers. Informatics experts created a generic data model based on an existing metadata repository. In order to establish a national knowledge management system for standardized cancer documentation, a prototypical tumor wiki was designed and implemented. Requirements engineering techniques were applied to optimize this platform. It is targeted to user groups such as documentation officers, physicians and patients. The linkage to other information sources like PubMed and MeSH was realized.

Keywords. Oncological documentation, knowledge management, meta-data-repository (MDR), Kano model, wiki.

1. Introduction

Tumor documentation in Germany is very heterogeneous [1], which results in different documentation practices depending on the clinic, region or information system used. This is also underlined by the German Hospital Federation in their research concerning quality in the national cancer plan for Germany [2, 3]. Possible uncertainties in the interpretation of terms (e.g. primary tumor, diagnosis date) lead to problems in analyses created by clinical and epidemiological cancer registries. These differences are a result of the respective specialization of cancer registries, varying quality assurance requirements and diversely used documentation systems.

Existing resources like handbooks for oncological documentation are mostly limited to technical parameters, such as field definitions and value domains [4]. But evaluation and also re-use of existing routine data for analyses require conceptual agreements on terms [5]. Up until now, knowledge systems, which provide structured,

---

[1] Corresponding Author.

free and independent information access to oncological terms, hardly exist. An international approach, which addresses this topic, is the terminology system of the National Cancer Institute (NCI) with their Enterprise Vocabulary Services [6]. Due to the increasing need for valid information, it is necessary to have one single repository as a national reference for routine cancer documentation, quality assurance documentation and scientific purposes. This repository should contain terms, definitions, comments about usage and interpretation - but no individual patient data. We designed and implemented a content delivery portal with commenting functionality and semantic links to international term definitions to increase transparency in medical documentation and to contribute to a common understanding for physicians, documentation officers and for laypersons. This system behaves similar to a wiki, although the creation of new content is limited to experts in the field of oncological documentation to assure a high quality of information.

Our objectives were to collect and analyze user requirements to improve the existing system from the user's point of view, to recognize and classify user requirements with regards to their effect on user satisfaction and to increase transparency of the oncological documentation for physicians, documentation officers and for laypersons. Requirements engineering provides many techniques for defining and prioritizing requirements [7]. The evaluation and classification technique suggested by Kano is well suited for prioritizing requirements artefacts.

2. Methods

To create a user-focused concept for the system, we analyzed the existing documentation handbooks (GEKID, ADT), coding guidelines for oncological documentation (OnkoZert) and information repositories. Together with partners from four German Comprehensive Cancer Centers (Münster, Hamburg, Dresden, Frankfurt), we defined an approval and validation process for the submission of new terms. First, terms from the existing sources were collected and analyzed concerning representation, comprehensibleness, evidence, confirmability and availability of source data. Second, a common data field definition with value domain, plausibility checks and documentation notes was created.

The Samply.MDR [8] was used as a technical base. This metadata repository already contained a raw structure of the ADT/GEKID-terms. The system is based on common web technology and its design consists of a layered architecture with data access, service and presentation layer. Within the latter one, a flexible design for different views (depending on the target group) was realized. The graphical user interface was created with JavaServer Faces 2.2 [9] and has been extended by portal-specific functionality, such as a navigation tree and a navigation bar to recognize the classification order for a term. We implemented new Java classes for the commenting functionality and extended the generic slot functionality with specific multiline text fields to ease the collection and management of term characteristics containing continuous text.

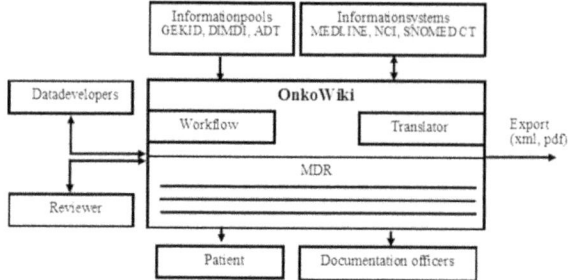

Figure 1. Architecture of the content delivery portal. Three layers allow independent access from different user groups to data from oncological information pools.

Figure 1 shows a simplified, high-level representation of the system architecture and the interaction with users and other applications, which calls services implemented within the application's service layer.

One focus was a user-oriented design, suitable especially for the main target group of documentation officers. There are physicians and scientists who have own requirements. To involve users and to implement their requirements, different methods were conducted: a pre-test in July and August of 2016, the Kano method for the prioritization process, requirements collection in an internal content management system and a main test in February 2017.

The questionnaire, which was specifically developed by the medical experts for the pretest, was based on the reference model for process description PAS[2] 1032-1, published by the German Institute for Standardization (DIN). We received complete questionnaire replies from six users.

Following a user-oriented design with focus on the documentation officers in the university hospitals with clinical cancer registries, we got insight regarding technical requirements definitions and prioritization of user requirements with Kano-classification. These requirements definitions are mainly based on contact with project workers and analysis of scientific literature. The requirements data collection comprised of an e-mail survey among medical experts and documentation officers in addition to telephone interviews. In the beginning, a set of 46 system features and requirements was identified. Informatics experts drafted a questionnaire based on the results of structured surveys with six categories: functions for compilation of terms, term usage, data, ergonomics, interfaces and documentation. A questionnaire related to the Kano model contains a set of question pairs for each requirement. The question pair includes a functional question, which captures the user's response if a product has a certain attribute, and a dysfunctional question, which captures the user's response if the product does not have that attribute. Questionnaires are presented to the future users, project partners from four German Comprehensive Cancer Centers (Munster, Hamburg, Dresden and Frankfurt) and a group of medical documentarists from Essen. The corresponding requirement class was identified by using statistical analysis of the survey results for each requirement.

After prioritization and application of changes to the user interface, we analyzed the common design and requirements again. To avoid unstructured proceeding during realization of requirements, we collected the newly arrived requirements and suggestions

---

[2] Publicly Available Specification

to alter the design provided by the users and summarized their feedback. In an internal content management system we analyzed more than 50 requirements. For each requirement, users filled in the category (preference, must be, bug) and prioritization of that item (high, medium, low). The comments of web application developers and the time required for the realization was captured. Agreement by all four centers was required to implement the specified offer.

Having the revised version of the web application available after the pre-test, medical experts started the main evaluation in February 2017. The user feedback was considered during the adaptation of the questionnaire, which was reduced to seven categories. The maximum number of questions was set to five per category.

3. Results

The developed data model is generic and enables the detailed specification of terms. The repository currently contains 126 oncological terms in different grades of complexity, definitions and comments about usage stored in 16 additional attributes. The terms are divided in 18 groups based on the ADT/GEKID dataset. Each term is described by its data type, domain, category and code. It is also possible to add synonyms and links to other data sources. The first prototype contains the management of terms (term creation, term representation) and user management. Currently it is possible to manage and view existing terms and review specific information about data type, plausibility checks and documentation hints with focus on medical experts. A flexible model with different views as a part of the web application's environment was developed and is available at: www.onko-wiki.de.

Usability evaluation in the pre-test phase resulted in a heterogeneous picture. The responses varied considerably and showed the importance of a structured approach that involves all key actors in the requirements analysis.

The Kano survey was planned to be distributed within the oncological network in order to receive enough answers and to prioritize the requirements from a technical point of view. Four out of ten interviewed persons (one physician, two documentation officers and one person in the field of education) returned completed questionnaires. We identified the corresponding requirement classes for each requirement. The most relevant category is the "Must-be"-category, currently containing 23 items. According to the Kano method an absence of these requirements will lead to user dissatisfaction. Seven items belong to the A-category, correlates linearly with user satisfaction. A low degree of fulfilment of these attributes reduces user satisfaction.

During the development phase, the users remained informed. The 45 proposals of their communicated feedback or change requests collected in the internal content management system were recorded within three months. All 13 requirements with high prioritization were implemented. Jointly agreed changes led to an adjustment of the system and the structure of the portal. The evaluation based on the answers of 23 persons obtained to the present show that the user acceptance score increased significantly.

4. Discussion

We implemented a prototype of the tumor wiki, which allows information retrieval of existing terms as well as adding new elements by a selected number of medical experts.

A pre-test with a limited number of medical experts assessed the software and gave valuable input for further optimization to follow a user-oriented design. A disadvantage of the Kano classification is the length of the questionnaire. Each requirement is represented so that a complex application will result in a longer list of questions. There might also be a misunderstanding while reading the requirements. Therefore, it is important to discuss the results in the user group while offering them the chance to give feedback. This study will help to establish a wiki featuring moderation and an approval concept to provide oncological terms in a quality-assuring way. The integration of the MDR helps to establish the nation-wide character of the platform as (1) further possibly relevant data elements can be retrieved from the MDR and included into the approval process and (2) portal-specific information (e.g. documentation hints) can be helpful for any other third party, which is using the MDR.

With regards to the content, the ADT-datasets build a very good source for our portal, but have to be extended to fulfil all subordinated purposes. We aim to connect it to other important knowledge bases, such a link to MEDLINE, which display other studies using the same term definitions. All terms are mapped to concepts defined by the NCI [6]. In addition, all terms should contain references to international terminology systems (especially to SNOMED CT or LOINC) to allow international comparisons. A term submission process should be extended. Medical societies can suggest new terms to be included into the wiki. After formal evaluation of a coordinator, the term will be provided to a team of medical oncology experts to rate and comment on the new entry. After a two-stage commentary phase and a final approval of experts and coordinator, the term will be added to the wiki and can be accessed by the different target groups.

References

[1]   Blatt K, et al. Aufwand-Nutzen-Abschätzung zum Ausbau und Betrieb bundesweit flächendeckender klinischer Krebsregister. *Gutachten Prognos AG* (2010).
[2]   German Hospital Federation, Quality assurance, http://www.dkgev.de/dkg.php/aid/7691/cat/42 (last access 13.03.2017).
[3]   Beckmann M, Sell C, Aydogdu M, Brucker SY, Fehm T, Janni W, Kreienberg R, Kümmel S, Neumann M, Scharl A, Schleicher B, Wallwiener D, Wöckel A, Fasching PA, Lux MP, Documentation Time and Effort and Associated Resources for Patients with Primary Breast Cancer from Diagnosis to End of Follow-Up - Results of a Multicentre Validation. *Gesundheitswesen* (2015).
[4]   Altmann U, Handbuch für die Anwendung der Basisdokumentation basierend auf den neuen ADT-Bögen, https://www.uni-giessen.de/fbz/fb11/institute/imi/ag/akkk/datAkkk/BAsisdoku (last access 23.03.2017).
[5]   Ries M, Prokosch H U, Beckmann M, Bürkle T, Single Source Tumor Documentation. Reusing Oncology Data for Different Purposes, *Onkologie* **36(3):136-41** (2013)
[6]   NCI Enterprise Vocabulary Services (EVS) http://www.cancer.gov/research/resources/terminology (last access 01.02.2017).
[7]   Pohl K, Requirements Engineering. Fundamentals, Principles and Technics, *Springer-Verlag Berlin Heidelberg* (2010), 632-643.
[8]   Kadioglu D, Weingardt P, Ückert F, et al., Samply.MDR – Ein Open-Source-Metadaten-Repository, *German Medical Science GMS Publishing House* 2016, doi:10.3205/16gmds149.
[9]   JavaServer Faces http://www.javaserverfaces.org/specification/ (last access 08.03.2017).

German Medical Data Sciences: Visions and Bridges
R. Röhrig et al. (Eds.)
© 2017 German Association for Medical Informatics, Biometry and Epidemiology (gmds) e.V. and IOS Press.
This article is published online with Open Access by IOS Press and distributed under the terms
of the Creative Commons Attribution Non-Commercial License 4.0 (CC BY-NC 4.0).
doi:10.3233/978-1-61499-808-2-185

An Abstraction Layer to Facilitate Technical Interoperability Between Medical Records and Knowledge Modules

Martin STAUDIGEL [a,1], Hans-Ulrich PROKOSCH [b] and Stefan KRAUS [b]

[a] Medical Center for Information and Communication Technology, University Hospital Erlangen, Erlangen, Germany.
[b] Medical Informatics, Univ. of Erlangen-Nürnberg, Erlangen, Germany.

Abstract. Integrating clinical decision support (CDS) functions into an existing hospital information system (HIS) is often a tedious task. This problem area is so pervasive that the Arden Syntax, a widely used standard for CDS functions, assigned a specific designation, the so-called "curly braces problem". It derives from a pair of curly braces used to encapsulate any parameters required for the interactions with a HIS. The traditional approach is to leave the problem area of technical interoperability entirely to the specific institution, possibly entailing a considerable amount of initial programming work. This study describes a reusable and expandable solution to this problem in the form of an abstraction layer. Our study comprised an analytical phase in which we investigated the data source access capabilities of five Arden Syntax environments. Building on the results, we implemented a working prototype that is capable of querying heterogeneous data sources, which facilitates a straightforward connection of new data sources with existing and future communication protocols and standards. From our point of view, the technical aspects of the "curly braces problem" with respect to data source access have changed over the years, insofar as technical progress lead to defacto standards for data storage, data querying and inter-system communication. An agreement on such a convention, together with the supply of commonly used data source adapters could promote the further dissemination of the Arden Syntax as a standard for representing and sharing medical knowledge.

Keywords. Clinical decision support, Arden Syntax, interoperability, curly braces problem

1. Introduction

Integrating clinical decision support (CDS) functions into an existing hospital information system (HIS) is often a tedious task. Technical interoperability presupposes suitable interfaces, and semantic interoperability may require controlled vocabularies. This problem area is so pervasive that the only widely used standard in clinical routine for CDS functions, the Arden Syntax for Medical Logic Systems, assigned a specific designation, the "curly braces problem" [1]. This term derives from a pair of curly braces used to encapsulate any parameters required for the interaction with a HIS. In clinical routine, the vast majority of HIS are commercial solutions. Their

---

[1] Corresponding Author: martin.staudigel@uk-erlangen.de

interfaces to third party components are often insufficient for the integration of CDS functions. Some institutions solve this problem by replicating EMRs into external databases, or duplicating streams of Health Level Seven (HL7) messages at their communication server. In case of successful data replication, as well as in self-developed EMRs, the actual database access is usually straightforward. In such cases, one might expect that integrating Arden-Syntax-based CDS functions should be seamless. However, this is not necessarily the case, as the specification of this standard does not govern the actual EMR access at all. As a result of its historic development, the Arden Syntax standard leaves the problem area of technical interoperability entirely to the specific institution, possibly entailing a considerable amount of initial programming work in the early stages of an integration process. This study describes an expandable approach that, if provided by an Arden Syntax environment, may eliminate the need for tedious preliminary programming work. Moreover, by providing a simple abstraction layer, it would enable a knowledge engineer to access data items from the electronic record without knowledge of the specific database schema.

2. Methods

In Arden Syntax, knowledge is processed in the form of Medical Logic Modules (MLMs). MLMs access EMR items by means of the READ statement, followed by an expression enclosed in curly braces. The retrieved data items are returned as a list of values, associated with their clinical timestamps. The content of a curly braces expression is not specified by the standard. In practice, it may be quite complex, depending on the characteristics of the interface to the storage system. Multiple examples from the literature use SQL queries, such as in [2].

We investigated the data source access capabilities of multiple Arden Syntax environments. Our analysis included a commercial Arden Syntax server, which is in routine use at our largest intensive care unit [3], an open source Arden compiler [4], an Arden Syntax engine which is an integrated part of our HIS, a prototypical decision support framework developed during a project for standards-based drug safety functions [5], and an experimental Arden Syntax environment used for research on further development of the standard. Based on this analysis, we designed and implemented a prototype of an abstraction layer, introducing a template concept with placeholders for the content of the curly braces to abstract from specific query languages. We designed our approach in a generic way insofar as we enabled the simultaneous use of heterogeneous data sources and query languages within an MLM. The technical aspects of the implementation were separated from the institution specific information by storing the latter inside of a human readable configuration file. We based the first version of our prototype on SQL access, as this is the most widespread query language at our local institution. To prove the general applicability of our concept, we added another adapter, which is able to retrieve data from a Fast Healthcare Interoperability Resources (FHIR) [6] interface.

3. Results

Our analysis revealed different levels of database abstraction. The HIS-integrated Arden engine is restricted to the application-specific database, requiring deep knowledge of the underlying storage concept. The other systems provide a higher level of flexibility. All of them are capable of connecting different types of SQL databases. Concerning versatility, two systems are limited to one SQL database at a time by default, while the two other systems are able to simultaneously access multiple databases. Concerning usability, one system provides a graphical user interface to switch between different SQL data sources, the others use text based configuration. Two implementations are limited to the use of SQL statements within the curly braces, the other two provide a concept to hide SQL, considerably simplifying the curly braces expressions. All systems provide means to insert the contents of predefined variables into curly braces expressions. Furthermore, all systems besides the HIS-integrated solution support the integration of interface components to arbitrary data sources. These components must be implemented by the customer.

The implemented prototype constitutes such an interface component. It was designed with a layered architecture, comprising (in top-down order) a template layer, a distribution layer and an adapter layer. The template layer includes a convention for the content of curly braces expressions. We identified the following parameters for a generic but easy-to-use abstraction layer. A data source, the name of a data source specific template, and a list of arguments to be inserted into the template, if necessary. The last item of the argument list is the patient context, typically in form of a case number. It constitutes a special case insofar as typical MLMs have a single patient context, which is implicitly adopted from the triggering event message, but can be altered on demand. This enables straightforward READ statements as illustrated in figure 1. If data source or patient context are omitted, the corresponding default values are used.

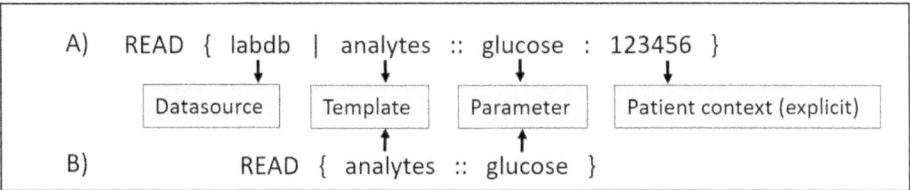

Figure 1. - Read statement: A) with a full set of parameters, B) only with obligatory parameters. The default data source will be queried with the implicitly adopted patient context.

Figure 2 illustrates the steps from the curly braces expression to a data source query. While an expression is passed through the layers, elements are replaced by their low-level counterparts. The template layer selects a specific adapter by the given data source identifier. The selected adapter translates the template name into a technically oriented query with placeholders. The placeholders are replaced by the given parameters. The adapter layer handles different technical connections (e.g. databases, email) by means of adapter classes that use connection specific query languages and protocols. Each adapter instance handles exactly one physical connection. In the example the adapter communicates with a SQL data source. The retrieved result set is sent back to the distribution layer, and finally transformed into Arden Syntax datatypes by means of the application programmer interface of the specific Arden Syntax environment.

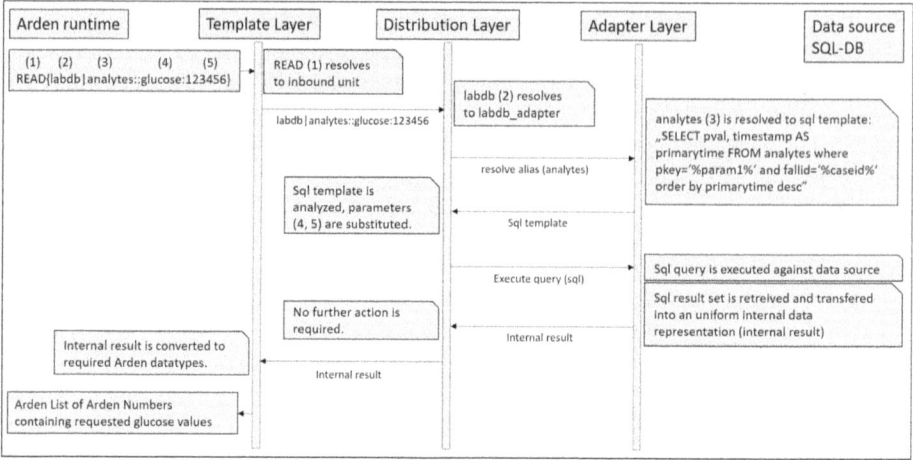

Figure 2. - Data flow and responsibilities with respect to the processing of a curly braces expression.

4. Discussion

The traditional approach to solve the curly braces problem is to leave its solution to the specific institution. As a consequence, with respect to data source connectivity an institution may have to "reinvent the wheel", just like in case of our local integration [3], when the interface component had to be implemented from scratch, including database access and messaging. Many institutions likely repeat the same basic programming tasks, although this could be avoided, at least in large parts. Some parameters, however, will always remain institution specific, thus a completely seamless "out of the box" Arden Syntax integration is unlikely; examples are connection parameters, data models, rarely used data sources or specific vocabularies. A compromise can be to define a framework in terms of a simple but flexible means of configuration that enables the user to adapt the interfaces behavior. From the system integrators point of view, presupposed a system with capabilities of an abstraction layer is available, the effort of an integration is reduced to providing the content of the configuration file and filling a database with templates to translate expressions into institution specific queries.

Multiple aspects concerning the curly braces problem with respect to data source access have changed over the years, insofar as technical progress has led to de facto standards for data storage, data querying and inter-system communication. This enables CDS vendors to establish interoperability on a level that spares customers the recurring effort of creating interface components to widely used data storage systems. Our study may outline the possibility to perform an integration without recurring programming tasks and without requiring institution specific knowledge in advance. The design goals of the Arden Syntax – knowledge transfer between institutions and ease of use – would be supported, if the traditional approach "The rest of a query is enclosed in curly brackets, and is specific to the authoring institution" [7] would be reconsidered, and possibly replaced by a convention that allows to specify data sources, queries and other parameters in a regulated manner. An agreement on such a convention, together with the supply of commonly used data source adapters could promote the dissemination of the Arden Syntax standard.

Broad adoption of communication standards in medicine is often a long-term process. Accessing EMRs by means of ab abstraction layer that does not presuppose query language skills or architectural knowledge can be seen as a key feature for fast integration. A convention for integrating heterogeneous data sources has to be comfortable in use, but furthermore has to be adaptable and principally capable of connecting new data sources with future communication protocols and standards. Currently, the emerging FHIR standard is widely acclaimed. Although FHIR uses common standards and protocols like JSON and HTTP, any query result has still to be transformed to the data type system of the Arden Syntax. This task can be done by an adapter component. Our prototype is capable of integrating different data sources and communication endpoints, and currently it handles all data-driven MLMs in clinical routine at our hospital. With a modular approach to cover the technical differences, and a straight forward configuration to serve the institutional specifics, responsibilities for technical interoperability can be clearly assigned either to the vendor or the customer. Moreover, as technologies like databases and email are everyday standard in hospital IT infrastructures, the developed interfaces may be, at least in large parts, re-used at other institutions. Thus, the difficulty that "even if it is possible to share the medical knowledge, the link to the database will have to be redone by each institution" [8] might be considerably simplified.

5. Acknowledgements

The present work was performed in (partial) fulfillment of the requirements for obtaining the degree "Dr. rer. biol. hum." of MS from the Friedrich-Alexander-Universität Erlangen-Nürnberg.

References

[1] Hripcsak G, Wigertz OB, Clayton PD. Origins of the Arden Syntax. *Artif Intell Med* 2015. doi:10.1016/j.artmed.2015.05.006.
[2] Johansson B, Bergqvist Y. Integrating decision support, based on the Arden Syntax, in a clinical laboratory environment. *Proc Annu Symp Comput Appl Med Care*. 1993:394–8.
[3] Kraus S, Castellanos I, Toddenroth D, Prokosch H-U, Burkle T. Integrating Arden-Syntax-based clinical decision support with extended presentation formats into a commercial patient data management system. *J Clin Monit Comput*. 2014;**28**:465–73. doi:10.1007/s10877-013-9430-0.
[4] Gietzelt M, Goltz U, Grunwald D, Lochau M, Marschollek M, Song B, Wolf K-H. ARDEN2BYTECODE: a one-pass Arden Syntax compiler for service-oriented decision support systems based on the OSGi platform. *Comput Methods Programs Biomed*. 2012;**106**:114–25. doi:10.1016/j.cmpb.2011.11.003.
[5] Sojer R, Bürkle T, Criegee-Rieck M, Neubert A, Brune K, Prokosch H-U. Knowledge modelling and knowledge representation in hospital information systems to improve drug safety. *Journal on Information Technology in Healthcare*. 2006;**4**:29–37.
[6] Benson T, Grieve G. Principles of FHIR. In: *Principles of Health Interoperability: SNOMED CT, HL7 and FHIR*. Cham: Springer International Publishing; 2016. p. 329–348. doi:10.1007/978-3-319-30370-3_18.
[7] Hripcsak G, Ludemann P, Pryor TA, Wigertz OB, Clayton PD. Rationale for the Arden Syntax. *Comput Biomed Res*. 1994;**27**:291–324.
[8] Nadkarni PM. *Metadata-driven Software Systems in Biomedicine: Designing Systems that can adapt to Changing Knowledge*. London: Springer-Verlag London Limited; 2011.

190   *German Medical Data Sciences: Visions and Bridges*
R. Röhrig et al. (Eds.)
© *2017 German Association for Medical Informatics, Biometry and Epidemiology (gmds) e.V. and IOS Press.*
doi:10.3233/978-1-61499-808-2-190

Analysis of Annotated Data Models for Improving Data Quality

Hannes ULRICH [a,b,1], Ann-Kristin KOCK-SCHOPPENHAUER [a],
Björn ANDERSEN [b], Josef INGENERF [a,b]
[a] *IT for Clinical Research, Lübeck (ITCR-L), University of Lübeck, Germany*
[b] *Institute of Medical Informatics, University of Lübeck, Germany*

Abstract. The public Medical Data Models (MDM) portal with more than 9.000 annotated forms from clinical trials and other sources provides many research opportunities for the medical informatics community. It is mainly used to address the problem of heterogeneity by searching, mediating, reusing, and assessing data models, e. g. the semi-interactive curation of core data records in a special domain. Furthermore, it can be used as a benchmark for evaluating algorithms that create, transform, annotate, and analyse structured patient data. Using CDISC ODM for syntactically representing all data models in the MDM portal, there are semi-automatically added UMLS CUIs at several ODM levels like *ItemGroupDef, ItemDef,* or *CodeList item*. This can improve the interpretability and processability of the received information, but only if the coded information is correct and reliable. This raises the question how to assure that semantically similar datasets are also processed and classified similarly. In this work, a (semi-)automatic approach to analyse and assess items, questions, and data elements in clinical studies is described. The approach uses a hybrid evaluation process to rate and propose semantic annotations for under-specified trial items. The evaluation algorithm operates with the commonly used NLM *MetaMap* to provide UMLS support and corpus-based proposal algorithms to link datasets from the provided CDISC ODM item pool.

Keywords. CDISC ODM, UMLS, Semantic Interoperability, Natural Language Processing

1. Introduction

To prove effectiveness and efficiency of medication and medical therapies, clinical studies are performed. The results are documented in Case Report Forms (CRFs), which can easily consist of hundreds of documentation items, e. g. weight in kg. The Meta Data Models (MDM) Portal [1] developed by the Institute of Medical Informatics at the University of Muenster provides a huge collection of documentation items out of CRFs and routine care documentation with the aim to improve sharing and reuse of items. All forms and items are provided in the Clinical Data Interchange Standards Consortium Operational Data Model (CDISC ODM) format [2], can be downloaded in various formats, and are publicly available. For the majority of data items, semantic annotations from the Unified Medical Language System (UMLS) were added [3].

---

[1] Corresponding Author: **Hannes.Ulrich@itcr.uni-luebeck.de**

Sharing and reuse of documentation items is deeply dependent on the understanding of the meaning of such an item. This meaning can be expressed using coding systems such as UMLS or SNOMED Clinical Terms (CT). Our approach aims for a method to check whether semantically similar datasets are processed and classified similarly. The MDM Portal therein serves as the source system for documentation items.

2. Methods

This work describes an automatic approach for the analysis and assessment of the semantic codes assigned to items, questions, and data elements. It uses a hybrid evaluation process to rate and propose semantic annotations for under-specified, non-annotated trial items. The implemented evaluation algorithm utilises the commonly used National Library of Medicine's (NLM) MetaMap API [4] to provide UMLS support and extends it by corpus-based proposal algorithms to link datasets from the provided CDISC ODM item pool.

2.1. Text and String Similarity

Information about the pairwise similarity of terms and sentences is required for further processing of text and plays an important role in the field of information retrieval and text classification. The given terms can either be lexically or semantically similar. The former denotes that the given inputs share a common sequence within their respective string representations, whereas the latter signifies whether the inputs represent the same cognitive concept and is more difficult to determine. The field of string similarity and the measurement thereof is well explored and is divided into three major types of algorithms: string-based, corpus-based, and knowledge-based approaches [5].
This approach proposes a similarity algorithm that combines two string-based measurements: the *five-gram* algorithm and the *metric Longest Common Subsequence* (mLCS) [6]. The first splits the given terms into subsequences of five characters and measures their similarity based on correspondence. The mLCS is based on the longest subsequence that both terms share. The subsequence differs therein from the substring that for the subsequence it is not mandatory to have the same position in the terms. In order to minimise false positives, a quality threshold rejects proposals with a low score.

2.2. Unified Medical Language System and MetaMap

UMLS is a linked collection of the majority of biomedical vocabularies. The NLM initiated the project in 1996 to help researchers to retrieve and integrate electronic biomedical information. One of the most well-known programmes for natural language processing of biomedical texts is *MetaMap*, which is also developed and published by the NLM. It provides access to UMLS by analysing a given biomedical text and mapping it to the corresponding concepts. Hence, a link between unstructured free text and the rich knowledge of UMLS is established, including all synonymy relationships and further references from other medical knowledge systems.

2.3. Processing Pipeline

In order to analyse given items, a processing pipeline was designed and implemented as a modular Java project, containing eight submodules with distinct functionality to minimise overlapping source code and to support reusability, see Figure 1.

In addition, a data pool was generated that contains 250 trial forms, provided by the MDM portal. The fields of the clinical forms are heterogeneous to broaden the applicability and reliability. The forms contain 4240 items and are annotated with 3291 different UMLS concepts. The most frequently used item describes the patients' age and the most frequent concept is "Date in time" as a temporal concept.

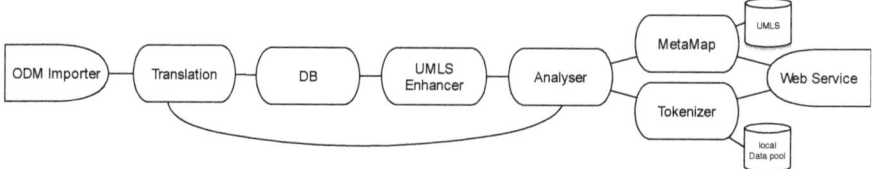

Figure 1 Central modules are the database access, ODM processing, UMLS querying, *Tokenizer*, and the web service. Special, customised services are the MetaMap access, *Translation*, and *Importer*.

The given ODM-XML file is read and split into sections of items grouped by their corresponding *ItemGroup*. The new trial items can enter the pipeline in two different manners: (1) in order to expand the data pool or (2) to be analysed. If they are to expand the information base, it is reviewed whether they are already known and can be linked. The UMLS querying module then enhances the item by adding UMLS semantic concept descriptors in addition to the corresponding Medical Subject Headings (MeSH) and SNOMED CT reference, if existing. The entered item is also checked for the languages it provides and is translated if no English translation is already given. The English version is necessary to use the *MetaMap* module and to be able to find further UMLS concepts to enhance the given item and therefore the quality of the data pool. The translation module benefits from Google's translation API. If the given item is to be analysed, two major criteria are determined: (1) Is the item or a related one already in the data pool and (2) does the item contain any UMLS references. Based on these criteria, the item is either reviewed or new UMLS concepts are proposed. Upon review, for the item and its included references it is tested as to whether *MetaMap* can confirm the connection or whether a related item in the curated pool contains the same references. For the concept proposal, the algorithm uses *MetaMap* to link the term and the previously described similarity measurement to determine related items in the database, see Figure 2. The entire data pool is examined by the analyser component and shown next to the pipeline health status, e. g. connection to the database, *MetaMap,* and the Google Cloud services.

```
PROPOSE to Allergies (text)

Tokenizer
Allergens( text )
[5289] C0002092 - Allergens
Allergies( text )
[5698] C0020517 - Allergies

MetaMap
[-1000] C0020517 - Allergies
```

Figure 2 Example output for the underspecified trial item *Allergies* of datatype *text:* The tokenizer finds similar items in the data pool and *MetaMap* generates a corresponding proposal.

3. Results

The herein described environment was successfully implemented and tested to measure the overall benefit of the approach. To evaluate the implementation, 25 trial forms containing 639 items were randomly chosen from the MDM portal and assessed. The system exhibits good performance at proposing UMLS concepts based on the similarity results of the tokenizer and *MetaMap*, as shown in Table 1.

Table 1 Proposal of under-specified trial items based on the pipeline.

	proposal		no proposal	total
	correct proposal	wrong proposal		
abs. number	64	0	17	81
ratio	79%	0%	21%	100%

The good hit ratio of 79% demonstrates that the system provides reliable proposals for the 81 under-specified trial items. After expert review, it was stated that the algorithm did not suggest a single wrong proposal, but for 17 items the system could not provide any proposal. The reasons are two-fold: the system could either not identify any concepts by processing the term or the results were not satisfying the quality threshold. The quality check of given 764 UMLS concepts in relation to the *item name* provided a 62% correspondence ratio, see Table 2.

Table 2 Evaluation of the accuracy of UMLS code and *item name*.

	correct match	incorrect match	total
CUIs	474	291	764
ratio	62%	38%	100%

The mismatch of 291 items has various reasons: additional domain-specific knowledge that could not be determined by the name, e. g. an item named "Date" has the additional concept "Date of Death", the composition of long and rich item names, e. g. "maintenance treatment tablets Injection Infusion", or names like "Unequivocalprogressivediseaseinnontargetlesionsisbasedon: (pleasedecribe)".

4. Discussion and Conclusion

The system meets the specified requirements and provides good results in proposing and analysing the given trial items. However, during implementation and evaluation some limitations were discovered. The most challenging is the need for a curated and well-structured item pool to provide good and reliable results. But the acquisition of high-quality data sources is difficult: Whereas the MDM portal provides a reliably good data pool, additional resources – ideally covering a broad range of clinical disciplines – are needed for the similarity algorithm to process the majority of items.

The combination of mLCS, nGram, and quality thresholds is an improvement over previous approaches: It achieves better results than simple annotation comparison and Levenshtein distance [7]. Due to the introduction of a quality threshold, the results could be optimised and the output refined. The use of *MetaMap* to identify UMLS concepts corresponding to the given trial item increases the data quality significantly. The gained link between term and UMLS is an enabler for linking further medical concept knowledge, e. g. relations to anatomy or drugs from *Snomed CT* or *MeSH*. However, MetaMap does not always provide suitable results for a given term.

Regarding UMLS, another problem was discovered: Older forms are annotated with concept codes that are not included in the current UMLS version, which raised errors processing them. As the given ODM forms do not contain any version information regarding UMLS, solving this conflict remains difficult [8]. The processing of non-English forms could be realised using the Google Translation API, but due to occurring inaccuracies an alternative approach would be desirable [9]. Nevertheless, the prototypical pipeline already supports the identification of candidates for an independent review of the quality and consistency of annotations.

Dugas et al. [3] reused known concepts from their repository to minimise the concept variability in large terminologies in their ODM data pool. But sometimes the concept choice appears to be arbitrary. For coding "Height" they prefer "Patient height" (C0005890) instead of the more general "Height" (C0489786). However, temperature items are most often annotated with "Temperature" (C0039476, i. e. in the sense of bio-specimen characteristics), and "Body Temperature" (C000590). In general, the pipeline based on two different knowledge bases yields good and reliable results. The modular software design enables the integration into existing study and metadata repositories as well as the reuse of the developed tools. The semi-automatic approach can accelerate the process of curating item annotations, e. g. by externally and independently enhancing the repository provided by the MDM portal [10]. A predicted mismatch shall not perturb, but encourage the user to review the items and either modify or rather improve the actual items and annotated concepts.

5. Conflict of Interest/Acknowledgment

The authors state that they have no conflict of interests. The authors express their gratitude to Martin Dugas and the MDM portal team for their kind support!

References

[1] Dugas M: „Metadata Repository for Medical Forms Portal". *Medical-data-models.org*. Retrieved from http://www.medical-data-models.org (17. 03. 2017).
[2] Operational Data Model (ODM)-XML".
    Retrieved from https://www.cdisc.org/standards/foundational/odm. (17. 03. 2017)
[3] Dugas M, Neuhaus P, Meidt A, Doods J, et al. (2016): „Portal of medical data models: information infrastructure for medical research and healthcare". *Database (Oxford)*. 2016 10.1093/database/bav121.
[4] MetaMap - A Tool For Recognizing UMLS Concepts in Text". *Metamap.nlm.nih.gov*. Retrieved from https://metamap.nlm.nih.gov/. (17. 03. 2017)
[5] Gomaa WH, Fahmy AA: „A Survey of Text Similarity Approaches". In: *International Journal of Computer Applications*. 68 (13), 2013), 13-18.
[6] Bakkelund D. "An LCS-based string metric" *University of Oslo* (2009).
[7] Ulrich, H., et al. "Metadata Repository for Improved Data Sharing and Reuse Based on HL7 FHIR." *Stud Health Technol Inform.* 2016, 228: 162-6.
[8] Seerainer C, Sabutsch SW: "eHealth Terminology Management in Austria" in *Studies in Health Technology and Informatics 2016, 228: 426-30*
[9] Schlegel DR, Crowner C, Elkin PL: "Automatically Expanding the Synonym Set of SNOMED CT using Wikipedia". *Stud Health Technol Inform.* 2015; 216:619-23.
[10] Varghese J, Dugas M: Frequency analysis of medical concepts in clinical trials and their coverage in MeSH and SNOMED-CT. *Methods Inf Med.* 2015; 54(1):83-92.

7. Biomedical Informatics, Innovative Algorithms and Signal Processing

German Medical Data Sciences: Visions and Bridges
R. Röhrig et al. (Eds.)

doi:10.3233/978-1-61499-808-2-197

Optimizing a Query by Transformation and Expansion

Katrin GLOCKER[a,1], Alexander KNURR [b], Julia DIETER[a], Friederike DOMINICK[a],
Melanie FORCHE[a], Christian KOCH[a], Analie PASCOE PÉREZ[a], Benjamin ROTH[a]
and Frank ÜCKERT[a]

[a] *Division of Medical Informatics for Translational Oncology,*
Deutsches Krebsforschungszentrum
Heidelberg, Germany
[b] *National Center for Tumor Diseases (NCT), Heidelberg, Germany*

Abstract. In the biomedical sector not only the amount of information produced and uploaded into the web is enormous, but also the number of sources where these data can be found. Clinicians and researchers spend huge amounts of time on trying to access this information and to filter the most important answers to a given question. As the formulation of these queries is crucial, automated query expansion is an effective tool to optimize a query and receive the best possible results. In this paper we introduce the concept of a workflow for an optimization of queries in the medical and biological sector by using a series of tools for expansion and transformation of the query. After the definition of attributes by the user, the query string is compared to previous queries in order to add semantic co-occurring terms to the query. Additionally, the query is enlarged by an inclusion of synonyms. The translation into database specific ontologies ensures the optimal query formulation for the chosen database(s). As this process can be performed in various databases at once, the results are ranked and normalized in order to achieve a comparable list of answers for a question.

Keywords. Data Mining; Information Storage and Retrieval; Information Management; Medical Informatics

1. Introduction

The daily routine of physicians includes an intensive research of information beyond clinical records and documents retrieved at the hospital. This research is a time consuming and complicated task as different databases have to be addressed with appropriate ontologies in order to receive relevant information. The formulation of the query plays a very important role in this process. Queries with too little information may lead to an overwhelming amount of results, which are not valuable for the user (false positives), while a too detailed formulation may lead to false negatives, as important information may be missed. Thus, with the query term "breast cancer", the terms "neoplasm of the breast" or "mammary carcinoma" may be marked as false negative. Therefore, automated optimization of a query is a crucially needed feature to provide the best possible treatment for patients. A technique to increase the efficiency

---

[1] Corresponding Author, G230, Im Neuenheimer Feld 280, 69120 Heidelberg, Germany, E-Mail: k.glocker@dkfz-heidelberg.de

of humanly implemented search strings is the method of automated query expansion. Here, additional query terms are added in order to specify the question [1]. This can be accomplished by using unstructured data such as documents or publications, or by structured data like synonym databases or ontologies.

Another form of query expansion is the documentation of previous queries. The analysis of these queries can detect term co-occurrences. Terms, which are often searched in the same context as a term from the original query can be included. This principle is used by a variety of search engines on the web, like Yahoo! and Google.

Because of the vast spread of biomedical knowledge in the web, the possibility to compare results of different databases is essential. In order to save time the best results have to be ranked and assessed at one glance.

In this paper we introduce a new workflow, which combines the described query expansion methods (semantic co-occurrences and synonyms). However, the function of the Common Query Database gets expanded as terms, which were never used in the given context get ignored in the query. Furthermore, we translate the query terms into appropriate ontologies for different databases. Via a ranking of the received results, a pseudo relevance feedback would be possible to even further improve the query. However, in this work we will concentrate on the steps of query expansion and formulation, which are necessary for forming a query optimized for the user's needs.

2. Methods

2.1. Semantic Co-occurrences

The potential of term co-occurrences in improving information retrieval was already demonstrated in 1960 by Maron and Kuhns and is part of many studies since then [4]. These co-occurrences were shown to be computed by a non-linear weighting function or by using the previous queries [10].

2.2. MetaMap

MetaMap is the most extensive thesaurus in the biomedical field. As MetaMap creates a distance score and a history for related terms within the UMLS Metathesaurus, this tool can be used to identify synonyms for a query term. The introduction of these two features allows an easy display of the similarity of the proposed synonym [5].

2.3. Ranking Algorithms

The most frequent applied algorithms are Okapi BM25 and TF-IDF. Both algorithms, compute the relevance of a document by the frequency of a term in the document, while the relevance is offset by the frequency of the term in the document collective. While BM25 is a probabilistic model, TF-IDF is a vector space model [7–9].

3. Results

Searches in external data sources play an increasingly important role in the medical daily routine. As the optimal formulation of a query is a crucial task in obtaining the best possible results we constructed the concept for a workflow containing various methods for an automated expansion and formulation of queries. Since this automation can lead to a change of direction of the question, human interaction cannot be completely avoided. Nevertheless, our theoretical approach on automated query optimization is designed to require as little human interference as possible.

After defining attributes by the user, the search string consisting of sub-queries connected with logical operators (AND, OR or NOT), will be transferred to the Common Query Database. Here, all queries are documented and summed up in a database, in which the current query can be compared with all previous queries. Terms, which are never mentioned in context with the rest of the query can be considered as not appropriate in this question and can be excluded. Furthermore, the query terms are analyzed for terms with semantic co-occurrences. These additional terms can be included to the query as new attributes. After the analysis the user can choose to reject or accept the elimination of a defined attribute or the expansion of the query and can allow the addition of single terms by using logical operators (AND, OR or NOT).

> *Example: defined attributes: Mutation in ER, Mutation in APC, ICD50, Therapy*
> *Common Query Database:*
> *suggested exclusions: Mutation in APC (used in 0,5% of queries with this context)*
> *suggested addition: Mutation in PR (used in 18% of queries with this context)*
> *suggested addition: Mutation in HER2 (used in 23% of queries with this context)*
> *resulting query: Mutation in ER, Mutation in PR, Mutation in HER2, ICD50, Therapy*

Figure 1: Transformation of the query in the Common Query Database.
The user defines the sub queries "Mutation in ER", "Mutation in APC", "ICD50" and "Therapy". Previous queries are compared and analyzed for semantic co-occurrences. As APC is only used in 0,5% of queries in this context this attribute can be excluded. PR and HER2 are used more often in this context and are suggested to be added to the query. The user can decide if he wants to exclude/add the attributes and if the added terms are added with AND, OR or NOT. (ER= estrogen receptor, APC=adenomatous polyposis coli, ICD50=breast cancer, PR=progesterone receptor, HER2=human epidermal growth factor receptor 2.) [2]

The transformed query will then be supplemented by synonyms for each keyword extracted from the query. For this, the keywords are mapped to the UMLS using MetaMap. The utilization of MetaMap bears the advantage of an integrated system of computing distances and histories of possible synonyms. With these distances and histories the relation of terms is defined [5]. While "limb" functions as a direct synonym for "extremity", "arm" and "leg" have a greater distance, but can also be used for query expansion. Vice versa, "extremity" cannot always function as a synonym for "arm" (depending on the question of the query). As the usability of the synonyms is very variable, the user can confirm or refuse the inclusion of synonyms as of a defined distance or history.

---

[2] Percentages were computed by analyzing the number of Pubmed results received for the original query, expanded with the MeSH terms for either "APC", "PR", or "HER2". The analysis was conducted on 02.03.2017.

> *Example: Query: Mutation in ER, Mutation in PR, Mutation in HER2, ICD50, Therapy*
> *Synonyms "ER": estrogen receptor 1; ESR1; ESR; ESRA; ESTRR; Era; NR3A1*
> *Synonyms "PR": progesterone receptor; NR3C3*
> *Synonyms "HER2": human epidermal growth factor receptor 2; ERBB2; CD340;*
> *HER-2; HER-2/neu; MLN 19; NEU; NGL; TKR1*
> *Synonyms "ICD50": breast neoplasms; tumors, breast; breast cancer; mammary*
> *cancer; malignant neoplasm of breast; malignant tumor of*
> *breast [extract]*
> *Synonyms "Therapy": therapeutic; therapies; treatment; treatments*

Figure 2: Expansion of the query with synonyms.
Keywords are extracted from the question and used for the mapping. The keywords are mapped to UMLS via MetaMap. With this, synonyms can be added to the query.

With all synonyms added, the query can be transformed into database-specific ontologies or thesauri. As these ontologies can have an enormous impact on the quality of the results, the accurate translation in the appropriate ontology for the desired database(s) is a crucial part in this workflow.

> *Example: MeSH: Estrogen Receptor alpha [MESH] AND Receptors, Progesterone [MESH]*
> *AND Receptor, ErbB-2 [MESH] AND Breast Neoplasms [MESH] AND*
> *Therapeutics [MESH]*

Figure 3: Translation of the query into the MeSH ontology.
The query terms are translated into the appropriate ontologies for the databases. In this example, the query is converted into MeSH for an optimal search in MEDLINE.

In some queries the amount of results can still be overwhelming. To get easy access to the most important results, a ranking is essential. For this purpose the two most frequently used ranking algorithms will be used (BM25 and TF-IDF) [7–9].

As more than one database can be addressed at once, the delivered results can be in different formats. Via APIs these outcomes can be collected and normalized in one format. This facilitates the comparison of results of different databases.

All the introduced features will be developed to help the user to optimize a query, but will not be mandatory. As most features need human feedback, the user will be able to disable components of the workflow to reduce the need of user interference. However, this may have influence of the quality of optimization.

4. Discussion

The introduced workflow provides the opportunity to place a simple query in various databases, while the query gets optimized in the process. Despite the successful performance of similar, separately used, query expansion features, the combination will likely lead to better results. However, all features bear problems which are to be considered more closely. To minimize the time consumption for researching a biomedical question transformation of the query can help, but can also be complicated when too much human interaction is necessary. This can be avoided by the possibility to disable single features in the workflow, which are not necessary for less complicated queries. Especially the Common Query Database will require human interference, but can lead to a notable improvement of the query. The approach of using sematic relationships between terms for query expansion has been used since 1977. However, Peat and Willet demonstrated the limitations of this technique [10,11], by stating that terms with a close semantic relationship are likely to retrieve the same results in a query. Since in our work the Common Query Database is not exclusively restricted to a weighting algorithm, but also to the accumulated knowledge of all users, the problems mentioned by Peat and Willet are avoided [11]. A similar approach was successfully conducted within the PONTE project, which was completed in 2013. The "Decision Support" component communicates with a predefined queries templates database, which stores human readable descriptions and ontologies [12].

The addition of synonyms poses the challenge of requiring huge databases. The mapping of terms within the ULMS with MetaMap provides a solution for the problem for the English language. As English is the most used scientific language, the use of other languages is not planned to be considered at this stage. Although the MetaMap concept bears problems in recognizing chemical names or acronyms and in the resolution of ambiguity even in English, previous experiments showed an improvement of queries [5].

With the proposed work process it is feasible to receive the best possible answer to a question with a saving of the user's time and effort. The automated query expansion enables the user to optimize the formulation of a query only by accepting or declining of suggested changes. Thereby the user is still able to steer the questions in the intended direction. Since the workflow allows to inquire more than one information source at once, the information of different sources is presented to the user in a comparable way. As the user is able to gain great insight on a topic in a short time, we want to help physicians and researchers to improve their way to find important information.

Conflict of Interest

The authors state that they have no conflict of interest.

References

[1]   Carpineto C, Romano G. A Survey of Automatic Query Expansion in Information Retrieval. ACM Comput. Surv. 2012;44:1–50.
[2]   Khennak I, Drias H. Bat-Inspired Algorithm Based Query Expansion for Medical Web Information Retrieval. J Med Syst. 2017;41:34.
[3]   Alipanah N, Parveen P, Menezes S, Khan L, Seida SB, Thuraisingham B. Ontology-driven Query Expansion Methods to Facilitate Federated Queries. IEEE International Conference on Service-Oriented Computing and Applications, SOCA 2010. 2010.
[4]   Maron ME, Kuhns JL. On Relevance, Probabilistic Indexing and Information Retrieval. J. ACM. 1960;7:216–244.
[5]   Aronson AR. Effective mapping of biomedical text to the UMLS Metathesaurus: the MetaMap program. Proc AMIA Symp. 2001:17–21.
[6]   Furnas GW, Landauer TK, Gomez LM, et al. The vocabulary problem in human-system communication. Commun. ACM. 1987;30:964–971.
[7]   Singhal A. Modern Information Retrieval: A Brief Overview. IEEE Data Eng Bull. 2001:35–43.
[8]   Kwak M, Leroy G, Martinez JD, et al. Development and evaluation of a biomedical search engine using a predicate-based vector space model. Journal of Biomedical Informatics. 2013;46:929–939.
[9]   Robertson SE, Walker S, Jones S, Hancock-Beaulieu MM, Gatford M. Okapi at TREC-3. 1996.
[10] Van Rijsbergen CJ. A theroretical Basis for the Use of Co-Occurrence Data in Information Retrieval. Journal of Documentation. 1977:106–119.
[11] Peat HJ WP. The Limitations of Term Co-Occurrence Data for Query Expansion in Document Retrieval Systems. Journal of the American Society for Information Science. 1991:378–383.
[12] Tsatsaronis G, Mourtzoukos K, Andronikou V, Tagaris T, Varlamis I, Schroeder M, Varvarigou T, Koutsouris D, Matskanis N. PONTE: A Context-Aware Approach for Automated Clinical Trial Protocol Design. Proc. Of the 6th International Workshop on Personalized Access, Profile Management, and Context Awareness in Databases (PersDB), Microsoft Research. 2012.

German Medical Data Sciences: Visions and Bridges
R. Röhrig et al. (Eds.)
© 2017 German Association for Medical Informatics, Biometry and Epidemiology (gmds) e.V. and IOS Press.
This article is published online with Open Access by IOS Press and distributed under the terms
of the Creative Commons Attribution Non-Commercial License 4.0 (CC BY-NC 4.0).
doi:10.3233/978-1-61499-808-2-202

Deep Learning for Magnetic Resonance Fingerprinting: A New Approach for Predicting Quantitative Parameter Values from Time Series

Elisabeth HOPPE[a,b,1], Gregor KÖRZDÖRFER[a,c], Tobias WÜRFL[b], Jens WETZL[b],
Felix LUGAUER[b], Josef PFEUFFER[a] and Andreas MAIER[b]

[a] *MR Application Development, Siemens Healthcare, Erlangen, Germany*
[b] *Pattern Recognition Lab, Department of Computer Science, Friedrich-Alexander-Universität Erlangen-Nürnberg, Erlangen, Germany*
[c] *Friedrich-Alexander-Universität Erlangen-Nürnberg, Erlangen, Germany*

Abstract. The purpose of this work is to evaluate methods from deep learning for application to Magnetic Resonance Fingerprinting (MRF). MRF is a recently proposed measurement technique for generating quantitative parameter maps. In MRF a non-steady state signal is generated by a pseudo-random excitation pattern. A comparison of the measured signal in each voxel with the physical model yields quantitative parameter maps. Currently, the comparison is done by matching a dictionary of simulated signals to the acquired signals. To accelerate the computation of quantitative maps we train a Convolutional Neural Network (CNN) on simulated dictionary data. As a proof of principle we show that the neural network implicitly encodes the dictionary and can replace the matching process.

Keywords. Convolutional Neural Networks, Deep Learning, Machine Learning, Magnetic Resonance Fingerprinting, Supervised Machine Learning

1. Introduction

Previously presented methods for generating parameter maps in MRF are time-consuming and require a dictionary of time series for every possible combination of parameters like T1 and T2 relaxation times [1, 2]. Furthermore, such a dictionary will only have discrete entries for reasons of efficiency. This can lead to errors in MRF parameter maps [3]. To overcome these time and storage limitations, we train a Convolutional Neural Network (CNN) to predict quantitative T1 and T2 values from MRF time series. Deep leaning has recently been shown to be a promising technique for many applications in medical imaging, e.g. reconstruction in X-ray computed tomography [4, 5]. Two advantages of this method are i) fast computation of the quantitative parameter maps and ii) a better representation of the dictionary data (our trained model requires about 2 MB compared to 210 MB for a dictionary with e.g. 8750 T1/T2 combinations). Moreover, the CNN can predict values for time series

---

[1] Corresponding author, Pattern Recognition Lab, Department of Computer Science, Friedrich-Alexander-Universität Erlangen-Nürnberg, Erlangen, Germany, E-Mail: elisabethhoppe@web.de

continuously. This study investigates the execution time and accuracy of predicted parameters using a CNN compared to the conventional dictionary matching approach using simulated data from a FISP MRF implementation [6].

2. Methods

Experiments were performed on a head-shaped gel phantom, a NIST phantom [7] and healthy subjects on a MAGNETOM Skyra 3T (Siemens Healthcare, Erlangen, Germany). 2D MRF-FISP [6] data served as the experimental basis of the dictionary simulation. It was acquired using a prototype sequence with the following parameters: Field-of-view (FOV) 300 mm, resolution 1.17x1.17x5 mm^3, variable repetition time (TR, 12-15 ms), flip angle (FA, 5-74°), number of repetitions (Nrep) 3000. A dictionary with high resolution was simulated to obtain a large amount of training and testing data. Relaxation parameters present in normal human tissues [8, 9, 10] and in the NIST phantom [7] were selected for the simulation (T1: 50 to 4500 ms, T2: 20 to 800 ms, with steps from 2 to 50 ms, with relative B1+ magnitude values ranging from 0.7 to 1.3, step: 0.05, overall about 120,000 time series). Implementation and testing were run on GPU using the machine learning library TensorFlow [11]. The architecture of the network (Figure 1) was inspired by neural networks used in the domain of speech processing [12], as these problems are similar to our problem. We tested different architectures using different numbers of convolutional and fully connected layers. We found that the network model with smallest average error for validation data consists of 3 convolutional layers (kernel size = 3, stride size = 2), each followed by a rectified linear unit (ReLU) activation function. The number of the feature maps per convolutional layer is increasing, from 32 in the first to 128 in the last. After convolution an average pooling layer follows with the same size as the stride size. The last layer is fully connected, with 2 outputs. The simulated time series data was randomly partitioned into disjunct sets for training, validation and testing (80/10/10 %). The weights were initialized uniformly randomly distributed. Training was done with the ADAM [13] optimization method with an initial learning rate of 5*10^-4, by minimizing the Mean Squared Error. Batch size was set to 5 time series. The model was trained for maximal 200 epochs. Early stopping was performed using the validation data. The training was stopped when the validation average error of current epochs increased in comparison to the past epochs.

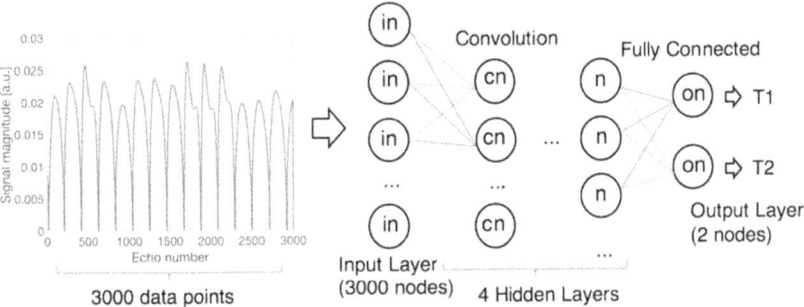

Figure 1. Schema of the CNN. The input is one simulated time series, the outputs are the estimated quantitative values for T1 and T2.

3. Results

The range of T1 and T2 values was chosen to be close to values present in the NIST phantom [7] and in human tissues, especially brain regions [8, 9, 10]. Estimated values of our proposed method show only small average deviations from ground truth values (Figures 2 and 3): The mean absolute deviations (standard deviation, SD) are 0.29% (0.44%) for T1 and 1.22% (2.04%) for T2 for relevant NIST values (T1: 80-1500, T2: 20-450), and the mean absolute deviations (SD) for complete test data (T1: 50-4500, T2: 20-800) are 0.18% (0.44%) for T1 and 1.3% (2.23%) for T2. The comparison between estimated parameters from the network and the simulated dictionary time series for some T1 and T2 values and their deviations are shown in Figures 4 and 5. The comparison of execution time was carried out on a 2.7 GHz Intel Core i5. While the estimation for one time series using the matching method proposed by [1] took about 100 ms, the CNN approach vastly improves this by a factor of 30 (or about a factor of 100 on a GPU).

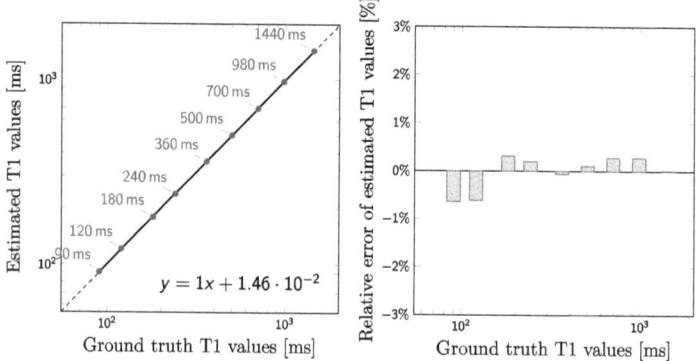

Figure 2. Left: Estimated T1 values for some typical NIST values (90, 120, 180, 240, 360, 500, 700, 980 and 1440 ms). The dashed line is the x = y line, the solid line is the linear regression, with its formula in the bottom right corner. Right: The relative deviations of the estimated values from ground truth values.

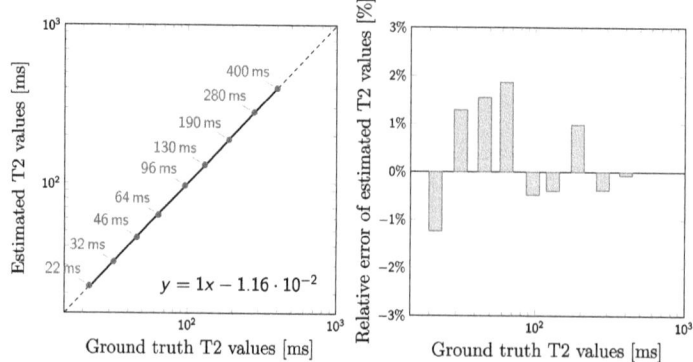

Figure 3. Left: Estimated T2 values for some typical NIST values (22, 32, 46, 64, 96, 130, 190, 280 and 400 ms). The dashed line is the x = y line, the solid line is the linear regression, with its formula in the bottom right corner. Right: The relative deviations of the estimated values from ground truth values.

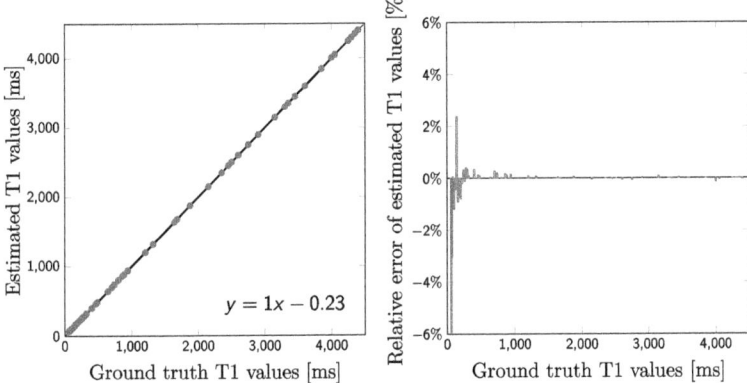

Figure 4. Left: Quantitative examples for estimated T1 values. The solid line is the linear regression, with its formula in the bottom right corner. Right: The relative deviations of the estimated values from ground truth values.

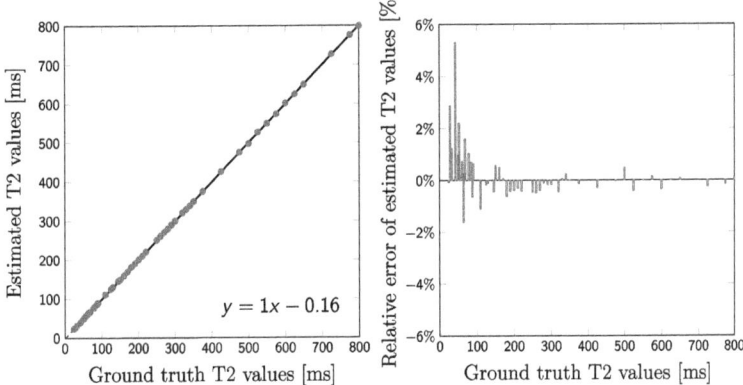

Figure 5. Left: Quantitative examples for estimated T2 values. The solid line is the linear regression, with its formula in the bottom right corner. Right: The relative deviations of the estimated values from ground truth values.

4. Discussion and conclusion

A CNN, trained with simulated time series from a MRF dictionary, is shown to produce accurate predictive results for quantitative parameters like T1 and T2 times. Thus the CNN is able to detect the relevant features and differences between time series for the different T1 and T2 times and can learn these features by itself during training. A CNN model works well as an alternative approach for prediction of quantitative values from time series in MRF. Besides providing accurate results for simulated time series, it also has the following two advantages compared to state-of-the-art matching methods: Firstly, the computation time can be greatly reduced. Secondly, the neural network also provides a very efficient representation of the model when compared to a dictionary. Future work will include the adaption of the proposed concept to real measured time series for generating quantitative parameter maps of human tissues.

References

[1]   Ma D, Gulani V, Seiberlich N, Liu K, Sunshine JL, Duerk JL, et al. Magnetic Resonance Fingerprinting. Nature. 2013;495(7440):187-92.

[2]   Cauley SF, Setsompop K, Ma D, Jiang Y, Ye H, Adalsteinsson E, et al. Fast group matching for MR fingerprinting reconstruction. Magn Reson Med. 2015;74(2):523-8.

[3]   Wang Z, Zhang Q, Yuan J, Wang X. MRF denoising with compressed sensing and adaptive filtering. In: 2014 IEEE 11th International Symposium on Biomedical Imaging (ISBI 2014): Proceedings of the 11th International Symposium on Biomedical Imaging; 2014 Apr 29-May 2; Beijing, China. IEEE; 2014. p. 870-3.

[4]   Würfl T, Ghesu FC, Christlein V, Maier A. Deep Learning Computed Tomography. In: Ourselin S, Joskowicz L, Sabuncu M, Unal G, Wells W, editors. Medical Image Computing and Computer-Assisted Intervention -- MICCAI 2016. MICCAI 2016. Lecture Notes in Computer Science. Vol 9902. Cham: Springer; 2016. p. 432-40.

[5]   Hammernik K, Würfl T, Pock T, Maier A. A Deep Learning Architecture for Limited-Angle Computed Tomography Reconstruction. In: Maier-Hein K, Deserno T, Handels H, Tolxdorff T, editors. Bildverarbeitung für die Medizin 2017. Informatik aktuell. Berlin, Heidelberg: Springer Vieweg; 2017. p. 92-7.

[6]   Jiang Y, Ma D, Seiberlich N, Gulani V, Griswold MA. MR fingerprinting using fast imaging with steady state precession (FISP) with spiral readout. Magn Reson Med. 2014;74(6):1621-31.

[7]   Calibrate MRI Scanners with NIST Referenced Quantitative MRI (qMRI) Phantoms (QIBA DWI and ISMRM) [Internet]. Boulder(CO): High Precision Devices, Inc.; c2017 [cited 2017 Feb 16]. Available from: http://www.hpd-online.com/MRI-phantoms.php.

[8]   Bojorquez JZ, Bricq S, Acquitter C, Brunotte F, Walker PM, Lalande A. What are normal relaxation times of tissues at 3 T?. Magn Reson Imaging. 2017;35:69-80.

[9]   Stanisz GJ, Odrobina EE, Pun J, Escaravage M, Graham SJ, Bronskill MJ. T1, T2 relaxation and magnetization transfer in tissue at 3T. Magn Reson Med. 2005;54(3):507-12.

[10]   Li Y, Xu D, Ozturk-Isik E, Lupo JM, Chen AP, Vigneron DB, et al. T1 and T2 metabolite relaxation times in normal brain at 3T and 7T. J Mol Imaging Dynam S. 2012;1:2.

[11]   Abadi M, Barham P, Chen J, Chen Z, Davis A, Dean J, et al. TensorFlow: A system for large-scale machine learning. In: 12th USENIX Symposium on Operating Systems Design and Implementation: Proceedings of the 12th USENIX Symposium on Operating Systems Design and Implementation; 2016 Nov 2-4; Savannah(GA), USA. USENIX Association; 2016 [cited 2017 Feb 16]. p. 265-83. Available from: https://www.usenix.org/sites/default/files/osdi16_full_proceedings.pdf.

[12]   Zhang Y, Pezeshki M, Brakel P, Zhang S, Bengio CLY, Courville A. Towards end-to-end speech recognition with deep convolutional neural networks. In: Interspeech 2016. Proceedings of Interspeech 2016; 2016 Sep 8-12; San Francisco(CA), USA. 2016 [cited 2017 Feb 16]. p. 214-16. Available from: http://dx.doi.org/10.21437/Interspeech.2016-1446. doi: 10.21437/Interspeech.2016-1446.

[13]   Kingma D, Ba J. Adam: A method for stochastic optimization. arXiv preprint [Internet]. 2014 [cited 2017 Feb 16]. Available from: https://arxiv.org/abs/1412.6980.

German Medical Data Sciences: Visions and Bridges
R. Röhrig et al. (Eds.)
© *2017 German Association for Medical Informatics, Biometry and Epidemiology (gmds) e.V. and IOS Press.*
doi:10.3233/978-1-61499-808-2-207

Evaluation of an Interactive Visualization Tool for the Interpretation of Pediatric Laboratory Test Results

Johannes HIRSCHMANN [a], Brita SEDLMAYR [a], Jakob ZIERK [b], Manfred RAUH [b],
Markus METZLER [b], Hans-Ulrich PROKOSCH [a] and Dennis TODDENROTH [a,1]

[a] *Medical Informatics, Univ. of Erlangen-Nürnberg, Erlangen, Germany*
[b] *Department of Pediatrics and Adolescent Medicine, University Hospital Erlangen*

Abstract. The physiological age-related development of pediatric laboratory results interferes with pathological derangements, which can complicate the interpretation of test results. Recently proposed continuous reference intervals (RIs) promise to be beneficial, although their clinical use may depend on graphical presentations. To estimate the clinical utility of continuous RIs, we developed and evaluated an interactive visualization tool, and examined the differentiation of hemoglobinopathies that is attainable based on the underlying innovative RI model. The implemented web application allows users to easily enter laboratory test results, and displays various visualizations in conjunction with the corresponding RIs, such as charts and personalized Z-scores. To evaluate the usability of the visualization tool, we conducted concurrent think-aloud sessions with four physicians, who were prompted to solve a set of typical interpretation tasks, and acquired additional information through a questionnaire including the System Usability Scale (SUS). We used 85 de-identified clinical cases for an exemplified assessment of how well model-based interpretations of blood count parameters reproduced previously diagnosed hemoglobinopathies. Usability tests as well as questionnaire responses indicated that the developed tool was well received by the physicians. Results from the think-aloud evaluation revealed only minor problems and the tool reached an average SUS score of 86.9, suggesting good usability. Hemoglobinopathy discrimination depended on the considered subtype, although the overall performance of the novel method rivaled the one of the conventional approach. The interactive visualization of innovative continuous reference intervals demonstrated promising results, which justifies further testing on the path towards clinical routine.

Keywords. Technology assessment, evaluation studies, medical informatics application

1. Introduction

Clinicians commonly interpret laboratory tests in relation to established reference intervals (RIs). These limits serve to differentiate between normal and pathological findings, and to gauge the severity of any abnormal increases or decreases. In healthy children, several laboratory parameters are known to characteristically vary with age,

---

[1] Corresponding Author, Dr. Dennis Toddenroth, Medical Informatics, Friedrich-Alexander-Universität Erlangen-Nürnberg (FAU), Erlangen, Germany, dennis.toddenroth@fau.de

so pediatric test results are usually interpreted in relation to these physiological dynamics. Pediatricians have a particular interest in carefully analyzing available findings, because obtaining blood samples can be more stressful for younger patients.

Conventionally, RIs for pediatric patients have been calculated by partitioning data from a healthy reference population into age groups, so that the corresponding subset-specific percentiles would form step functions of age. More recently proposed statistical approaches instead derive continuous models of the physiological development, which seem biologically more plausibly. The resulting graphical appearance of these modern RIs resembles the familiar steadiness of established anthropometric growth curves [1]. Visual representations of clinical time series generally promise to support diagnostic considerations, for example by promoting a faster recognition of gradual trends [2, 3].

Even if automated graphics creation may theoretically facilitate medical decision-making, practitioners frequently experience that the involved electronic data processing can also introduce tedious obstacles [4]. For a systematic analyses of such intricacies, research on human-computer-interaction has defined usability as *'the extent to which a product can be used by specified users to achieve specific goals'*, which for software applications can depend on the *'capability [...] to be understood, learned [and] operated [...] under specific conditions'* [5]. To evaluate usability, concurrent think-aloud (TA) prompts representative users to verbalize their thoughts while accessing the studied system for typical tasks. This instrument requires that user comments and activities are recorded, but may permit inferences about cognitive processes [4].

The diagnostic constellations where laboratory tests can be relevant include the identification of hemoglobinopathies, which are oxygen transport diseases that can result in anemia of variable severity. The analysis of the complete blood count usually constitutes only the first step, and further classification of these conditions involves more specific tests [6]. To explore their potential utility for assessing pediatric hematology test results, we thus analyzed how well these next-generation reference intervals reproduced a set of formerly diagnosed hemoglobinopathies in comparison to conventional discrete RIs, and evaluated the usability of a functional visualization prototype.

2. Methods

The previously published method for inducing novel-type continuous RIs leans on estimating the composition of normal and abnormal values in data from routine care; uninterrupted percentiles are then interpolated from overlapping age strata [1]. Our prototypical tool for interactively visualizing such percentile charts together with user-entered blood count values from individual patients was implemented as a web application based on conventional server-side technical platforms. Frontend interactivity was realized via jQuery, while PHP scripts dynamically generate chart graphics and downloadable multi-page PDF files.

Users can enter the patient's sex, birth date and test results from a set of measurement series. Each series includes up to nine hematological analytes as well as the corresponding measurement dates, which can be easily entered via a specialized calendar widget. Besides the plotted percentiles (see figure 1), age-adjusted Z-scores are dynamically calculated for each value and are embedded in the form of „micro-graphics" next to the input fields. A simple color coding scheme highlights pathological results. All user-entered data can be encoded as and later recalled from Uniform Resource Locators (URLs). An English version of the visualization tool can be accessed at http://www.pedref.org/.

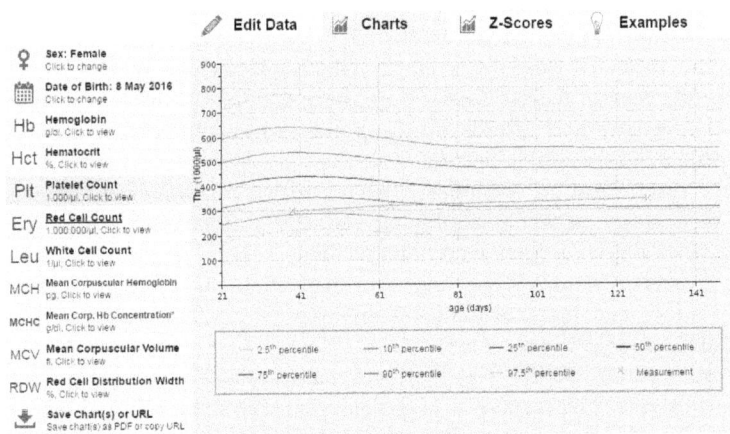

Figure 1. Screenshot of an English version of the visualization tool showing the „Charts" view for the platelet count. Age-dependent percentiles are presented in shades of blue, while current patient measurements are shown in red.

To assess how well the underlying continuous percentile models discriminate between relevant pathology and physiological variation, we considered the exemplary setting of hemoglobinopathy classification based on blood count analysis. The ground truth of our investigation was a de-identified dataset of blood count parameters, taken from initial blood draws of approximately 100 patients including diagnoses. According to the pertinent literature on hemoglobinopathies, we developed simple classification rules, such as „*Is the Hb value below the 2.5th percentile of the standard RI?*" To statistically compare classifier performance, we calculated sensitivity, specificity, as well as receiver operating characteristic curves.

For the usability analysis, we prepared two interpretation tasks of intermediate difficulty; these scenarios required that the test persons access different functions of the visualization tool for interpreting given clinical cases. The test setup consisted of a laptop and a webcam with a microphone. Besides audio and video records, we also captured their onscreen activities to gather task-specific information about possible usability flaws.

Four pediatricians with professional experience ranging between 5 and 14 years participated in separate TA sessions of approximately 30 minutes, held in the pediatrics hospital in Erlangen. During the TA sessions, we tried to keep the level of interference as low as possible, only reminding subjects to think aloud after longer phases of not verbalizing [7]. To gather physician perceptions of the interactive visualizations, we prompted participants to fill out a questionnaire that contained 32 multiple choice items regarding usability, required effort, as well as perceived benefits of the application. From the responses, we calculated system usability scale (SUS) [8] scores.

3. Results

After excluding 15 of the 100 cases due to certain missing blood count values or diagnoses, we analyzed hemoglobinopathy differentiability based on the remaining 85 cases. Inspecting blood count parameters in relation to the RIs revealed that thalassemia diseases might be differentiated from all other observed diagnoses by evaluating the mean corpuscular volume, which seemed to be sharply decreased especially in the case of thalassemia minor. Minor and major forms of thalassemia, as well as homozygosity and heterozygosity of the sickle cell disease, appeared to be distinguishable in a comparable fashion.

In these discrimination scenarios, high classifier performances were achieved. However, differences between employing standard reference intervals, continuous reference intervals and Z-scores were diminishingly small. For example, the resulting area-under-the-curve values regarding the distinction between the 25 cases of thalassemia minor and the remaining 60 diseases were 0.949 (standard RIs), 0.945 (continuous RIs) and 0.912 (Z-scores).

Observations from the TA tests indicated that test subjects were able to complete most tasks with ease. The responses to the questionnaire indicated that our developed application is by and large usable. The items that concerned the data entry options and the Z-score micrographics, for example, were rated very well. However, the evaluation also yielded suggestions for improving certain features, such as connecting it to the hospital information system in order to automatically retrieve patient data via technical interfaces.

Two users had difficulties with the save function, because they were unaware of the German word for „clipboard" (copy-to-clipboard button). This can be seen as a minor issue that could be addressed via various possible solutions. Another suggestion for a potential optimization was given in a comment that implied that the colors of the different percentiles in the charts were not very easy to discriminate.

In total, however, an average SUS score of 86.9 with a standard deviation of 8.5 was obtained, indicating good overall usability. The expert interpretations of the clinical cases often did not match our previously specified diagnoses exactly, although their responses were very close to our expected solutions, and trends were recognized correctly. The additional feedback gathered after the TA sessions stated that the visualization tool could be especially beneficial for assessing more complex clinical cases.

4. Discussion

Our analyses demonstrate that all three models achieved a similar capability to reproduce previously diagnosed hemoglobinopathies. However, a detailed differentiation does not seem to be possible without more advanced tests that involve modern medical apparatus. Furthermore, the sample size was limited, and some patients might even have received blood transfusions before the blood draw, which could have distorted some findings. The good classification performance of all three reference models, on the other hand, indicates that an automated differentiation might be feasible in some scenarios. Further studies of a broader spectrum of hematological data could plausibly reveal additional benefits in other settings.

In order to assess the usability of our visualization tool prototype, we applied the TA protocol, a user-based usability evaluation method. Expert-based methods are seen as more suitable for earlier stages of development [4]. The standardized SUS score that we had measured was considerably above SUS scores that are often referenced in the literature about healthcare sector products [9; 10]. We interpret our obtained results as rather satisfying, and although test subjects were novice users, the visualization tool was well received. The additional feedback can be seen as a sign of interest in the modern visualization of continuous RI. While the usability assessment was done under controlled circumstances, investigations in clinical settings in various institutions could be a reasonable next step to possibly confirm and widen the findings from our experiments.

5. Conclusion

A highly usable tool for visualizing innovative continuous RI was developed. The promising results call for further research, especially towards the impact of integrating such a tool into daily routines.

6. Acknowledgement

Some of the results that are reported here have been previously submitted as part of JH's Master's thesis at Erlangen University. The physicians from the Department of Pediatrics and Adolescent Medicine of the University Hospital Erlangen are gratefully acknowledged for their precious time and effort in participating in this study.

References

[1] Zierk, J.; Arzideh, F.; Haeckel, R.; Rascher, W.; Rauh, M. & Metzler, M. Indirect determination of pediatric blood count reference intervals Clinical Chemistry and Laboratory Medicine, 2013;51:863–87
[2] Torsvik, T.; Lillebo, B. & Mikkelsen, G. Presentation of clinical laboratory results: an experimental comparison of four visualization techniques J. Am. Med. Inform. Assoc., 2013;20:325 - 331
[3] Bauer, D.; Guerlain, S. & Brown, J. The design and evaluation of a graphical display for laboratory data J Am Med Inform Assoc., 2010;17:41 6- 424
[4] Jaspers, M. A comparison of usability methods for testing interactive health technologies: Methodological aspects and empirical evidence Int J Med Informatics, 2009;78:340–353
[5] Fernandez, A.; Insfrana, E. & Abrahãoa, S. Usability Evaluation Methods for the Web: A Systematic Mapping Study Information And Software Technology, 2011;53:789-817
[6] Kutlar, F. Diagnostic Approach to Hemoglobinopathies Hemoglobin, 2007; 31:243-250
[7] Boren, T. & Ramey, J. Thinking Aloud: Reconciling Theory and Practice IEEE Transactions on Professional Communication, 2000;43:261-278
[8] Brooke, J. SUS - A quick and dirty usability scale, Digital Equipment Co Ltd., Reading, United Kingdom, 1986
[9] Kortum, P. & Peres, C. S. Evaluation of Home Health Care Devices: Remote Usability Assessment JMIR Human Factors, 2015, 2, e10
[10] Brooke, J. SUS: A Retrospective Journal of Usability Studies, 2013;8:29-40

212

German Medical Data Sciences: Visions and Bridges
R. Röhrig et al. (Eds.)
© 2017 German Association for Medical Informatics, Biometry and Epidemiology (gmds) e.V. and IOS Press.
This article is published online with Open Access by IOS Press and distributed under the terms
of the Creative Commons Attribution Non-Commercial License 4.0 (CC BY-NC 4.0).
doi:10.3233/978-1-61499-808-2-212

Machine Learning Models of Post-Intubation Hypoxia During General Anesthesia

Philipp SIPPL [a], Thomas GANSLANDT [b], Hans-Ulrich PROKOSCH [a,b],
Tino MUENSTER [c] and Dennis TODDENROTH [a,1]

[a] *Medical Informatics, Univ. of Erlangen-Nürnberg, Erlangen.* [b] *Medical Center for Information and Communication Technology, University Hospital Erlangen.* [c] *Dept of Anaesthesiology & Intensive Care, University Hospital Erlangen.*

Abstract. Fine-meshed perioperative measurements are offering enormous potential for automatically investigating clinical complications during general anesthesia. In this study, we employed multiple machine learning methods to model perioperative hypoxia and compare their respective capabilities. After exporting and visualizing 620 series of perioperative vital signs, we had ten anesthesiologists annotate the subjective presence and severity of temporary post-intubation oxygen desaturation. We then applied specific clustering and prediction methods on the acquired annotations, and evaluated their performance in comparison to the inter-rater agreement between experts. When reproducing the expert annotations, the sensitivity and specificity of multi-layer neural networks substantially outperformed clustering and simpler threshold-based methods. The achieved performance of our best automated hypoxia models thereby approximately equaled the observed agreement between different medical experts. Furthermore, we deployed our classification methods for processing unlabeled inputs to estimate the incidence of hypoxic episodes in another sizeable patient cohort, which attests to the feasibility of using the approach on a larger scale. We interpret that our machine learning models could be instrumental for computerized observational studies of the clinical determinants of post-intubation oxygen deficiency. Future research might also investigate potential benefits of more advanced preprocessing approaches such as automated feature learning.

Keywords. Machine Learning, Anesthesia, General, Hypoxia, Medical Records Systems, Computerized

1. Introduction

While modern anesthetic procedures already achieve considerable clinical safety, electronic documentation promises to computerize the analysis of perioperative complications in order to identify preexisting complication-predisposing constellations. Among critical situations that may occur during general anesthesia, hypoxia after endotracheal intubation can be difficult to investigate systematically, insofar as such episodes can produce polymorphic patterns in recorded time series. Studying such phenomena requires that analytical algorithms are closely adapted to the particular clinical problem as well as to the specific structure of the input data [1].

---

[1] Corresponding Author, Dr. Dennis Toddenroth, Medical Informatics, Friedrich-Alexander-Universität Erlangen-Nürnberg (FAU), Erlangen, Germany, dennis.toddenroth@fau.de

While machine learning (ML) methods are already widely accepted for various medical data-processing tasks, the peculiar data format of time series inputs with their repeated measurements does not naturally conform to the column-based structure processed by conventional machine learning algorithms. This demonstrates the need for suitable methods for converting and processing time series in order to be usable by machine learning algorithms. In this study, we thus adapt and evaluate ML methods for modeling post-intubation oxygen desaturation in perioperative time series.

2. Methods

To gather expert annotations of post-intubation hypoxia as a starting point for model development and evaluation, we exported and visualized de-identified perioperative time series from 2015 from the clinical data warehouse of Erlangen University Hospital. As our analyses were exclusively geared to optimizing and evaluating analytical methods based on de-identified clinical data, informal consultation with a representative from the local ethics committee indicated that no formal review was necessary. Since the overall incidence of relevant cases was expected to be low, an oversampling method was chosen to optimize the relevance and information content of each manually annotated label. This oversampling was implemented by deliberately selecting those perioperative series with lower global SaO_2 minima with a higher probability.

Afterwards a group of ten specialist physicians accessed each individually allocated set of graphics in a customized web application (see figure 1) and entered the subjective presence and severity of temporary oxygen desaturation during anesthesia induction and intubation. Severity was thereby measured on a four-stage ordinal scale (light, moderate, severe, not existent), which corresponds to the one used in [5].

Each expert was given approximately one hundred time series graphics that displayed the timestamps for anesthesia and intubation as well as the trends of arterial oxygenation (SaO_2), mean arterial pressure and heart rate (HR) from the initial 30 minutes of each anesthesia induction episode. About 20 percent of episodes were annotated by three experts, so that the performance of ML models could be evaluated in comparison to the mutual agreement between human experts. For training and testing phases these duplicates were consolidated via a majority decision. In total, 1576 labels were gathered for 620 unique time series. We then split these annotations into disjunctive subsets for training and testing ML models according to a ratio of 80 to 20.

Dynamic Time Warping (DTW) as implemented in the R library *dtwclust* was used as one of the methods geared towards processing clinical time series, which seemed suitable due to its invariance under time shifts and differences in scale or noise [2]. DTW-based distance measures were used in combination with two clustering techniques, namely *TADPole* and KNN, with the former one being an algorithm specialized on time series [3], and the latter a simpler clustering method used as a comparison.

To estimate the relevance of other input variables for hypoxia models, including basic patient attributes such as demographics, Random Forest and deep learning methods in form of multi-layer neural networks were also applied to the available dataset. This was realized via the R library *cforest* and the R implementation of the *H2O* Framework. In practice, certain case-specific clinical attributes were simply copied from the original data exports, while some were computed with these dedicated preprocessing methods from the time series structure. The resulting intermediate column-based representation that was then passed on to the ML algorithms consisted of 17 different features in total. To identify suitable feature constellations for Random Forest models and multi-layer neural networks, we employed the wrapper method [4] for more than 1000 unique feature constellations and subset sizes. Automatically trained models were then ranked by their respective sensitivity, specificity and Youden's index on the same separate test data.

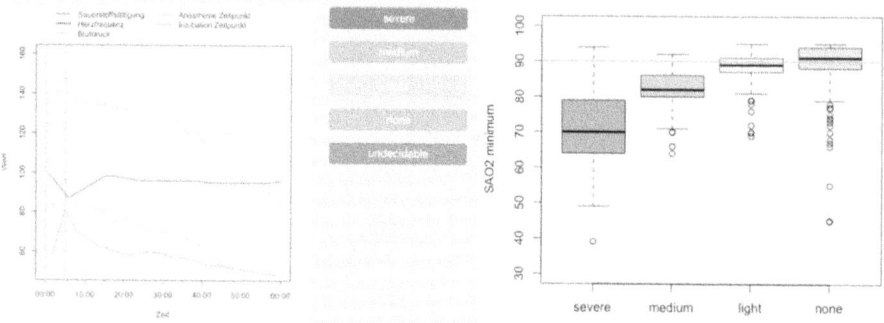

Figure 1. Annotation tool with scale for example time series (left), distribution of SaO2 minima (right).

3. Results

3.1. Descriptive distribution of annotation data

Annotation results showed that assessments of any oxygen desaturation (either light, medium or severe) were entered nearly as often as the absence of any hypoxia. Due to our intentional oversampling, however, this distribution cannot be seen as representative for the overall incidence of oxygen desaturation among all episodes. As expected, the medians of the SaO_2 minima of each group showed clear associations with hypoxia labels, and seemed to correspond to the threshold values used for differentiation in [5], although the substantial overlap between the boxplots also indicates that SaO_2-minima alone do not achieve a satisfactory discrimination (see figure 1). This points to the potential additional benefits of more advanced methods and of using further information than just SaO_2 minima.

3.2. Building machine learning models

Based on this annotated data, we evaluated how well a conventional threshold from the literature of a minimum of 90% SaO_2 [5,6] reproduced the labeled presence or absence of oxygen desaturation. This simple criterion achieved a sensitivity of 67,9% and a specificity of 62,7%, which corresponds to a Youden's index of 0,31. Interestingly, the more complex and computationally expensive DTW method did not substantially outperform this approach as measured by Youden's index, neither in combination with TADPole, which demonstrated a sensitivity of 51,8% and specificity of 81,9% in conjunction with 3 clusters, nor with KNN (k=5), which reached a sensitivity of 60,7% and specificity of 70,0%. Random Forest models outperformed all previously described methods using a combination of six different features. These feature sets included basic patient attributes such as weight, but were mostly derived from the available time series, including mean arterial pressure, HR and SaO_2. All tested Random Forest models attained high specificity, but only relatively low sensitivity.

The best overall results were achieved by a multi-layer neural network with three hidden layers that each consisted of 50 nodes. The automated feature selection process resulted in overall model scores of 74% sensitivity and 93% specificity, while using a subset of seven features, including the area of the SaO_2 curve below a presumed threshold of 95%-saturation, the global drop of SaO_2, the latency between intubation and the observed SaO_2 minimum, patient age, Cormack-Lehane scores of expected intubation difficulty [7], the 'awake intubation' flag, and ratio of HR at time of SaO_2 minimum to the global HR maximum.

3.3. Comparison to medical experts and model application

According to the overlapping annotations from three physicians, it could be shown that all three experts reached exact agreement for 52% of the cases. While this full consensus within the gold standard may seem small, one should take into consideration that perfect alignment within three or more experts on a four-stage scale is itself relatively hard to attain on a task that allows considerable room for interpretation and furthermore, while another 39% of our labels only differed by one level on our ordinal scale. Thereby, most disagreements arose due to discrepancies between light and no hypoxia. For comparison, our best ML models aligned exactly with consolidated annotations in 71% of all cases. In a second comparison for each of the overlapping annotations, one label was picked randomly and compared to the combined version of all. This should simulate the performance of a single random physician, who achieved an alignment of 79% and therefore slightly beat the model according to this comparison method.

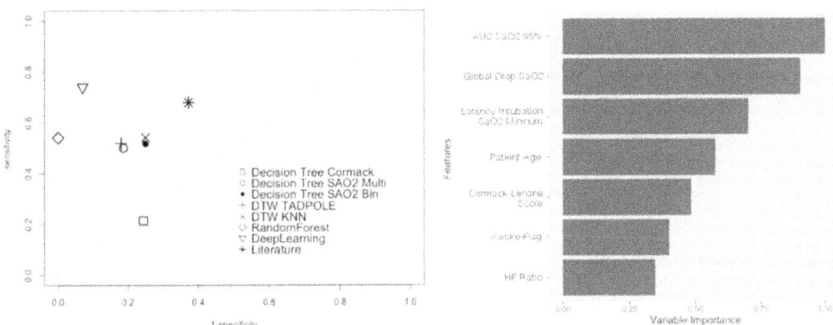

Figure 2. Results of all different models in ROC chart with each model being displayed by corresponding sensitivity/specificity pair (left), all features used by the neural network sorted by importance (right).

Using the best neural network to compute desaturation classes in the unlabeled dataset of 17.000 perioperative episodes from 2015, we were able to estimate that any form of oxygen desaturation occurs during less than 10% of episodes, while severe or medium hypoxia affects 3-5% of anesthesia inductions and intubations. These plausible figures point to the fundamental feasibility and to the potential scientific utility of these automated model-based annotations.

4. Discussion

Our findings indicate that DTW in combination with special clustering algorithms did not perform better than the SaO_2 threshold criterion from the literature. This suggests that these methods have not derived any time series patterns that would be more informative for reproducing hypoxia annotations than just the plain SaO_2 minima. Multi-layer neural networks achieved the best overall agreement with expert assessments by including additional patient information.

Observed accuracy for clinically relevant oxygen desaturation was quite high, whereas a lower model performance in the class of light desaturation cast some doubt on the practical utility of automatic identifications for this class. A similar problem of a reliable discrimination between milder forms of hypoxia also affected the original annotations from the medical experts, which suggests that this uncertainty was rather transferred to and not inherent to our ML model. Neural-network-based models far outperformed the threshold-based criterion from the literature and resembled the mutual agreement within the physician control group, which points to the potential scientific utility of this ML application.

Since some ML models use data that in practice would only become available after surgery, our methods would not be appropriate for real-time prediction scenarios, although the approach could be usable for computerizing large-scale retrospective observational studies of clinical determinants of post-intubation desaturation. Other potential clinical use cases could include quantitative reviews of the quality of care, or automatically monitoring the incidence of subtle clinical phenomena over time.

5. Conclusion

In this work we demonstrate the development of an ML model that is able to classify oxygen desaturation on a level that resembles the mutual agreement between human experts. These techniques are not inherently limited to analyzing SaO_2 patterns, but could in principle be applicable to other types of time series. Future research on the evolving methods might investigate the potential benefits of more advanced preprocessing approaches for clinical time series such as automated feature learning.

References

[1] Bellazzi R, Zupan B. Predictive data mining in clinical medicine: Current issues and guidelines. Int J Med Inform. 2008;77(2):81–97.
[2] Sardá-Espinosa A. Comparing Time-Series Clustering Algorithms in R Using the dtwclust Package. 2015;1–41.
[3] Begum N, Wang J. Accelerating Dynamic Time Warping Clustering with a Novel Admissible Pruning Strategy. 2015;49–58.
[4] Guyon IAE. An Introduction to Variable and Feature Selection 1 Introduction. 2003;3:1157–82.
[5] Hansjörg Aust et al. Impact of medical training and clinical experience on the assessment of oxygenation and hypoxaemia after general anaesthesia: an observational study. J Clin Monit Comput (2015) 29:415–426
[6] Dunford et. al. Incidence of Transient Hypoxia and Pulse Rate Reactivity During Paramedic Rapid Sequence Intubation. 2003;(December):1–8.
[7] Cormack RS, Lehane J. Difficult tracheal intubation in obstetrics. Anaesthesia. 1984;39(11):1105–11.

German Medical Data Sciences: Visions and Bridges
R. Röhrig et al. (Eds.)
217
© *2017 German Association for Medical Informatics, Biometry and Epidemiology (gmds) e.V. and IOS Press.*
This article is published online with Open Access by IOS Press and distributed under the terms
of the Creative Commons Attribution Non-Commercial License 4.0 (CC BY-NC 4.0).
doi:10.3233/978-1-61499-808-2-217

Considering Information Up-to-Dateness to Increase the Accuracy of Therapy Decision Support Systems

Jan GAEBEL[a,1], Mario A. CYPKO[a], Steffen OELTZE-JAFRA[a]

[a] *Innovation Center Computer Assisted Surgery, University Leipzig, Faculty of Medicine, Leipzig, Germany*

Abstract. During the diagnostic process a lot of information is generated. All this information is assessed when making a final diagnosis and planning the therapy. While some patient information is stable, e.g., gender, others may become outdated, e.g., tumor size derived from CT data. Quantifying this information up-to-dateness and deriving consequences are difficult. Especially for the implementation in clinical decision support systems, this has not been studied. When information entities tend to become outdated, in practice, clinicians intuitively reduce their impact when making decisions. Therefore, in a system's calculations their impact should be reduced as well. We propose a method of decreasing the certainty of information entities based on their up-to-dateness. The method is tested in a decision support system for TNM staging based on Bayesian networks. We compared the actual N-state in records of 39 patients to the N-state calculated with and without decreasing data certainty. The results under decreased certainty correlated better with the actual states (r= 0.958, p=0.008). We conclude that the up-to-dateness must be considered when processing clinical information to enhance decision making and ensure more patient safety.

Keywords. Clinical Decision Support Systems, Cancer Staging, Probabilistic Models

1. Introduction

The primary tumor stage classification is recognized as the most important prognostic factor in oncological diseases. The TNM staging is derived from multiple different diagnostic findings and consists of three parameters: extent of primary tumor (T), infiltration of surrounding lymph nodes (N) and existence of distant metastases (M) [1]. Based on all diagnostic findings, the tumor stage is then interpreted by clinicians in tumor board meetings to find the most suitable therapy for a patient. Advanced stages are associated with a higher mortality and thereby influence the applicable therapy [2].

Usually the diagnostic process for patients with suspected head and neck tumors takes place in an outpatient setting. Therefore, the time span until a therapy decision is reached can take several weeks; known as the diagnostic delay. Caused by a longer delay, diagnostic findings may lose validity which could lead to suboptimal therapy decisions. In a meta-review, Gómez et al. combined the results of nine studies of head

---

[1]Jan Gaebel, Innovation Center Computer Assisted Surgery, Semmelweisstraße 14, 04277 Leipzig, Germany; E-mail: jan.gaebel@medizin.uni-leipzig.de.

and neck cancers. In average, they measured a diagnostic delay for non-advanced stages of 70 days and 73 days for advanced tumor stages. They found a significant correlation between diagnostic delay and advanced tumor stages [2]. However, it is hard to find suggestions or recommendations for tolerable delays. Jensen et al. claim that it is not possible to define thresholds for acceptable time intervals [3].

To support physicians in finding the best treatment decision for laryngeal cancer, we are developing a treatment decision support system (TDSS). The TDSS is based on a Bayesian network (BN). A BN describes a decision by a directed, acyclic graph (DAG) with conditional probabilities [4]. A DAG consists of a set of variables and direct causal dependencies between pairs of these variables. Each variable has at least two states, from which one can occur in a specific situation. Clinical information can be assigned to the states of a subset of the network's variables, and an inference algorithm infers the probabilistic occurrence for all states of the remaining, unobserved variables. We developed a disease model for laryngeal cancer with over 900 variables and 1200 dependencies [5]. From this model, a subset with 303 variables and 334 dependencies describes the TNM staging. The system has an accuracy of 89% in calculating the tumor stage [6]. With empirical studies, we recognized that incorrect calculations are based on at times outdated and therefore inconsistent information. By itself, a Bayesian network is not capable of evaluating individual information entities based on aspects like their up-to-dateness. Technical methodologies for information applicability, e.g. fuzzy sets in Arden Syntax [7], have deficits in complex decision inference, but are suitable frameworks for information preprocessing and evaluation. In this paper, we propose a method to assess the diagnostic delay of patient information.

2. Methods

We retrospectively analyzed 39 cases of patients with laryngeal cancer from 2013 that were treated in our specialized otolaryngologic clinic. The data was provided by this clinic and contained all finding results with the respective date of the procedure. A physician pre-structured and anonymized it beforehand. For the exemplary evaluation of the up-to-dateness, we focused on calculating the N-state of the tumor. Determining the N-state of laryngeal cancer requires information from radiological examinations (CT or MRI scan of the neck and sonography) and histopathological analyses.

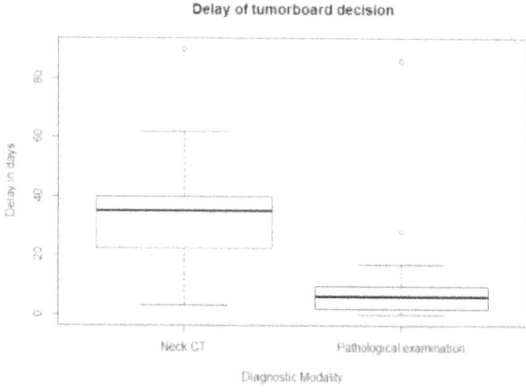

Figure 1. Delays of diagnostic examinations relative to the respective tumor board meetings.

All 39 cases contained findings from radiology and pathology, which were expressive enough to evaluate the N-state. We calculated the delay of each procedure relative to the date of the respective tumor board meeting that the patients were discussed at. In Figure 1, the delays of CT scans and histopathological examinations relative to the tumor board meeting are presented. The two outliers at over 80 days are two patients that were transferred from a primary care physician after initial anamnesis and diagnosis. The median delay for the neck CT scans is 35 days, for the histopathological reports the delay is 6 days. Hence, as a subgroup of a complete diagnostic process the data in general coincides with the average values (around 70 days) stated by Gómez et al. in [2]. For the application in the BN-based TDSS, we chose these median delays as thresholds beyond which the information is no longer considered reliable.

Each variable in the Bayesian network is defined with different states, representing the possible values of the real world patient situation. For example, they contain the different aspects of infiltration that are necessary for the determination of the N-state, as illustrated in Figure 2. The state "unknown" represents the uncertainty inherent to the diagnostic modality or as declared by the physician. We employ the unknown state to reflect outdated information. To answer the question of how the impact of information should be reduced when it is too old, we iteratively calculated the behavior of our system with different probability values for the unknown state.

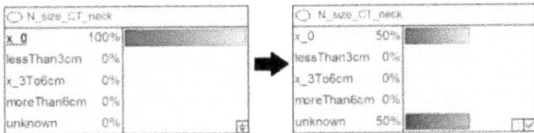

Figure 2. Adaptation of certainty values for outdated data in a node of the BN model.

We implemented a Java program that processes the BN decision model using the framework *SMILE*; a reasoning engine for graphical models. The data of the 39 test cases was copied to a local MySQL database for easier access by the program. For information that is older than the calculated median value (35 days for CT, 6 days for pathology), we iteratively decreased the certainty of the respective finding by 10%. This change was entered into the Bayesian network as the value of each single state within one node, representing the probability of occurrence of the respective state (see Figure 2). We started with 100% for each observed state and then reduced the input values by 10% and simultaneously increasing the "unknown"-state, since the sum of all input values in one node must add up to 100%.

We compared the calculated N-state with the declared N-state in the patient record. For the initial correlation between the documented N-state in the patient record and the computed N-state of our system, we calculated the Pearson correlation coefficient. To be able to calculate correlations between ordinal data, like stages in the N-state, we substituted them with numerical values, e.g. "N1"=1, "N2a"=2.0, "N2b"=2.3 etc.

3. Results

Without any preconditions, our system computed 35 out of 39 N-states correctly (accuracy $a = 0.897$) with a correlation coefficient $r = 0.877$ ($p = 2.43 * 10^{-13}$). For all 39 cases, we computed the N-state with iteratively decreasing certainty. In 14 cases no reduction was necessary because the information entities were not delayed. Figure 3 shows the trend of the accuracy depending on the certainty that is associated with the information entities. With a certainty of $c = 0.4$, the system correctly calculated 36 N-states; using $c = 0.3$, 37 correct N-states were calculated. The set of cases with an already correctly computed N-state was stable and growing across the iterations from $c = 1.0$ down to $c = 0.1$. Hence, an adjustment of the certainty c did not corrupt prior correct results. Only when an information was discarded completely ($c = 0.0$), the accuracy dropped drastically (23 out of 39, $a = 0.589$).

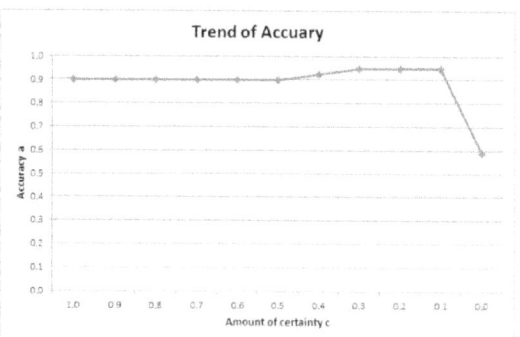

Figure 3. Distribution of certainty values for delayed data

With a correlation coefficient of $r = 0.877$ and an accuracy of 35 out of 39 results, the decision support system for TNM staging correlates well with the real world status of the patient. With the application of reduced certainty $c = 0.3$, we reached an accuracy of $c = 0.948$ (37 out of 39 cases) and a correlation of $r = 0.958$ ($p < 0.05$). The two remaining cases suffered from data inconsistency in the patient record, so that a correct TNM stage could not be calculated. We performed a Fisher z-transformation to transfer the sample pairs into a normal distribution. Conducting a right-sided Steiger's Z-test shows that our method results in a significantly better correlation ($p < 0.05$).

4. Discussion

This paper introduces a method to consider diagnostic delay in a decision support system. Individual information entities are evaluated by the time between the performed diagnostic procedure and the tumor board meeting in which the information is assessed. However, the sample size of our study is rather small (39 cases). We analyzed the influence of the amount of certainty of an information entity on the calculation results of our decision support system. With 30-40%, the information certainty is reduced to a reasonable amount so that the results of the decision support system are improved. The correlations of the computed results to the actual N-state of laryngeal cancers are significantly better than with no consideration of the delay.

The application with respect to other clinical facets, e.g. other types of tumors, is not assured. Tumors, different from laryngeal cancers, may grow at different rates, so that the diagnostic delay needs to be reevaluated. We are sure however, that the general method can be expanded to other oncological aspects or even different clinical fields with the necessary adjustments.

The method of dealing with medical uncertainty in a clinical decision support system based on probabilistic models can be translated to other kinds of uncertainty. Different diagnostic modalities entail different types of uncertainty, e.g. blur or noise in radiological images. Experiences and states of knowledge of physicians (e.g. resident vs. specialized physician) could also be represented by quantification of uncertainty.

It is also very important to notify the clinical users about the fact that information entities are being evaluated as outdated and their certainty is therefore reduced. They must in the end understand the decisions that the system proposes and choose the most suitable therapy. However, the use of an adjusted certainty for other technical environments, e.g. onscreen notifications, must be reconsidered. The main issue would be the corresponding consequence of such an adjusted information certainty.

5. Conclusion

We propose an approach to considering information up-to-dateness. The evaluation of the diagnostic delay and the definition of a possible threshold for the application in decision support systems are necessary methods to understand and objectify the coherences of diagnostic delays. We will conduct another study with additional patient data to validate the calculated temporal thresholds and applicable amount of certainty.

We plan to extend our therapy decision support system with additional functionalities that assess the up-to-dateness of the clinical information from the electronic patient records. The interpretation of the information certainty will be implemented as intelligent agents. We plan to use Arden Syntax since it is a language for medical decisions. In individual medical logic modules, we will define the assessment of the up-to-dateness. The system of agents can be implemented into systems and act as an interface between the hospital information system and the TDSS.

6. Conflict of Interest

The authors state that they have no conflict of interests.

References

[1] National Cancer Institute. Cancer Staging [Online]. Available: https://www.cancer.gov/aboutcancer /diagnosis-staging/staging. [Accessed: 07-Dec-2016].
[2] I. Gómez, J. Seoane, P. Varela-Centelles, P. Diz, B. Takkouche, *Is diagnostic delay related to advanced-stage oral cancer? A meta-analysis*, Eur. J. Oral Sci., **117**:5 (2009), 541–546.
[3] A. R. Jensen, H. M. Nellemann, J. Overgaard, *Tumor progression in waiting time for radiotherapy in head and neck cancer*, Radiother. Oncol., **84**:1 (2007), 5–10.
[4] J. Pearl, *Probabilistic Reasoning in Intelligent Systems: Networks of Plausible Inference*. San Francisco, CA, USA: Morgan Kaufmann Publishers Inc., 1988.
[5] M. Stoehr, M.A. Cypko, K. Denecke, H.U. Lemke, A. Dietz, *A model of the decision-making process: therapy of laryngeal cancer*, Int J Comput Assist Radiol Surg., **9**:1 (2014), 217-218.
[6] M.A. Cypko, M. Stoehr, M. Kozniewski, M. Druzdzel, A. Dietz, L. Berliner, H.U. Lemke, *Validation workflow for a clinical Bayesian network model in multidisciplinary decision making in head and neck oncology treatment*, Int J Comput Assist Radiol Surg., (2017), 1-14.
[7] T. Vetterlein, H. Mandl, K.-P. Adlassnig. *Fuzzy Arden Syntax: A fuzzy programming language for medicine*, Artif Intell Med., **49**:1 (2010), 1–10.

222

German Medical Data Sciences: Visions and Bridges
R. Röhrig et al. (Eds.)
© 2017 German Association for Medical Informatics, Biometry and Epidemiology (gmds) e.V. and IOS Press.
This article is published online with Open Access by IOS Press and distributed under the terms
of the Creative Commons Attribution Non-Commercial License 4.0 (CC BY-NC 4.0).
doi:10.3233/978-1-61499-808-2-222

Processual Reasoning over Sequences of Situations in Endoscopic Surgery

Sebastian SIEMOLEIT[a,1], Alexandr UCITELI[a], Richard BIECK[b] and Heinrich HERRE[a]

[a] *Institute for Medical Informatics, Statistics and Epidemiology (IMISE), Leipzig University, Germany*
[b] *Innovation Center for Computer Assisted Surgery, Leipzig University, Germany*

Abstract. Minimally invasive surgery is a highly complex and technically demanding alternative to open surgery. Surgical procedures based on this method are characterized by small incisions and allow for a fast recovery of the patient. Such techniques are challenging for surgeons since they do not have a direct view of the surgical area. Systems that provide surgical navigation are well established in clinical practice but depend on external markers allowing a mapping between a surgeon's tools and a patient's medical images. As of today, these systems are prone to inaccuracies, the reasons of which lie in their extensive technical requirements. The BIOPASS project aims to develop an alternative that works without external markers and indirect computation of locations. An ontology has been used to provide an adequate vocabulary describing situations and their temporal relationship. This ontology is expected to relate real time multimodal sensor data and static surgical process models in order to infer movement directions, subsequent actions and hidden anatomical structures that inhere risk for surgical interventions. However, the Web Ontology Language is not capable of modelling temporal conditions, which are necessary to provide such exhaustive situational descriptions as expected by a surgeon. This paper concerns an ontology design pattern developed to overcome this issue by the integration of dynamic ontological classes that are assigned according to the temporal relations between situations.

Keywords. Surgical Endoscopy, Computer-Assisted Surgery, Knowledge Bases, Decision Support Techniques, Situation Awareness

1. Introduction

Optical surgical navigation systems significantly reduce the cut-seam-time leading to improved post-operative results [1]. To gain further improvements in such systems, it is necessary to provide situational decision support for a surgeon based on information provided by endoscopic images these instruments capture. In the BIOPASS Project [2], we aim for a solution that comprises surgical process knowledge and multimodal sensor data to establish this goal. A set of highly specialized classifiers are incorporated to process these data to identify anatomical structures visible in an endoscopic image. To support a surgeon during a surgical intervention, the results have to be processed, unified and shown immediately to provide navigation information and suggestions about the next steps, which have to be taken according to the surgical process model.

---

[1] Sebastian Siemoleit, Institute of Medical Informatics, Statistics and Epidemiology, University of Leipzig, Härtelstraße 16, 04103 Leipzig, Germany; E-mail: ssiemoleit@imise.uni-leipzig.de

The BIOPASS Situation Ontology (BISON) has been implemented in the Web Ontology Language (OWL), which is the state of the art modelling language for ontologies [3], and is applied to a continuous stream of classification and sensor data. BISON consists of a complex vocabulary which formalizes these streams as sequences of situations, as well as axioms to infer knowledge about the most current surgical situation. Unfortunately, it is not possible to infer processual information from singular situations only. Thus, it was necessary to reference different states of individuals in axioms. However, to express that these states are exhibited by the same individual, the axioms must concern this individual and no other individual.

This problem of modelling in OWL is referred to as the *uncle problem* [4] and solved from a general perspective also in [5]. These approaches are applicable for many use cases since they use complex OWL constructs, but in our special case of changing data and streams that describe a sequence of situations, it is more elegant to use temporal information to approximate these constructs. We want to present such a novel approach that relies on temporal information that are encoded in simple OWL classes. This work was supported by the BMBF sponsored project BIOPASS (FK: 16SV7254K).

2. Methods

2.1. BIOPASS Situation Ontology

The General Formal Ontology (GFO) [6] provides a complex vocabulary describing processes as well as participating actors and their change during these processes [7]. In comparison to other top level ontologies [8,9,10] that only offer rudimentary process modelling capabilities, GFO can express concepts and relations that are necessary to describe the interrelations between surgical interventions and endoscopical images.

Surgical interventions belong to the class of *Situoids* and thus, are coherent and comprehensible as wholes. Situoids itself are processual entities since they describe entities that can be restricted to certain timepoints. The entities describing the state of the situoid at a timepoint are referred to as *situations*. The type of situations that are exhibited by surgical interventions are referred to as surgical situations and describe endoscopical images. The parts of a surgical interventions are anatomical objects, e.g. anatomical features, internal organs, or blood vessels. They belong to the class of *material continuants* because they persist through time and have a lifetime. At each timepoint of this lifetime they exhibit *presentials*. The type of presentials that are exhibited by anatomical objects are referred to as anatomical structures. These structures are the *constituents* of surgical situations if they occur in an endoscopic image.

In GFO, each individual participates in a spatiotemporal reality. Thus, there is a spatial and a temporal order between the individuals that we have defined. Situations are temporally ordered and we say a situation *a temporally_follows* a situation *b*. This temporal order is a strict linear ordering. Anatomical objects are spatially ordered according to a surgeon's expectancy of them to occur in an intervention. We say that an anatomical object *a spatially_follows* an anatomical object *b*, if *a* is located farther from the entrance of a surgical intervention than *b*. It is obvious that such expectancy is specific to each type of surgical intervention. This spatial order is a strict partial ordering.

BISON in its entirety will be published elsewhere and thoroughly discussed regarding approaches like [11] that focus on a different level of reality since they are based on activities in processes rather than the spatiotemporal relations of their actors.

2.2. Modelling of Situational Knowledge

Despite the tasks to determine hidden anatomical structures that inhere a risk for the surgical intervention, i.e. risk structures, and to indicate which anatomical objects will exhibit an anatomical structure in following situations, the most important task was to infer the direction in which the endoscope has been moved. The sensors of the endoscope can detect the direction of movements, such that data of image classifiers can be validated. If detected anatomical structures in the endoscopical image imply a backwards movement and the sensors registered a forwards movement, the classifier data represent false results and must be disregarded.

If there had been only one visible anatomical structure in each endoscopical image, the rule which infers the directions of its implied movement would have been a simple formula. Because this case is highly unlikely, we had to model the following two propositions that exhaustively describe forwards movements and can be expressed analogously for backwards movements. (a) If an anatomical object o is visible in a situation s, but was not visible in the temporally preceding surgical situation s' of s, and o is spatially following any of the anatomical objects which were visible in s', s participates in a forwards movement. (b) If an anatomical object o is not visible in a surgical situation s, but was visible in the temporally preceding surgical situation of s, and o is spatially preceding any of the visible anatomical objects of s, s participates in a forwards movement. We assume, that situations fulfilling (a) and (b) are participating in a movement that is prolonged into the future, although this cannot be inferred from presential information. In fact, if the surgical situation that is directly following temporally does not fulfill (a) and (b), the movement has come to its end.

$$
\begin{aligned}
\forall x \exists u (Surgical\_situation(x) \wedge Anatomical\_structure(u) \\
\wedge\ has\_constituent(x, u) \\
\wedge\ \exists v, w (Surgical\_situation(v) \wedge Anatomical\_structure(w) \\
\wedge\ has\_constituent(v, w) \wedge temporally\_follows(x, v) \\
\wedge\ \exists s, t (exhibited\_by(u, s) \wedge exhibited\_by(w, t) \\
\wedge\ spatially\_follows(s, t)) \\
\wedge\ (\neg has\_constituent(v, u) \vee \neg has\_constituent(x, w))) \\
\rightarrow \exists y (Forwards\_movement(y) \wedge participates\_in(x, y)))
\end{aligned} \tag{1}
$$

Eq. 1 generalizes (a) and (b) formally. It includes a syntactical diamond as described in [5] and, thus, is not expressible in OWL, which is restricted to tree syntax only.

3. Results

We introduced the classes *Current_situation* and *Last_situation*, which are specific surgical situations. The current situation is the unique surgical situation that describes the most recent endoscopical image. The last situation is its direct temporal predecessor. Both classes have exactly one member changing with every new set of classification and sensor data. Since this behaviour is counterintuitive to the character of OWL classes, which generally do not lose members but rather grow monotonically, we call them dynamic classes. The usage of these classes allows for an alternative definition of Eq. (1) without the clause *temporally_follows*(x, v). Furthermore, we can define the classes *Occurring_anatomical_object* and *Last_occurred_anatomical_object*.

However, OWL is based on the open world assumption, which states that if a fact is not given resp. inferred, its negation is necessarily true. Thus, a reasoning engine is not able to decide if an anatomical structure is not constituent of a surgical situation if this fact is not asserted in the dataset. The negation of such a fact would have been defined as a negative object property assertion. Likewise, the engine is not able to falsify the existence of another current situation if this class is no nominal. Both constructs increase the DL expressivity of our constructs, which implies a higher reasoning complexity and hence have a tremendous impact on the system's performance with respect to the implementation of state of the art reasoners [12]. Thus, we decided to approximate both constructs with the introduction of the classes *Not_occurring_anatomical_object* and *Not_last_occurred_anatomical_object*, enabling us to formulate axioms (figure 1) that completely define the participation of the current situation in forwards movements.

```
Current_situation                                      Current_situation
   and (has_constituent_part some (Anatomical_structure    and (temporally_follows some (Surgical_situation
   and (exhibited_by some (Anatomical_object               and (has_constituent_part some (Anatomical_structure
   and Not_last_occurred_anatomical_object                 and (exhibited_by some (Anatomical_object
   and (spatially_follows some Last_occurred_anatomical_object)))))     and Not_occurring_anatomical_object
     SubClassOf participates_in some Forwards_movement        and (spatially_precedes some Occurring_anatomical_object)))))))
                                                            SubClassOf participates_in some Forwards_movement
```

Figure 1. General Class Axioms that define the most recent situation to participate in a forwards movement.

This argument forced us to assert the members of these dynamic classes according to the stream of classifier and sensor data rather than inferring them from the temporal relation of the current resp. last situation, such that each new set of data defines a unique dataset. Without dynamic class membership, all datasets could be unified into a coherent whole; if this membership is included, they are mutually contradictory. This has no impact on our system, since it is only necessary to keep a set of two situations in memory to infer the direction of movement resp. three situations if changing directions need to be inferred.

4. Discussion

Compared to the pattern proposed in [4], our approach has the advantage that no nominals must be used, which decreases the DL expressivity. One might argue that such effect is marginal after a restriction to OWL EL [13] because this profile allows singleton nominals with a lowered reasoning complexity. However, if we expressed dynamic concepts as nominals, each new situation had to be formalized as a Tbox change rather than an Abox change, resulting in repeating reclassifications of the ontology.

The even more complex pattern proposed in [5] is far too expressive in our context. The approach disqualifies itself for our purpose by the mere amount of additional information it presupposes to be applied. As surgical situations are coherent wholes they can be bound to dynamic classes, such that there is no need to implement a complex vocabulary build around *owl: sameAs*.

One might argue that given problem could be solved by temporal reasoning engines as described in [14]. However, the individuals are not only ordered temporally but also integrated in a spatiotemporal process. Moreover, since temporal reasoning as needed in BIOPASS, i.e. PTL constructs necessary to encode preceding states of individuals, has been proven undecidable [15], approximations like the one presented in this paper seem more feasible for the given use case of representing real-time data streams.

5. Conclusion

We presented an approach that empowered us to infer the direction of movement from a stream of classifier and sensor data that have been formalized as a sequence of surgical situations. Although the introduced dynamic classes were intended to be used in the context of sequences of surgical situations only, we believe that there is a more abstract concept behind this ontology design pattern. Such abstraction will be analyzed as an application of the ontological axiomatizations of Space and Time in GFO. Furthermore, the discussed dynamic classes have been used to simplify existing axioms in BISON, e.g. the detection of risk structures with respect to the current situation.

6. Conflict of Interest

The authors state that they have no conflict of interests.

References

[1] G. Strauß, E. Limpert, M. Strauß, M. Hofer, E. Dittrich, S. Nowatschin and T. Lüth, "Untersuchungen zur Effizienz eines Navigationssystems für die HNO-Chirurgie: Auswertungen von 300 Patienten", *Laryngo-Rhino-Otologie*, **88** (2009).

[2] Leipzig University, ICCAS, BIOPASS: Bild-, Ontologie- und Prozessgestützte Assistenz für die minimal-invasive endoskopische Chirurgie, https://www.iccas.de/forschung/weitere-projekte/biopass/

[3] P. Hitzler, M. Krötzsch, B. Parsia, P.F. Patel-Schneider and S. Rudolph, eds., *OWL 2 Web Ontology Language: Primer*. W3C Recommendation (27 October 2009).

[4] M. Krötzsch, F. Maier, A. Krisnadhi and P. Hitzler, A Better Uncle for OWL: Nominal Schemas for Integrating Rules and Ontologies, in: *Proc. 20th International Conference on World Wide Web (WWW'11)*, ACM (2011), pp. 645–654.

[5] R. Hoekstra and J. Breuker, Polishing Diamonds in OWL 2, Knowledge Engineering: Practice and Patterns: 16th International Conference, Springer, Berlin (2008), pp.64–73.

[6] H. Herre, General Formal Ontology (GFO): A Foundational Ontology for Conceptual Modelling, *Theory and Applications of Ontology: Computer Applications*, Springer Berlin (2010), pp. 297-345.

[7] H. Herre, Persistence, Change, and the Integration of Objects and Processes in the Framework of the General Formal Ontology, *Dynamic Being*, Cambridge Scholar Publishing (2015), pp. 337–354.

[8] A. Gangemi, N. Guarino, C. Masolo, A. Oltramari , L. Schneider, Sweetening Ontologies with DOLCE, *Knowledge Engineering and Knowledge Management: Ontologies and the Semantic Web*, , Springer Berlin Heidelberg (2002), pp. 166–181.

[9] R. Arp, B. Smith and A.D. Spear, *Building ontologies with basic formal ontology*. Mit Press, Cambridge MA, 2015.

[10] A. Pease, I. Niles and J. Li, The Suggested Upper Merged Ontology: A Large Ontology for the Semantic Web and its Applications, *Working Notes of the AAAI-2002 Workshop on Ontologies and the Semantic Web* (2002), p.2002.

[11] D. Katic, C. Julliard, A.-L. Wekerle, H. Kenngott, B.P. Muller-Stich, R. Dillmann, S. Speidel, P. Jannin and B. Gibaud, LapOntoSPM: an ontology for laparoscopic surgeries and its application to surgical phase recognition, *International journal of computer assisted radiology and surgery*, **10**, 9 (2015).

[12] E. Sirin, B. Parsia, B.C. Grau, A. Kalyanpur and Y. Katz, Pellet: A practical OWL-DL reasoner, *Web Semantics: Science, Services and Agents on the World Wide Web*, **5** (2007).

[13] M. Krötzsch, Efficient Inferencing for OWL EL. *Logics in artificial intelligence*. Springer (Lecture notes in computer science Lecture notes in artificial intelligence, 6341), Berlin, 2010, pp. 234–246.

[14] S. Batsakis, K. Stravoskoufos and E.G.M. Petrakis, Temporal Reasoning for Supporting Temporal Queries in OWL 2.0, *Knowledge-based and intelligent information and engineering systems*, Springer, Berlin, 2011, pp. 558–567.

[15] A. Artale, C. Parent, and S. Spaccapietra. Evolving objects in temporal information systems. *Annals of Mathematics and Artificial Intelligence*, **50**, 2007, pp. 5–38.

Subject Index

German Medical Data Sciences: Visions and Bridges
R. Röhrig et al. (Eds.)
© 2017 German Association for Medical Informatics, Biometry and Epidemiology (gmds) e.V. and IOS Press.
This article is published online with Open Access by IOS Press and distributed under the terms
of the Creative Commons Attribution Non-Commercial License 4.0 (CC BY-NC 4.0).

Author Index